PRAISE FOR *INTO THESE HANDS*

Bringing midwifery back to life once it has been forgotten or severely marginal-ized requires recognition of the sacredness of birth, boldness, creativity, and an abiding determination to return birth to women's domain. Geradine Simkins' collection of twenty-five stories of some of the women who have devoted their lives to this work is entertaining, inspiring, and unforgettable. I am proud to be one of them.—Ina May Gaskin, author of *Birth Matters, Spiritual Midwifery, Ina May's Guide to Childbirth*

A must read for every woman who has experienced the miracle of birth. A fitting tribute to the legacy of midwifery.—Byllye Y. Avery, Founder of Black Women's Health Imperative

What a very welcome treat it is to have this book delivered into our hands! It is a book to be savored, to be read for inspiration, hope, encouragement—to keep us pushing when we feel like the movement's stopped. For our sisters, our mothers, our daughters and our midwives, this is the book to bring us the strength to keep on going.—Barbara Katz Rothman, Professor of Sociology, City University of New York, co-author of *Laboring On: Birth in Transition in the United States*, author of *Recreating Motherhood: Ideology and Technology in a Patriarchal Society*

These are stories of remarkable women who are fully engaged in the profession and art of midwifery. Inspiring.—Eugene R. Declercq, PhD, Professor of Maternal and Child Health, Boston University School of Public Health, lead author on two national surveys, *Listening to Mothers I and II*, producer of educational video, *Birth by the Numbers*

Into These Hands offers intimate insight into the world of midwifery and midwives through personal stories that transcend ethnic, cultural and professional bound-aries that too often divide us. The stories reflect the personal dedication, sacrifice and challenges of those who have chosen to serve women and children.—Michael E. Bird, past President of the American Public Association, Vice Chair of Kewa Pueblo Health Board

Simkins has gathered the remarkable stories of twenty-five extraordinary midwives. They so eloquently remind us of why we must keep working to ensure that every community offers women the option of midwifery care—in the home, birth center, and hospital settings.—Judy Norsigian, Executive Director of Our Bodies Ourselves, co-author of *Our Bodies Ourselves: Pregnancy and Birth*

During the twentieth century the practice of obstetrics made many advances in the treatment of high risk pregnancies. As a result, the individualized event of birth moved from the guidance of the hands of midwives assisting women laboring and birthing in their beds at homes, to an institutional event with physicians using technology and instruments to deliver women of their newborns on operating tables in hospitals. This is a powerful collection of stories about the reemergence of midwives as the guardians of normal birth in America. It tells about the lives of individual midwifery leaders and Geradine Simkins weaves them together to tell the larger story of a quiet revolution. Although quiet, this revolution is filled with politics and passion. At the heart of these stories is birth, and the right for women to choose with whom and how they wish to give birth. Based on the leadership and courage of these midwives, and thousands of others working alongside, women across America can now once again experience birth safely into the hands of a midwife. This is the story of midwives in America, but it exemplifies the critical need for the stories of midwives around the world to also be told. Together our voices, our passion and our work will continue to improve the lives of all childbearing women and their newborns, wherever they live. Gera's book is a critical and timely event in modern midwifery. It is about more than the lives of these midwifery leaders, it is about history in the making.—Bridget Lynch, President of International Confederation of Midwives

Into These Hands is an important contribution to the literature on childbirth. Midwives always have and will continue to attend the vast majority of births and have been proven scientifically to be the safest and best birth attendant for most births. Midwives have a vast wisdom about childbirth and this book gives us an opportunity to learn from this wisdom.—Marsden Wagner, MD, perinatologist and perinatal epidemiologist, author of *Born in the USA: How a Broken Maternity Care System Can Be Fixed to Put Women and Children First*

Every woman and baby has the right to a respectful, safe and deeply fulfilling birth experience. *Into These Hands* doesn't just assure us that this can be achieved, it shows us how.—Elan McAllister, Founder of Choices in Childbirth, co-chair of *The Birth Survey*

What does birth mean for the midwives who attend it? Why choose a path and a practice that lead to years of getting up in the middle of the night, missing family holidays and birthdays, coming home exhausted from one birth only to catch two hours of sleep to get up and attend another? What should an aspiring midwife know about the practice of midwifery? And most importantly, why does midwifery matter—why should a woman choose a midwife when obstetricians are so widely available? This thrilling book shows us all why midwifery is the vanguard of the best possible future for women, families, birth, and the economy and effectiveness of maternity care.—Robbie Davis-Floyd, author, cultural/medical anthropologist and Senior Research Fellow at University of Texas, Austin

With the United Nations Population Fund's recent recognition of the importance of strengthening midwifery worldwide to save lives and promote the health of women and newborns, the words of these wise women who birthed modern midwifery couldn't be more timely. This collection is a testament to the skill, dedication, and love with which midwives approach their work. It will undoubtedly be an inspiration to future generations of midwives, who support pregnant women and in doing so, promote social justice.—Farah Diaz-Tello, staff attorney of National Advocates for Pregnant Women

The remarkable midwives who tell their interesting personal stories in *Into These Hands* have all played significant roles in bringing home birth and midwifery back into existence in the U.S. They are real individuals, who each in their own way realized that something was wrong with maternity care back in the '60s and '70s and decided to offer something that made more sense. Now there are more serious problems with this country's maternity care, and inspired midwives and committed citizen advocates are needed more than ever. Whether you are a woman looking at childbirth options, a health care provider, or someone thinking about becoming a midwife, this is an important, fascinating, informing and inspiring book.—Susan Hodges, Founder and past President, Citizens for Midwifery

Birth, power, politics—all of which are inseparable from the story of midwifery—as told by the amazing women who have forged the her-story in *Into These Hands*. Each memoir takes us deeper so that we can witness the insights, wisdom and transformation that these women have experienced becoming and living as midwives. There are lessons for all of us in how to live our passions and make a difference.—Debra Pascali-Bonaro, filmmaker, doula, director of documentary films *Orgasmic Birth: The Best Kept Secret* and *Organic Birth: Birth is Natural*

Some of my most cherished moments as a student midwife involved sitting mesmerized along with my fellow apprentices, often into the wee hours of the morning, as our senior midwives launched into one of their famed storytelling moods. We all loved these times and often tried to draw them out, asking to rehear our favorites. *Into These Hands* somehow captures these magical moments, making them available to all. This is a gift beyond measure. As a medical anthropologist and midwife, specializing in cross-cultural maternal child health, I am convinced that the twenty-five remarkable women chronicled here provide all the key ingredients needed for contemporary North American childbirth reform. Thank you Geradine!—Melissa Cheyney, PhD, CPM, Department of Anthropology, Oregon State University

The moment my daughter reached down to hold her son as he emerged from her body, at home, under the watchful eye of a midwife, I felt an instant, awesome connection to all my women ancestors. I had written about the superior care by midwives, knew many as friends, watched many DVDs, but never personally experienced a midwife-attended birth, though I had given birth to my daughter at home with a family practitioner in attendance. What a wonderful personal confirmation of everything I knew to be true. *Into These Hands, Wisdom From Midwives* distills all that truth in a book you'll be hard pressed to put down, once you start reading. Buy it and give to every woman you know—Roberta M. Scaer, co-author of *A Good Birth, A Safe Birth*

into these hands

into these hands

wisdom from midwives

edited by Geradine Simkins

Spirituality
& Health
BOOKS

With deepest gratitude for the never-ending lineage of midwives—
past, present and future.

And in honor of all the mothers and babies,
most especially my own,
Margaret, Maya, Leah and Sean.

Contents

Acknowledgements

I love when the Universe arranges the puzzle into the best possible configuration. Looking back, that is the gift I was given, step-by-step. I am grateful to my dear friend and writer, Barbara Gentry, who wisely advised, "You need a mentor for your project; you need Max." I did not know Max Regan—writer, internationally published poet, and teacher—when I asked him to be the literary midwife for this anthology. As it turns out, he possessed everything you'd want in a midwife: exquisite observational skills, meticulous attention to detail, brilliant knowledge of his craft, innate kindness, unending patience, and a fabulous sense of humor. From our very first phone call in 2007, in which I proposed this monumental project, he passionately dedicated himself to seeing it manifested. He collaborated with me in shaping the authors' texts so that each voice rang clear while blending into a harmonious chorus of voices. He skillfully guided me through the arduous process of getting this book born and in the process has become a cherished friend.

It is difficult enough to create a first book, much less with twenty-four contributing authors. In my naïveté I thought this would be no big deal. I underestimated what it would take to midwife these midwives into telling their tales. The twenty-four memoir authors were as hard to herd as Royal Siamese cats, but every bit as elegant and beautiful. I am grateful for their willingness to share their remarkable life-stories. Their memoirs weave together a multicolored fabric connecting the strands of modern midwifery and childbirth in America. I believe that their voices and insights are critical to the discourses on contemporary women's health, the politics of childbirth in the United States, and social movements. To these amazing authors I say: Thank you, dear ones. I am also deeply grateful to the 35,000 women whom we have tended in our 800 collective years of midwifery service. These women's stories are entwined into our lives. I am also grateful to our mentors and partners who are integral to our stories. And I am grateful to each baby-spirit who was born into our hands, for they are our teachers.

Two women generously helped with the early manuscript—Cristina Alonso and Jo Anne Myers-Ciecko, and I thank them for their keen insights in suggesting revisions for the Introduction. Sairy Franks, a doula and one of "my babies," typed early versions of the manuscript. Tina Williams painstakingly formatted the final manuscript to make it shine for the publishing review process. I am grateful for several colleagues who encouraged me and shared book-writing tricks of the trade, including midwife and author Carol Leonard.

During the arduous final editing of the manuscript in autumn 2009, Max and I took a break and went to Lake Michigan. We walked along the shore and Max gathered a handful of beach stones. When we returned home, he set up a small altar in my workspace. Twenty-five stones were placed in an outer circle, one for each author, one stone each for him and me, and a bowl was set in the very center with eight stones and a candle. He said, "the stones in the center are for the people who are unknown at this moment but who will help us get this book to publication." We lit the candle and spoke words of gratitude. Now a year later, I know who those mysterious other people are. It was serendipitous luck that I passed journalist, Lissa Edwards, in the hallway of our Pilates studio one day. I told her I was despairing of ever getting my book into print. She said, "talk to Victoria Sutherland." And that was the most fortuitous tip I had gotten all year. For reasons still unknown to me, Victoria, Publisher of Spirituality & Health Books, instantly believed in my project and me. She has been an enthusiastic and skillful shepherdess of the entire process. Matt Sutherland, Managing Editor of *Spirituality & Health* magazine, has been the quiet but steady force behind the scenes for this project. Thank you to Brian Lewis, for being a supportive partner in this process; Sandra Salamony for brilliantly designing a book cover I could truly love; Barbara Hodge for her expertise in design and layout; Gary Klinga for his diligent copyediting; and Amanda Campbell for her tips on social media. I feel very fortunate that 'my baby' landed in the hands of tremendously supportive and conscientious professionals in the publishing world. And I am honored that my friend, Web site wizard, Andy McFarlane, let me collect on an old offer. Seventeen and a half years ago, in the excited blush of his firstborn's emergence into my hands, he offered to build me a Web site. I did not need a Web site then, but I needed it now for my book. I am grateful for his generosity and creative know-how.

Numerous friends nurtured this project into fruition with prayers and encouragement and I thank each of you. When the book was still a dream, my young friend, Rekia Jibrin, took a long walk with me and advised, "If you are going to write for my generation, you've got to inspire us." I took that sage advice seriously. A special thank you to my women's group who listened to my vision and supported my saga for four years. I am eternally grateful to my Pilates teacher and good friend, Jennifer Cutler, who helped me get out of my brain and into my body during this long creative process, and likewise my Zumba teacher, Martha Hubbell, who had me Salsa my worries away.

Thank you to the awesome partners and apprentices with whom I have worked as a midwife over three decades and those who helped me as I birthed my three children. You have inspired me so that this book could come into being. I especially cherish Nancy Curley, my soul-sister midwife-friend, who has walked this journey with me for over twenty-five years and with whom I have caught more babies than anyone else.

I have three amazing young-adult kids—Maya, Leah, and Sean—whose faith in me finishing this book never wavered, and who cajoled me with their wickedly funny humor throughout the process. These three extraordinary people have provided me with the profound gifts of truth, challenge, belonging, surrender, and unwavering love. Their births and their lives keep me connected to the rhythms of creation. I am grateful to my father, Earl, who rests beneath the plum tree outside my office window and comforts me daily from the Other Side. Finally, I say thank you to Margaret Mary Geradine Fitzpatrick Simkins, who keeps pushing me to write all of the books that are inside of me. What a rare and precious gift to have a mother who unconditionally believes in me and is my most enthusiastic advocate. Each of us has a mother, but I got the queen mother. At last, to Spirit at the center of it all, to the ancestors, the children, the generations to come, in an ever-connected spiral of life, I say *Ashe, Ashe, Ashe.*

Opening

The night is dark and the wind is howling. The moon is hidden behind snow clouds, but the lights are on in the small house in the woods. In the bedroom four candles are burning with a golden light, one for each of the birthing woman's grandmothers who she says "will guide me." She is deep in labor. She thrashes and howls with the wind, trying to get comfortable. Her own parents stand anxiously at the edge of the room waiting and watching. They have never seen a natural birth. The young woman does not notice them now. She is rocking her body rhythmically with each contraction, moaning her birth song, falling into a sleepy trance in between. She is in transition. Her partner sits very close, murmuring quiet words to her, holding their three-year-old daughter who is clutching her daddy's shirt. My midwife partner and I are preparing for the birth, moving silently in tandem, gracefully and efficiently.

I sit beside the birthing woman. Abruptly she snaps out of her trance, grabs my hand and says, "Here comes another one."

She squeezes my hand so hard that my rings cut into my fingers. When our eyes meet, she gives me the frightened look of a wild animal caught in a trap. But I simply stroke her and say, "You can do this," and I breathe with her and then she begins to find her rhythm again. She struggles to make it through her contraction. She sways her hips from side to side, and then when the contraction subsides, she rests her whole body against her partner. She relaxes for a moment. Then suddenly she squirms and says, "I have to push." I say, "Wonderful . . . push your baby out." She no longer needs my eyes to reassure her. She no longer needs to hold anyone's hand. Instinctively, she squats at the side of her bed and pushes, gently at first, then more rhythmically, and finally with a burst of energy like an athlete in the last few strides of a marathon. The baby crowns, its head emerges and rotates into my waiting hands, that exquisite moment of half in and half out. Time stops for everyone in the room. Perhaps time stops in the entire universe to make room for one more soul. We wait for the final contraction. Everyone is crowded around now, breathless, completely enraptured by being in the presence of such a miracle.

The three-year-old takes her thumb out of her mouth and says, "Is that my baby sister coming out?" Everybody laughs.

I say to the mother, "Reach down and touch your baby." When she touches the top of the wet slippery head an extraordinary calmness washes over her. She smiles. I say, "With the next contraction your baby will be born. Push gently." And she does. As the baby eases out, so does the rest of the amniotic fluid that always feels like a baptism to me. I whisper to the baby, "Welcome, little one," and in that holy moment the mother reaches down and brings her baby to rest against her naked chest, heart to heart.

Then she throws her head back and in an ecstatic litany she cries, "Oh my God, oh my baby, oh my God!" And then, "It's a girl!" The new big sister is clamoring to see better. The new grandparents are sobbing. The new daddy is weeping for joy. It is the ancient chorus of gratitude and relief. My midwife partner puts her arm around my shoulder and we just watch this sweet nativity scene, feeling blessed to be a part of it.

Several hours later, after the baby and the mother have been examined carefully, after everyone is cleaned up, after the herb bath, after the family has been served breakfast, and after the Champagne toast, we tuck the new family into their bed, pull the comforter up and hug them goodbye.

The new mother grabs our hands, pulls us to her chest, whispers sweet words of thanksgiving—like a prayer—into our ears, and kisses each of our cheeks. She lets go of our hands and we leave her gazing into the primordial pool of her newborn baby's eyes.

Introduction

Every new member of the human family arrives on Earth through the body of a woman. Each day on our planet, the majority of babies emerge from the waters of their mother's womb into the hands of a midwife. Since the dawn of time, midwives have been receiving the generations into their hands. Almost without exception, midwives exist in every culture, in every country. Midwifery may well be the oldest healing profession known to humans.

In Old English, *midwife* means "with woman." The Danish word for midwife, *jordmoder*, means "earth mother" and the Icelandic word, *ljosmodir*, means "mother of light." In French, *sage femme*, means "wise woman." Each of these words speaks to the broader roles that the midwife has played in various cultures—that of healer, counselor and practitioner in the realms of wellness and illness, birth and death—a constellation of ways of being "with woman." For this reason, it is sometimes difficult to find a singular translation for "midwife" in certain African, indigenous, and other languages because of the diverse roles in which these women serve their communities.

In most cultures midwives have enjoyed a place of honor, respected for their remarkable skills, wisdom and prowess as healers.[1] But in the United States midwives are as endangered as the spotted owl or the gray wolf. And like these animals, midwives face significant threats to their way of life. The United States is one of the few countries in the modern world to have ever outlawed midwives. In 1923 there were about 60,000 midwives practicing in the United States.[2] By the 1960s traditional midwives were all but extinct.[3] Slowly midwives have been making a comeback, but it has not been easy. Today there are roughly 10,000 practicing midwives. You are about to meet twenty-five midwives, key players who were influential in the revival of this ancient healing art and who have helped to shape the modern profession of midwifery as it is practiced today.

Telling Our Stories

As midwives, we have stories to tell. Our years are filled with tales worth telling and they will perish with us if they go untold. That is why I offered an invitation to these remarkable women to tell their unique stories about walking through the world in the shoes of a midwife. As many of us prepare to pass the torch on to younger protégés, we feel the urgency of sharing our wisdom and we have a longing to be heard. For the most part, these stories have been shared only in small circles, hence most people in this country have not yet been afforded a glimpse into the accumulated knowledge that midwives carry in their hands, hearts and souls.

The stories we need to tell are not only about pregnancy and birth, newborns and new parents, but also about the politics and power struggles that have shaped how we do what we do. Our stories are powerful not only because they speak of brushes with the law and with death, but also because they encompass a level of transcendence that many people long for but few ever actually experience. Midwives who assist in bringing babies into the world are aware that we bathe in the glow of a true miracle time and time again. And that baptism has conferred a kind of knowledge upon us that is profound, sacred and potent. So it is important that we tell our history—actually "herstory"— and that it be told with a decidedly feminine voice, recorded in our own words, authentically, powerfully, sensitively and accurately. Our stories must be told and remembered because whole new generations of young women are hungry for the hard-earned wisdom we have gathered over the years.

Regardless of our diverse spiritual backgrounds, many of us believe that we were "called" to midwifery, more as a vocation or a destiny than as a profession. That sense of calling may account for the extraordinary passion and dedication that we have brought to our work. This passion both enlivens and exhausts us.

A Diverse Chorus of Voices

The midwives in this anthology are all over fifty years of age and each has been a midwife for over twenty-five years, some for as many as forty years or more. Collectively, these women have over 800 years of experience and have assisted in approximately 35,000 births. They are not only pioneers but also accomplished professionals. They were chosen because I consider each of them to be a *Sage Femme*—a Wise Woman. They come from all across the United States, from California to New Jersey, Arkansas to Florida. They are racially and ethnically diverse—American Indian, Latina, African American, South Asian American, and European American. They come from diverse ideological and midwifery training backgrounds. They are self-taught, apprentice-trained, attended midwifery schools, and/or received a university education. They practice in a variety of settings—homes, clinics, birth centers, hospitals, tribes and global villages and some also work in other arenas such as education, research, public health and advocacy. Some have numerous professional credentials and licenses; some feel that midwifery should not be legislated at all.

Becoming a Baby Catcher

When we began "catching babies" in the '60s and '70s, most of us had no idea we would became part of an astonishing social movement that would influence and shape the discourse about reproductive rights and the content of maternity care in America.

I became part of the new era of midwives during the '70s in the midst of the Cultural Revolution, at a time when midwifery had nearly been stamped out in the United States. This was an era in which a number of social movements intersected—civil rights, feminism, gender equity, reproductive justice, anti-war, environmentalism, and, as women, we were fighting to regain control over our own bodies and reclaim our own experiences of pregnancy and birth.

It was 1976 when I attended my first home birth. I was twenty-six years old and in my fourth month of pregnancy with my first child. I had only begun to read about birth because I was pregnant, and my reading and conversations with other women led me to explore different topics. I began investigating different locations in which women gave birth, different birth practices and different birth attendants. I was introduced to the notion of midwifery by a friend who had a baby two years earlier in California. It was the first time I really heard the terms "home birth" and "midwife." It was a moment of epiphany for me, one of those uncommon times when something cracks open and you realize that there is an alternative to what you always thought was "normal."

My mother had told me about her four births. For the most part she was drugged, strapped down on her back, poked, shaved, cut through the perineum, and delivered of her infant, only to awaken in a haze and discover that her baby was no longer inside of her and not even by her side. That kind of birth was disorienting at best, highly disturbing at worst, but it was considered "normal" in my mother's generation. But the reality of coming of age in the '60s and '70s was that the status quo was inexorably transformed on most fronts amidst the social upheaval and moral scrutiny of the times. In fact, what was considered "normal" was changing all over the place.

Birthing a Vision

We were all young women in our twenties. One of our friends became pregnant. After doing some research and talking to a few other women, she went to the doctor and told him that she wanted to have a home birth. The doctor said, "Absolutely not; I can't participate in that." So our friend came back to the women's circle and said, "I am going to have my baby at home anyhow. I mean, after all, how hard can it be to have a baby? Women have been doing it successfully for centuries." That sounded logical to us, and she asked if we would help her give birth. After we bought some books and equipment and did some studying, we helped her birth her baby. And she was right. It wasn't all that tricky. Of course, there were those moments when she was panting and pushing hard that drew our undivided attention. But easily enough, the baby came out.

Over the course of the next year, each of us became pregnant and agreed to help one another. If we felt that we could not handle the situation, we would immediately seek medical assistance. Unlike obstetric texts that spelled out a specific process of labor and birth, we observed that there were many different possible ways to have a "normal" birth. We became familiar with what was in the normal range and what was not. And when something was not in the normal range, we learned to discern whether it was truly dangerous or just uncommon. Of course, we were met with challenges, even emergencies, but we were success-ful in managing them. And inevitably, birth after birth, babies came out.

I remember those early days of getting organized. They were charged with a level of excitement that tingled the spine as when something new is being created and you know that it is going to be powerful. I remember when we met in a hand-built cabin in the woods to write the articles of incorporation and by-laws for the newly-formed Michigan Midwives Association. There were six of us there from different parts of the state—Marta Hoetger and Diane Foss from the southeast,

Laura Slater and Cheryl Klug from the southwest, and Lori Cruden and I from the north. We each had a baby on the hip or at the breast and, although none of us had done such a task before, we still wrote a persuasive business plan and received non-profit corporate status from the State of Michigan in record time. At another meeting we spent a weekend together working night and day to draft bylaws and other foundational documents of the organization, as well as a midwife apprenticeship curriculum, standards for midwifery practice, peer review protocols, and midwifery certification procedural documents. Our babies could barely walk and were hanging onto our legs and drooling on our toes as we drafted our business documents; the energy and hope of our young motherhood infused everything we did. We learned how to hold a vision of where we wanted to go, and even though we didn't know how things were "supposed" to be done, holding that vision gave us a great sense of freedom and ascendancy. And it resulted in creative, innovative and dynamic outcomes. We were only vaguely aware of the history of childbirth and midwifery in America. In retrospect, it may have been a blessing that at that point in our development we had no idea what we were really up against.

Women's Work

In most societies worldwide, birthing is women's work and is therefore shaped and managed by women.[4] Historically birth has been a social event in which, for the most part, only women participated.[5-6] In the early 1900s nearly all births in the United States (over 95%) were attended by midwives in women's homes.[7]

By the mid-twentieth century, however, the U.S. diverged from the deeply rooted traditions of woman attending woman in childbirth. Four major social circumstances influenced this profound shift. First, emerging medical professions enjoyed rapid growth and prestige at the turn of the twentieth century and skillfully marketed modernity and the promise of a "better birth."[8] Women lacked a clear understanding about how their bodies' worked in the childbirth process and came to believe that doctors had the knowledge and ability to provide safer and speedier births than midwives.[9] The promise of a safer birth was a claim that lacked any proof, but the misperception persists even today. In fact, childbirth historians state that the increased presence of men and their "scientific methods" of the time caused more problems in childbirth than did traditional female midwives; neither women nor babies fared better.[10-11] Maternal mortality rates increased at the same time that women began birthing in hospitals.[12]

The second circumstance arose when, in order to access doctor-attended births with "man midwives" (as these doctors were called), women had to leave their homes and go to hospitals where doctors practiced.[13] While birth at home remained the norm even when doctors first began attending births, hospital birth soon became a fashionable status symbol for the middle and upper classes. Whereas in the late nineteenth century hospitals served the poor and rehabilitated the unfortunate,[14] by the early twentieth century hospitals boasted restful and clean environments with modern conveniences. What was "new," and at first only accessible to those with means to afford it, was perceived to be "better." Hospitals became "maternity hotels" that provided brand new amenities and a chance to recuperate away from home after giving birth. Also, the middle and upper class women who could afford hospitals came to believe that some medical attention would help ensure their survival through childbirth and the postpartum period.[15-16]

The third circumstance arose when licensure became synonymous with competence and university credentials became more valued than traditional experience.[17] While competence and skills varied among doctors just as among midwives, those midwives who were unlicensed and unschooled—no matter how competent—were at a disadvantage. Midwives were ill-equipped to compete with organized medicine that was becoming increasingly competitive and dominant. Licensure put midwives under the supervision of licensed doctors with whom they were in competition for business. Childbirth, for both midwives and doctors, was the entrée into caring for the whole family. As a result of this, competition stiffened.

The fourth circumstance arose as women grew more interested in newly developed pain relief medicines for childbirth. This invention trumped the attachment most women had to place of birth or birth attendant. Most women wanted to escape the pain of childbirth more than anything else.[18] Therefore, "since doctors and hospitals controlled anesthetics, they got the birth business."[19] And doctors believed they were offering the pain relief that women wanted and requested.[20] Women were making a choice. By 1939, half of all American babies were born in hospitals, and by 1970 that rate rose to ninety-nine percent.[21-22] Throughout the twentieth century, childbirth came under the control of men of medicine. As a result, women received the drug cocktail of narcotics and amnesiacs that they requested. Some women were given an injection, went to sleep, woke the next day, were presented with their babies and consequently remembered nothing of their births. Some women became semi-conscious patients, often so drugged or deranged that they had to be tied to their beds, lying flat on their backs so as not to fall or injure themselves. Women were delivered of their babies with the tools and procedures of the new obstetrics—drugs, forceps and episiotomies.

Thus over a period of about one hundred years, American women lost control over childbirth. What was sacrificed? In the shift from home birth to hospital birth, women not only lost the private and familiar domain of their own birthing rooms, but they also sacrificed their ascendancy in decision-making. They forfeited the use of female-ordained traditions and customs that made birth both a social and a sacred occasion. Birth was now seen through the eyes of medical men and enacted through medical procedures created *by* men. What women lost was significant: Women lost faith in their own bodies during the birthing process and trust in nature to take its course; they lost the powerful network of other women to provide the strength, companionship and comfort necessary to surmount the trials and ordeals of childbirth; midwives lost autonomy to doctors and lost control over their work; women lost the expertise and common sense of midwives as trustworthy birth attendants and community healers. In essence, the ability of women to shape, define and control the events of their own procreative lives was sacrificed.

Unlike the development of maternity care in Europe where male obstetrics and female midwifery developed side by side as complements to one another,[23] childbirth in the United States was marked by the rise of obstetrics, the fall of midwifery, and the outbreak of turf wars that persist to this day.

Until the late nineteenth and early twentieth centuries in America, doctors typically were only involved in abnormal births. But once they took control, all births were redefined as potentially or inherently abnormal. The rising medical model viewed birth as something that could be improved upon because it was perceived to be a process that was fundamentally pathological and dangerous. As a consequence, childbirth became increasingly mechanized and controlled. The shift from home birth with midwives to hospital birth with doctors was dramatic on many levels, most notably in its shift from "women's work" to "men's work." Men and women share accountability for this dramatic shift. Nonetheless, it became standard for a woman to lie back passively and succumb to a whole new set of labor and birth rituals and customs that were dominated by pharmacology, instrumentation and surgical procedures, provided by male doctors. Women were separated from the presence of supportive females during labor and from their babies at birth. Immediately after birth, newborn infants under the influence of potent drugs, were put into little metal boxes in another room to be medically managed and where they could be viewed by their mothers through a glass wall.[24]

Taking Birth Back

Then, a new era dawned. By the 1950s, some women began to question Twilight Sleep, forceps deliveries, separation from their infants and store-bought infant formula. By the 1960s, women began to realize that something precious and important had been taken from them and they were determined to get it back. As a result of the cultural revolution of the '60s and early '70s, birthing women finally reclaimed responsibility for their birth choices. A woman-centered, family-focused, social model of childbirth was popularized in which women sought family physicians and midwives to be primary birth attendants for their low-tech natural births. They rekindled the support and companionship of being surrounded by family and friends during childbirth. They learned how their bodies were designed to function in accommodating the natural processes of pregnancy, birth and lactation. And they discovered alternatives to drugs for dealing with pain and fear. In essence, they got off their backs and took charge. This was a radical departure from the way birth in the United States was conducted at that time. And as one might expect, this new model became a threat to the burgeoning competitive market in maternity care because it was a pretty simple, straightforward, and less costly model. Midwives and family practice physicians were perceived as threatening to the goals of the escalating corporatization and medicalization of maternity care, a system in which obstetrical specialists and an ever-increasing array of interventions for pregnant, laboring and birthing women and their infants were being developed and promoted.

Yet, nothing is ever black and white. Therefore, it is daunting to describe the events that changed maternity care into the model it is today: The quick progression from community midwives and country doctors as the norm to managed care via corporate and commercial enterprises; the rapid evolution of the profession of midwifery over the past century; and how midwives intersected with the evolving American healthcare system. This is a complex tale of multiple timelines, issues, trends and controversies that are still unfolding even today.

Maternity Care Goes Corporate

As women and their partners began to reclaim their birth experiences, a predictable backlash occurred. To understand this dynamic tension, it is important to recognize how the provision of medical care in the U.S. has become one of the biggest and most profitable industries in the world. As we are keenly aware in the United States, the health care industry typically focuses more on "industry" than "health care." The introduction and utilization of highly trained perinatal specialists and high-tech obstetrical interventions were necessary in order for the corporate model to succeed in the production and provision of maternity care. Dr. Barbara Bridgman Perkins' book, *The Medical Delivery Business*, provides an excellent analysis of the historical roots and contemporary consequences of applying an economic and industrial approach to childbirth.[25] Dr. Perkins stresses that there is a direct link between the rise of the assembly line and mass production (as in the automotive industry) and the rise of standardized, mechanized assembly line obstetrics. The assembly line is brilliant model for creating finished products much faster than with handcrafted methods, improving affordability, and increasing profits. I grew up in Detroit where Henry Ford not only rocked the world by revolutionizing automobile manufacturing, but also where his innovative methods inspired one of the first mother-baby assembly line hospitals in the country.

The shift from a low-tech social midwifery model of childbirth to the medicalization of childbirth was one significant trend, but the gradual and insidious corporatization of childbirth is quite another development. An awareness of the corporate business model that evolved in the mid-to-late twentieth century—the model that has come to dominate the U.S. maternity care system today—is essential to understand the big picture. Perinatal specialization changed maternity care—the workplace, the nature of birth work, its birth workers, what birth workers produced, and treatment of the subjects of the industry, i.e., mothers and babies. In routinizing childbirth, there was no longer an emphasis on the fluid (if sometimes chaotic) process of an individual woman's labor and birth, her needs, or continuity of care from a single practitioner. Rather, the corporate business model emphasized standard procedure-oriented tasks to be completed on all patients across the board at various antepartum, intrapartum and postpartum stages. Who would administer each procedure depended on the technical complexity of the task and the skill level of the staff member. But everything was done to ensure a "continuous operational flow of patients"[26] inspired by Ford's continuous moving assembly line. Underpinning the goals of corporatizing birth was what had to be done in order to shape women's thinking about the fundamental experience of giving birth so that they would be willing to buy the products and submit to the procedures of the new corporate maternity care industry, especially at a time when women had so recently achieved some success in taking birth back. It is necessary to be aware of the domination of corporatization in order to understand why midwives have had to continually struggle to maintain their ground within the healthcare system; why certain midwives chose to work completely outside of the system to sustain a different model altogether; and why some women actively sought out those alternatives.

A Captive Audience

In the past century, the role of medicine in improving maternal and child health status in many areas is undeniable, and for this we are grateful. But the fact is that indicators of health status and women's own stories reveal that our current maternity care system fails to meet the needs of women and infants in fundamental ways.[27] With over three-quarters of all American women becoming mothers and over 4.3 million births in the United States each year,[28] it is fair to say that maternity care affects large numbers of women and families. By the end of the first decade of the twenty-first century, more babies were born in the United States than ever before—about 15,000 more than the peak year of the Baby Boom.[29] On an average day in the United States, 11,120 babies are born.[30] This means pretty dependable work for obstetricians and hospitals where over 98% of all babies are born. Mothers and babies constitute a "captive audience."

Because pregnancy is not an illness but rather a healthy state of being, at least 85% of all women in the U.S. enter labor at low-risk for problems. Nonetheless, in a recent national survey women reported that they received at least seven to ten obstetrical interventions,[31] whether or not they needed them or were given full disclosure about them, and regardless of the scientific efficacy of the interventions. Forty-one percent indicated that their caregiver tried to induce their labor, and 55% were given a synthetic hormone to strengthen or speed up labor contractions.[32] Close to 90% of all women received spinal or epidural analgesia and/or narcotics in labor for pain management.[33] Use of narcotics can adversely affect mothers and their babies while non-drug therapies that are not dangerous are underused or ignored. Ninety-four percent of women were subjected to continuous fetal monitoring,[34] in spite of conclusive evidence that indicates the monitoring does not improve outcomes in either low-risk or high-risk women and, instead, definitely limits a woman's freedom of movement in labor and birth. Universal and continuous fetal monitoring is, however, easier for assembly-line obstetrics. One-third of all pregnancies end in major abdominal surgery (cesarean section) in the U.S.[35-36] And it is speculated that some teaching hospitals that train resident physicians have a much higher cesarean rate than the skyrocketing national average.

While the United States has the highest per capita spending on health care in the world, this has not led to optimal outcomes.[37] And if all of the technology and interventions made a substantial improvement in outcomes and quality of care, we might consider them necessary. But unfortunately, that is not the case. The U.S. has one of the highest infant mortality rates in the modern world, ranking about thirtieth among developed nations, and the rate is higher for infants of color.[38-39] Although the U.S. maternal mortality rate has improved over the past century, it has not improved at all since 1982 and appears to be increasing. Our maternal mortality rate is as dismal as some developing nations, and the rate is higher for women of color.[40-42] The safety, reliability, price and performance of our current maternity care system are issues of grave concern. And long overdue is a national maternal and child health agenda that recognizes that the well-being of women in their reproductive years affects the overall health status not only of women, but of children and families as well.

The Delivery Business

The common mainstream belief is that the safest place for birthing mothers and infants is in a hospital under the management of an obstetrician. While this perception has persisted since the early 1900s and has become the prevailing American viewpoint, it is neither factual nor supported by research. Low-risk women and infants who are under the care of midwives, regardless of the site of birth, have similar outcomes to low-risk women and infants under the care of obstetricians in hospitals.[43]

In order for the maternity care system in the U.S. to retain its prowess as a multi-billion dollar-a-year corporate enterprise and one of the largest and most successful for-profit industries out of all medical specialties,[44] some serious marketing has to be done. Consider the expenditures and the revenues. Hospital charges for the U.S. medical model of childbirth are enormous. In 2005, "combined hospital charges for birthing women (about $44 billion) and newborns (about $35 billion) totaled $79, 277,733,843 and far exceeded charges for any other condition."[45] If you were to ask a group of people to identify the most common reason for hospitalization and the most common surgical procedure in the U.S., they would probably think in terms of acute illnesses, serious accidents or chronic diseases. But they would be wrong. The most common reason for hospitalization in the United States is childbirth.[46] Cesarean section is the most frequently performed surgical procedure in the U.S., reaching an all-time high of 32% of all births in 2007 (the most current data available), marking the eleventh consecutive year of increase and the highest rate ever reported in the United States.[47] Of the most common hospital procedures, six out of fifteen involve childbirth.[48] The use of obstetrical procedures has doubled in the past fifteen years. Annually, one-quarter of all hospital discharges are for mother-baby healthcare related to childbirth.[49]

The U.S. maternity care system overuses expensive and often unnecessary medical practices such as surgery, pharmacology, and technology, and underuses other cost-effective practices and preventive healthcare modalities that are evidence-based and efficacious.[50] Maternity care expenditures play a significant role in healthcare costs that are spiraling out of control and are detrimentally impacting the families, businesses and governments that are footing the bills.[51]

Let me be clear: the problem is not that we have obstetrical practices available that can be useful in certain necessary or life-saving situations. The problem is that they are broadly applied to everyone without concern for necessity or efficacy. In a national survey, women reported that obstetrical interventions had been imposed on them without appropriate and timely discussions about the risks, benefits and alternatives and, in some cases, without their consent.[52] And at the same time almost 60% of women who wanted a VBAC (vaginal birth after cesarean) were denied that option.[53] In short, our maternity care system is driven by profit rather than driven by consumer choice or the best research evidence about childbirth practices. In light of this, it is clear why midwives—who not only espouse a low-tech, high-caring model and have the evidence to prove that the midwifery model is safe, satisfying, cost-effective and produces optimal outcomes—have become a threat to a system that advocates a costly high-tech biomedical model of childbirth. It is also clear why organized medicine is dedicated to discrediting the merits of the midwifery model, even seeking to eradicate midwives from the menu of choices for women seeking maternity care.[54]

The Model Matters

So what makes the difference in a maternity care system that works well and one that does not? Several contemporary social scientists who are experts in women's health, reproduction and maternity health care, state that it is the model of care that makes the difference. They have identified characteristics of models worldwide that work and don't work in terms of scientific, humanistic, economic, and outcome efficiencies and deficiencies, as well as effects on providers and recipients of these models of care.[55-58] In 1979, Rothman was the first to describe and contrast the medical model and the midwifery model of childbirth;[59] in 1992, Davis-Floyd described the technocratic model and the holistic model of birth.[60] Each model employs different tools, languages, skills, underlying beliefs, and power relationships. For example, the medical model would typically use the tools of narcotics and epidurals for pain relief, while the midwifery model would use water therapy, position change, or social support. In the medical model the physician "manages" the birth and the woman is "delivered" or "sectioned." In the midwifery model the midwife "attends" or "assists" and the woman "gives birth." One of the most important differences is that in the medical model the obstetrician is the central player and decision-maker. She or he controls and directs the course of events and continually focuses on averting potential pathology. By contrast, the midwifery model is woman-centered and directed by the mother in partnership with the midwife. This model focuses on the normalcy of the natural processes of pregnancy and birth and the instinctual rhythms of the individual mother-baby dyad. Practitioners in each model are highly skilled but possess (and value) very different skill sets.

For women who want an alternative to a highly medicalized model of birth, who believe that birth is a natural physiological process and even a celebratory event, choices are often unavailable. Normal birth that begins, proceeds, and concludes as nature designed it is so rare that most maternity care providers have never seen it, most resident doctors have not been trained to accommodate it, and most women have to go outside the hospital to find an experienced care provider if they choose it. Therefore, women who want to have a natural birth often choose their own home or a birth center. Fortunately, women have excellent choices in numerous areas of this country, but certainly not everywhere. And if you are a poor woman in America, your choices are even more limited and dependent upon what services and providers Medicaid will reimburse.

According to Davis-Floyd, the United States and Canada are the only two industrialized nations where professional midwives do not attend the majority of births and where midwives are not fully integrated into the system of care.[61] Throughout the twentieth century while America eliminated midwives, Europe generated them. Today in most of Europe, where the midwifery model coexists with the medical model, customers seem quite satisfied, healthcare delivery is less costly, and perinatal outcomes are better than in the United States. For example, Dutch midwives attend about 70% of all births, Danish midwives attend nearly all normal births, and Swedish midwives care for about 85% of all pregnant women and attend all normal births.[62]

In its quest to control the processes of pregnancy and birth, and thus control women, the model used by organized medicine in the U.S. has stripped pregnancy and birth of their magic and mystery. In a quest to make labor and birth more orderly for hospital protocols and personnel, the medical model has imposed routines on the most individualized and unpredictable process known to humans. Little else in the world is as unpredictable as birthing, except perhaps, dying. Just as the Hospice movement has crafted a space to return dignity and serenity to dying by taking end of life care out of the hospital and bringing it home to families, so too midwives shelter the same sacred space for birthing. In both cases the emphasis is on the importance of the whole process, not just on the final moments of birth or death. In the final analysis, what makes the difference is the model of care.

As we begin the second decade in the twenty-first century we stand at the cusp of the greatest potential for health care reform in decades. We have a chance to shift our U.S. healthcare system from "sick care" to "wellness care." Maternity care reform provides an opportunity to bring a wellness model to citizens at the moment when families are first begun. The midwifery model utilizes evidence-based maternity practices to provide optimal care with least interference in the body's natural processes. The midwifery model has proven to decrease unnecessary medical interventions without sacrificing safety, save money for taxpayers as well as private and public insurers, and increase satisfaction in the childbirth experience for women and their families.

Midwifing the Movement

With the organized efforts to supplant midwifery with obstetrics, midwives have had to be both clever and resilient in order to mount a movement of organized resistance. Social and legislative trends resulted in a variety of categories of midwives as they struggled to persist, and preserve the midwifery profession, amidst the cultural pressures. Two branches of the midwifery profession—nurse-midwifery and direct-entry midwifery—have been working as activists, often collaborating with midwifery supporters. Generally speaking, nurse-midwives have worked to make changes from within the system, while direct-entry midwives have worked to make changes from the periphery or outside the system. At times their strategies followed convergent pathways; at times their paths were divergent.[63]

In the following anthology, you will hear the authors speak of involvement with their professional midwifery organizations—the American College of Nurse-Midwives (ACNM), over fifty years old, and the Midwives Alliance of North America (MANA), nearly thirty years old. It is through these organizations that both advocacy for the survival and promotion of midwifery and assurance of women's choices in childbirth have been vigilantly pursued on a national level. What these two national professional organizations have accomplished is extraordinary in terms of influencing women's health care, shaping maternal and child health policy, and providing professional development for midwives, and thus, promoting the health and well-being of women and infants within their families and communities.

And while MANA and ACNM have been called by some, "sisters from a different mother," like sisters, they have worked cooperatively together and fought bitterly with one another. Unfortunately, midwives face threats from within as well as threats from the outside. While ACNM and MANA currently dedicate time and resources to collaborate more effectively each year, they have not been able to reconcile some key issues, and these differences and conflicts have kept them from forging a united front for all, threatening the stability of the profession.

Sisters on Different Paths

There is a diverse pool of midwives in this country, and those not in the inner circles are often confused by all of the various descriptors—traditional midwives, direct-entry midwives, nurse-midwives, community midwives, spiritual midwives—to name a few. In her 1997 book, *Sisters on a Journey*,[64] Penfield Chester described the "three strands of American midwifery"—Grand Midwives, Certified Nurse-Midwives, and Independent Midwives.

The Grand Midwives are sometimes referred to as "granny midwives," though some consider this a disparaging term. Grand Midwives are a group consisting of traditional midwives, including indigenous midwives, southern Black midwives, Latina *pateras* of the Southwest, and immigrant midwives. These women received midwifery knowledge through other women, usually via apprenticeship with a mother, grandmother, aunt or older women in the midwifery lineage. All across the continent indigenous, Black and immigrant midwives played indispensable roles as healers in their communities using traditional knowledge of herbs and tinctures, skills and techniques, rituals and prayers. They provided midwifery and other types of basic health care to women and their families who, in most cases, lacked access to formal medical services. Often, Grand Midwives were the only community health workers.

However, in the early twentieth century, as the medical establishment was getting organized in the U.S., state health departments began to train and super-vise the Grand Midwives. They came under public health regulations and, in a calculated campaign, were regulated out of business for being "ignorant" and "dangerous," finally supplanted with doctors who were "knowledgeable" and "safe."[65-67] The African American Grand Midwives were the last holdouts of non-medicalized midwifery. As important as the Grand Midwives have been to our country's history and to the well-being of villages, urban communities, tribes and remote areas across the nation, today they are virtually extinct.

Certified Nurse-Midwives (CNMs) came on the scene in the U.S. in the early twentieth century with origins in public health nursing. Just like the Grand Midwives, it was a struggle for them to survive at a time when organized medicine was trying to eliminate midwives of all kinds. The CNMs created a space for themselves amid a myriad of obstacles. They established themselves as well-educated health care providers and eventually gained a foothold in the American health care system because they were trained in two disciplines—nursing and midwifery. CNMs are required to complete accredited educational courses, pass a national certification examination, meet criteria established by the American College of Nurse Midwives (ACNM), and are certified by the American Midwifery Certification Board.[68] CNM's scope of practice includes all birth settings, although they work primarily in hospitals with over 95% of practicing CNMs working within the established health care systems where they have collaborative relationships with physicians. They are trained to provide primary health care for women and newborns, and some CNMs also work as educators, researchers and public health specialists. By working within the system CNMs are able to reach the large majority of women who choose to give birth in hospitals, including vulnerable and underserved women. They bring into the hospital the core midwifery beliefs in normal physiologic birth and a commitment to a woman's right to be engaged in her own care. Since the late twentieth century, CNMs have been able to practice legally in all fifty states. In the mid-1990s, the ACNM designed a direct-entry midwifery credential called the Certified Midwife (CM). The term "direct-entry midwife" implies that a person entered the midwifery profession directly without first being a nurse. CMs must meet the same educational requirements as described above for CNMs but without the requisite nursing component. Certified Midwives are legal to practice in only three states—New York, Rhode Island and New Jersey.

The category of Independent Midwives, as described by Chester, includes all other midwives such as lay midwives, direct-entry midwives (that are not CMs), community midwives, and spiritual midwives. Their emergence was a result of the counterculture fervor of the early 1970s and women's yearning to reclaim their birth experiences from an objectionable maternity care system. The grassroots movement of "lay" (self-taught and apprentice-trained) midwives spread across the country as women chose to give birth at home. Within a short time these practitioners created training courses, formal midwifery programs, midwifery schools, and organizations to support their autonomous style of practice. Their professional organization—the Midwives Alliance of North America (MANA)—was central to the development and evolving philosophy of contemporary direct-entry midwifery. In the late 1980s and early 1990s, MANA laid the groundwork for the establishment of the Certified Profession Midwife

(CPM), an innovative midwifery credential created by and for independent midwives. It was further developed by the North American Registry of Midwives (NARM) in collaboration with MANA, the Midwifery Education Accreditation Council (MEAC), and Citizens for Midwifery (a consumer-based group). The CPM credential requires that a candidate demonstrate successful mastery of didactic material and clinical skills, pass a national certification examination, meet criteria established by the North American Registry of Midwives and/or the Midwifery Education Accreditation Council, and be certified by NARM.[69] CPMs are trained via apprenticeship, independent midwifery schools or college-based programs. CPMs are unique among maternity care providers in the United States because their training requires experience and expertise in out-of-hospital birth. This expertise makes them perfectly positioned not only for women who choose home birth and freestanding birth centers, but also as providers of out-of-hospital services in times of natural disasters and disease epidemics. CPMs are a fast-growing segment of the midwifery profession; one in nine U.S. midwives is a CPM. Twenty-seven states now recognize direct-entry midwives in statute, twenty-five states have licensure, and about ten more states are currently pursuing licensing bills for direct-entry midwifery. In 2000, the National Association of Certified Professional Midwives (NACPM) was created as a professional organization. While many consider the CPM the gold standard for Independent Midwives, it should also be mentioned that not all Independent Midwives, such as some in the categories called "traditional" or "spiritual midwives," are in favor of midwifery certification and/or licensing.

Fusion Midwives

More than a decade after Penfield Chester's description of the three strands of American midwives—Grand Midwives, Nurse-Midwives and Independent Midwives—I propose that there is a fourth strand—the Fusion Midwives. The term "fusion" implies melding together or producing a union. Fusion Midwives had their roots as lay (direct-entry) midwives and later chose to become nurse-midwives. They did this for a variety of personal and professional reasons, including expanding their scopes of practice, earning more money, and gaining legal status. What resulted from this blending of midwifery genres is that Fusion Midwives cross the boundaries of that which divides the different types of midwives. Like bi-cultural people, they can walk in both worlds because they understand the language, traditions and values of both. Fusion Midwives honor diversity and see differences as strengths—not weaknesses or threats.

Consequently they are passionately committed to weaving all of the strands of midwives into a unified and sturdy tapestry that preserves the unique integrity and beauty of the individual fibers. They are much less interested in the numerous adjectives that describe midwives—traditional, lay, nurse, certified, licensed, direct-entry—and more interested in the one common noun—midwife. They emphasize that we are all midwives working to serve mothers, infants, families and our communities. They are ambassadors, bringing considerable hope to our profession because they espouse and work for unity among all of us.

Having "ambassador midwives" is important in order to promote diplomatic relationships among the different kinds of midwives and organizations. Fusion Midwives are typically members of both MANA and ACNM.

The key issues that have caused strife between midwife organizations and among practicing midwives of differing credentials revolve around training of midwives, autonomy of practice, and turf issues. Perhaps the specific trends that have caused the most conflicts are the following:

- Differing opinions regarding what constitutes bona fide midwifery education;
- Differences that result from contextual variations—working inside the established medical system versus working on the periphery or outside of the system;
- Creation of a direct-entry midwifery credential by both the ACNM (the CM) and MANA (the CPM) at nearly the same time in history with different degrees of success;
- Efforts to get the CM and CPM regulated, licensed and federally recognized that are perceived to cause a threat to the other; and
- Efforts to change laws that regulate the practice of midwifery in which nurse-midwives seek less restriction from medicine and more legislatively-mediated autonomy, while CPMs seek licensure as independent midwifery practitioners distinct and separate from the practices of medicine and nursing.

Regardless of the fact that recent research studies have demonstrated that midwives of all varieties are more alike than different in beliefs, attitude and practices,[70] conflicts still exist among the different strands of midwifery. These conflicts from within the profession pose almost as great a threat as the conflicts from outside, that is, from the medical establishment. At times in the past, these conflicts have sidetracked our ability to build a unified profession in the United States. Fortunately there are midwife activists—many of whom are authors in this anthology—who have been working to build bridges and create common ground among midwives and midwifery organizations towards strengthening, fortifying and unifying our profession. The Fusion Midwives, who can walk in both worlds, and talk both talks, often lead the pack in crafting meaningful communication and negotiating collaborative strategies.

Modern Day Heroines

The women whose lives are described in this book have an awareness of their place in history and the unique roles they have played in determining its course. They exemplify the indomitable spirit of consummate revolutionaries. But these midwives are not simply revolutionaries; they hold a vision for an overhaul of the health care system. They have generated new ideas, envisioned new paradigms and invented new systems in order to create change. They work to return birth to the domain of women; put average citizens in charge of family health decisions; replace unnecessary health care spending with cost-effective alternatives; utilize evidence-based protocols and practices; and restore normalcy to childbirth. They also work to ensure that transformation occurs within a social justice framework to enable all people to experience benefits of the system. Most importantly, these midwives form partnerships with women to assist them in discovering and recovering trust in their bodies and faith in the natural processes of pregnancy, birth, breastfeeding, mother-infant attachment, and parenting.

These are stories of women who have sought to forge an identity (in a health care industry shaped mainly by men) involving universal female events that have historically been in the hands of women and directly experienced only by women. These stories are studies in perseverance because the contemporary maternity care system has done its best, whether intentionally or unintentionally, to disempower women. Several authors in this anthology consider the mistreatment of women within the health care system to be a social justice issue. Each of the midwives whose stories you will find here has described her role in the ongoing contemporary social drama related to these struggles.

These are stories of women who have lived a demanding and unique lifestyle. They describe the everyday realities of being on-call twenty-four hours a day, seven days a week, and how that affects family responsibilities, time management, and personal relationships. They describe the necessity of becoming involved with politics in order to survive, the risks they took, the survival skills they developed, and how their political activities helped shape the course of recent history. Some lived in fear of being arrested; some were threatened with legal action; and some were brought to trial as criminals for practicing midwifery.

These are stories of women who are intensely dedicated to the work they do, and they describe both the rewards and what it cost them to do this work. While many of the midwives in this anthology are savvy entrepreneurs, none of them are in the profession "for the money." They are in it because they love the work and they love the women and families they serve. While many have learned to make a good living, they are, nonetheless, from the lineage of midwives who care for women and infants out of a deep sense of dedication and a calling to service.

These are women who have invested in building relationships and in serving their communities. The original word midwife, meaning "with woman," implies a relationship. And it has always been the investment in those relationships that have kept midwives passionate about their work and clients fiercely loyal to their midwives. These authors know that there is nothing quite like connecting intimately with one's community and being cherished by that same community.

These are stories of women who are practitioners, leaders, advocates, innovators and mentors. They are modern day heroines whose stories have escaped the contemporary history books, but whose contributions have not escaped the notice of their communities all across the country, and in some cases, across the world. These are women who stand on the shoulders of many generations of midwife ancestors. In turn, they are the new breed of "pioneer midwives" with generations of protégées now standing on their shoulders.

A Sheltered Place

With the unparalleled rise in cesarean sections and all manner of potentially injurious reproductive technologies, the space that midwives courageously hold for women and newborns is small but potent, sacred yet ephemeral. It is a space for women to trust their bodies and their natural cycles and processes. It is a space for a baby's first experience on Earth to be a peaceful one. It is a sheltered place for families to fall deeply in love with one another at the very beginning of life when new families are made and are magnificently vulnerable.

To watch the newborn infant unfurl its fetal body upon leaving water and entering air; to smell the salty oceanic aroma that fills a quiet room at the time of birth; to hear the first murmuring that a baby makes; and to watch a baby open its eyes and discover the face of its mother for the first time, is a true miracle. It is breathtakingly stunning. This sacred space that midwives hold for women and families is a temple, a sanctuary of initiation. This place is a hallowed haven you can call home.

Geradine Simkins
Northern Michigan
January 2011

Something ancient and new every time

MARINA ALZUGARAY

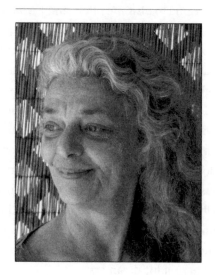

I was born after a very quick labor in Cienfuegos Cuba. Cuca, as I call my mom, tells me that her first labor started when I gave her a kick at 4 A.M., and by 6:30 A.M. I was born. She was nineteen years old then, and today we still go over the birth every year on my birthday. Every March 5th we celebrate our anniversary by talking about the experience, and we are mutually surprised. When recalling her labor, she fills in a new detail every single time, and I add to what she has forgotten to mention. I remember facts, like where my crib was positioned in relation to her bed the window where the light came from, and the sound of my father's footsteps. From Cienfuegos we moved to San Miguel de los

Baños, a spa close to Havana. It is there where I learned to walk at nine months of age on the cool tile floor, where the frogs were about the size of my head. For my two-year birthday, I was all dressed up in a starched dress with a big bow on my back like a gift-wrapped box. The itchy outfit was easy to forget about when I was riding the pony my dad had found for me. But it was a short ride. Soon my parents divorced, and I was never to be with my father again. I was raised in a whirlwind of change. My life has turned out to have many endings, just as it has had many unexpected beginnings. Maybe that is why I remember so many details, or perhaps it is because I was born with my eyes wide open. The rest of my early years before primary school were spent in Havana where I had night-mares, danced with a wonderful gay man, and had an imaginary friend. A Great Mother holding a child came to visit me often, and I would sing with her to the complete oblivion of the adults. When I was around three years old, I was given a duck that liked to play in a planter inside the house. A mirror lined the right, left and backside of that planter. There was no way I could learn not to play with my duck there, even though the adults asked me. I wanted to see myself in the crack between the mirrors. I contemplated images going on forever. While the duck made a royal mess, I was getting my first glance at infinity.

By the time I began elementary school I had a new father and a new town. My second father was a doctor, born a first generation Cuban of Lebanese parents. Tabouleh and hummus became a must-have in my diet from then on, and my lifelong affair with belly dancing began. That life lasted thirteen years in Santa Clara, where I lived through the exciting years of the Cuban revolution. I used to hike a hill close to my house that overlooks the town where Che Guevara now has his remains. It is a private spot for dreamers.

My maternal grandmother, Mama, as I called her, was my inspiration. She had eight successful home births even though she had diabetes and some of her babies weighed up to thirteen pounds at birth. "*Buenas tardes, Doña Cuca,*" echoes from my childhood memory as the customary greeting to my grand-mother from the people who passed by. Mama was a round woman with soft tender skin, big expressive brown eyes, and laughter that cascaded from deep inside her padded belly. She sat every afternoon in front of the verandah, saying hello to friends from her rocking chair and engaging her many grandchildren in long conversations about whatever the afternoon strollers inspired. Her stories ranged from her own childhood to the mischief of the world. Mama had a way with words. Her tone and manner of speaking was enrapturing. She would trans-fix her grandchildren for hours, transporting us into a multitude of adventures.

One warm Cuban afternoon she said, "Look, Mari," bringing me to full attention, "that *señora* is my *comadrona*, a midwife. She helped me with my births, right there in my bedroom, where I had your mother, aunt, and uncles."

The memory of the determined gait of my grandmother's midwife lingered, full of curiosity, in my mind as if awakening a calling; but back then, I was a little girl, not inclined to making future plans. I have asked my mother about the births of her sister and brothers. She told me that she recalled the noises in the middle of the night, the midwife arriving at the house, the other women boiling water, a table cleaned and rolled into the front bedroom, and her own quiet, as she listened to every sound. When the cry of a baby resonated throughout the house, she said, "Papo, my grandfather would say after each birth: 'A new baby always brings good fortune.'" The day after the birth, my mother would go into the bedroom to meet the little one. The baby would be nursing or sleeping quietly in the laced crib next to Mama's big bed. "Mama nursed all of her children until they were walking and swimming," my mother murmured, as if sharing a secret. "Swimming!" I exclaimed. "Yes Mari, Mama would nurse them in the water." She explained how her youngest brother had suckled, half floating, in the ocean.

I experienced the calling to be a healer on the night my grandmother passed on to the other side. She was my role model, curing the family with her own remedies. Walking the countryside with her and her husband—my grandfather—was a whole botany class lesson. They had set the stage for who I am by loving me easily. Along the way, the midwife inside of me awakened surprisingly naturally. It was as if midwifery was leading me on from the start, except that I was not aware of it.

Mama and I moved to the United States from Cuba during the late '60s, and what a blissful time it was for me to enter into sexual explorations. Confusing as it was, I was taken by a movement that encouraged my natural urges, leading me to find beauty in my own body, instead of guilt. I was part of a wave of people who traveled the world in search of answers. I went to California and there I met a lay midwife. She spoke about birth from a point of view of beauty, of the power life has to offer, of how a woman and her family can take the moment of birth as a journey of love and self-discovery. Her birth description had an old ring to it. I had never heard births described in that way before, but it was reminiscent of the pride with which my grandmother had spoken of births.

One night in northern New Mexico I sat on a mountaintop looking up at the swirling clouds over a full moon. The moon clouds were parading while sounds of chants from a Native American ceremony encircled me throughout

the night. At sunrise, I went into a *kiva*, a Native American underground structure, to meditate. I closed my eyes and saw my grandmother clearly. I was a small
girl sitting in a bathtub in her house in Cuba. Mama was sitting next to the old
fashioned tub bathing me, pouring water over my body with a large cup, while
she spoke in her romantic metaphors. She was counseling me about life as she had
done so many times before. "Stay out of deep waters," she said a few times while
dousing me. The water felt soothing, her voice rolled as smooth as water. The
scene was very clear and her speech was so real that I had to open my eyes several
times to see for myself that she wasn't standing in front of me. Her presence was
that strong, and all I had to do was to go back into my meditation again and there
the scene returned, until it melted away and the voice changed, moving directions, tone and language. Those last words I could not understand. They were in
a language I could not interpret. Then, it all stopped and I was no longer meditat-
ing. Her presence had warmed me during the crisp sunrise. Later that morning I
wrote Mama a long letter telling her about the sages in New Mexico, her presence
in my meditation, and that I had found my calling. I even included a few leaves of
sage in the envelope for her to smell, feel, and enjoy. The sage in New Mexico was
completely different from the one she knew and used, so I was sure she would be
pleased with the new variety. I added that the night had intoxicated me with the
chants and her presence, and it had clarified my thoughts. From that day forward
my life had a focus: I was going to follow the path of a healer.

After writing the letter to her, I packed up my backpack. During my hike
down the mountain that morning, I met a woman camping out. She was in early
labor and planning to birth her baby right there. There was much I needed to
learn, and with this woman I witnessed contractions for the first time in my life.
She sat up breathing loudly, practicing a type of yogic breath technique I had not
seen before. I wanted to help her, but I had no idea what to do. I stayed with her
for a few hours until someone who could help her arrived. I left thinking that
perhaps one day I would know what to do at a birth.

Soon I received an answer to the letter I had sent to Mama. I do not remember
exactly how they found me, but what I remember clearly is my conversation with my
aunt and how I stood at the public phone in Taos, crying loud enough to let the four
winds know that my grandmother, my love, had gone to the other side. "According
to the date of your letter," my aunt told me, "you wrote to her on the morning after
she passed away. Mama left during her sleep." That is how she had said she wanted
to die. She did not want to be ill or bedridden. She wanted to be well; she had gone
shopping that day and had gone to bed as usual. She was seventy-two years old.

I looked into going back to school and hitchhiked to Florida where my grand-mother had lived. I enrolled in a two-year associate degree nursing program. I was hoping that somehow becoming a nurse would help me to at least move closer to my goal to become a healer. During my nursing training, women were birthing their babies in desperation. I witnessed my first five births all during one night in the hospital where the student nurses trained. A full moon was shining through the open window, but there was nothing romantic about that night. Women were screaming, tied by their wrists to the bed railings, agonizing and delirious with medication making them incoherent. When it was time to birth, they were rolled into the delivery room, placed onto a delivery table, strapped down and given more medication to finally sleep. Their babies were pulled out with forceps. The infants were resuscitated and taken to the nursery while the moms woke up in the recovery room completely out of it and asking if they had had their babies yet. One after the other, I saw five different women go through it. By the time the sun came up, I had finished my intrapartum rotation.

No matter how bright the sun shone that day, I could not shake the darkness and the nightmares I had witnessed. I felt compassion towards the women, sadness for everyone, and anger at the misunderstanding and mistreatment of women during births. I refused to believe that this was what birth should be about. There had to be another way. The experience did not engulf me with fear of childbirth; instead I feared that the treatment of women had resembled torture. I could sense it, deep inside of me, and it was revolting. And just because this was the way it was being done by well-intended doctors and nurses, I was not favorably impressed. Pregnancy and birth were not illnesses, and medical interventions were not saving anything or anybody. What I had witnessed was an aberration not to be trusted. I had grown up in a family full of physicians. Hospital procedures, patient care, operative techniques and the importance of doctors were common subjects at lunch, dinner, and even parties. Physicians were people like anyone else.

I was deeply disappointed at what I had witnessed and decided to speak up about it at nursing school. Luckily one of my nursing instructors told me about The Farm in Tennessee. This was before we even knew that there was a home birth movement. All we knew was that there were women helping women to birth with the kind of care, understanding and bliss that was explained by Ina May Gaskin in her book *Spiritual Midwifery*. The "midwife's bible" I used to call it, proclaiming birth as a spiritual and loving process. I read it cover to cover several times. I memorized the language and ideas. The stories resonated in my heart unlike the births I had observed. I realized that if I was going to be a healer I did not need to take the medical focus on pathology seriously when it came to normal events. Pregnancy, childbirth and mothering are stages of women's lives that are meant to be nurtured.

Meanwhile, I graduated from nursing school, took my Registered Nurse (RN) board exams while living with my husband, Steve. I can still remember the smell of magnolias and the aroma of our bodies in our endless love embrace. I went about learning all I could about the reproductive system's anatomy and physiology, women's sexuality, and anything I could find on wellness, orgasms, massage, self-help, birthing, mothering, and enlightenment. The holiness of women is embellished by lovemaking. Conception and our reproductive powers are gifts that can culminate in the miracle of birth. Pregnancy is a time to be gently cared for. I firmly believe that just because women are vulnerable does not mean we should be mistreated.

With the RN license in my hand, we relocated to California in the mid-seventies. Steve worked as an artist, Sharin, our son, went to preschool, and I found the perfect job in Santa Barbara. I became part of a free clinic collective. At the community clinic I learned how to reorient medical services into wellness care. The collaboration between doctors and alternative health practitioners provided us with an opportunity to assist our clients holistically.

My first job was an experiment in the health care system. There I met a female physician who was integrating alternatives into her family practice. Doctors and healers worked side by side and shared their skills with the barefoot health workers like myself. We were demystifying the idea of the medical empire, creating a utopia within the fringes of the medical system. Soon I was able to create a healing environment, give a shiatsu massage, converse about herbs, do pelvic exams, and take care of simple problems on my own, or as part of the team. We gave information about self-help, herbs, massage, healing, and how to harmonize mind, body and spirit. It was the mid-seventies and the book, *Our Bodies, Ourselves,* from the Boston Women's Health Collective had just come out. The women's health movement was on the rise.

Assertiveness training for women, women's liberation, wellness and self-help were the core of the collective and what we offered at the Freedom Clinic. I facilitated groups of women interested in using their own speculum to examine their cervix. We took countless vaginal smears to look at vaginal mucus under the microscope to learn about our bodies, even our partner's sperm. The tadpole-like sperms had iridescent rainbow-like heads. We were following with excitement the discovery and application of alternative health and healing for our community and ourselves. Conception, pregnancy, birth, breastfeeding, children, parenting, womanhood, sexuality, and nurturing all fascinated me and seemed to fit into the very core of wellness. I wanted to be completely immersed in it. I prepared myself for my own pregnancy and focused on the study of my own fertile cycles. Motherhood forever! I was becoming a midwife. I attended a nurse practitioner program to become a women's health care specialist at the University of California at Long Beach. There I began to teach women about the menstrual cycle, ovulation, and the body's signs of fertility. It was not long before I realized I wanted to help women give birth. I applied to a midwifery educational program and was accepted with the very next class. As a consequence, we moved to San Francisco so I could attend class at the University of California (UCSF).

At the midwifery program I experienced bouts of diarrhea on my first few days on-call just by thinking of births. I wondered if I had the strength necessary to assist a woman in labor. Five days went by, but not a single woman in labor walked into San Francisco General Hospital. By the time of the first birth, my digestive nervous problems had stopped. After that experience, the midwife working with me asked if I had been a lay midwife, but added that my hands probably knew what to do. My body had known all along what my mind could not yet begin to comprehend. The body's natural intuition and the wisdom of women and midwives had been muted. An extraordinary gap of knowledge had to be rediscovered. Nancy, one of my classmates, made the point that we needed to deal with the emotional issues we had around birthing. These were either from our own upbringing, from our own experiences as women, or from what we were learning or experiencing in the program. She convinced us to do a form of counseling that focuses on emotional release. The idea was based on a theory that as long as a person is acting out of trauma with emotionally charged behaviors, it is impossible to be clear enough to open our minds to making new decisions or having a different outlook. My midwifery class accepted this type of counseling, and the results released old or new emotions and benefited us immensely. I learned that midwives have knowledge about life, living, birthing, and dying beyond what I had ever imagined, much of it seemingly stored in their genes or perhaps "genius."

I also learned that many of the doctors, nurses and even midwives were acting out of old fears. There was no way caregivers could shoulder so much stress in the hospital environment without protecting and distancing themselves. Or if they had been traumatized by a difficult complication, they were not going to allow the problem to recur. To prevent the problems they needed to intervene early. Cutting an episiotomy was done to avoid tears; yanking on a baby's head was done to avoid stuck shoulders; and resuscitating every baby was done to avoid breathing problems. And if asked, "Why do it?" because it did not look like the problem was imminent, the answer always came back to the fact that the caregivers had previously had a traumatic experience. The caregivers narrated in detail what had led them to their routine interventions. The caregivers were not about to go through that experience again, and women and infants, normal or not, were thus treated as if they were on the verge of a horrible mishap.

During my training I was also able to attend a few home births and witness the type of births I had always thought possible. The home births were intimate, hard but powerful, and at the end the family expressed a type of euphoria that I had never seen elsewhere. It became clear to me that I must safeguard the emotional and physical integrity of women and babies where the birth took place, and so I focused on developing the strength to heal within myself the shock of traumatic incidents. This endeavor has required me to participate in an endless path of self-healing to release traumatic experiences from the past and maintain a clear perspective to care for women as unique individuals, so that each woman will be able to birth wholesomely at home or even in a hospital.

I then began to understand and feel compassion for the kind of stress experienced by folks working in mainstream health systems. To lighten the load, I began to perform as a belly dancer and to teach Afro-Cuban dancing. Nurses, midwives, doctors, students, and families had all come together as a dance troupe to perform the Cuban "*Comparsa*" down Mission Street, all dressed up like Carmen Miranda during the San Francisco Carnival. We had a great time. The extra curriculum activity served to unite us in fun, bonding us with friendships that rippled into our work, opening a different level of communication and building solidarity. Uniting a diverse group in fun has a tremendous positive effect that can be used for healing. Since that very first dance troupe experience, I have proceeded to facilitate artistic expressions in groups everywhere. This includes expressions of birth in what I call "the birth dance," which combines storytelling and dance to create a feeling of "Ah…I get it," a realization for women about birthing.

As soon as I graduated as a Certified Nurse-Midwife, I went into private practice with Paula, one of my classmates. We planned to do home and hospital births in Washington State. One morning we were taking a big poster that said "Midwifery Services" to the hospital when a pregnant woman saw the sign and ran over to us. "Are you midwives? I am looking for one," she said. She became our first client, and two weeks later she was sitting by the fire pit during our home birth midwife initiation ceremony. She had carefully placed all of the special rocks to be heated in the fire—rocks that will not crack and shatter when the water sprinkled on them turns to steam—as well as arranging every single other item needed to run the ceremony. She was a Native American woman and was glad to facilitate the ritual in which we all were excited about participating. Before we began to attend home births on our own we needed to complete the ceremony. It was our blessing ritual, our rite of passage into a woman's sacred profession.

We gathered in a circle very early one morning, each of the women present sharing who they were and where they were in their journey as a woman. One woman was pregnant, so she was going to stay outside of the lodge and sit by the altar. Another was mensing, so for her we found a spot far away from the sweat lodge where she could run her own women's ceremony with her blood. Another woman was ovulating, another who did not menstruate anymore, another just past her monthly menstruation, and yet another some days before her menses. We realized that we were well represented, and so we proceeded with the ceremony. It was hard work. First we dug a pit and used the earth that we dug out to build an altar. We went about building the structure with long willow poles. And then we made the fire, cooked the rocks, and finally, almost by sunset, we were ready to go into the sweat lodge.

We blessed each of us before entering the sweat and all of our home birth midwifery tools. There were scissors for cutting the cord, a fetoscope for listening to the heart, and an assortment of items from our midwifery bag. We asked for blessings for our midwife hands, and said small prayers holding each object. We placed our midwifery kit close to the altar, wishing to establish a connection with spirit to guide our hands and the use of our tools. In the lodge we chanted and prayed for all women—for their healing, safety, and guidance. We asked for blessings for birthing women and for all of the future children. We gave thanks for that happy day, for being midwives, for the ceremony, and for the birth and life of the woman and the little Native American child within the woman who had brought us the rocks.

"I am now a midwife ready to serve women. May I listen carefully for what each woman needs, may I follow the guidance of spirit, and may I gently follow this path," I said. The group responded, "So be it." At the end of that evening we plunged into the cold and invigorating water of the Pacific Ocean. I felt alert and ready. We shared food by the fire, cleared the grounds, and received a light sprinkle from the sky as if the heavens had dropped a few joyful tears from witnessing the midwives' commitment and the beauty of our ceremony. This was the beginning of many such ceremonies.

Birthing is intense. It is unpredictable, it is powerful, it is work, but it is something a woman can do. Being a midwife of the unknown and laboring with each woman as if she is the only one ever to bring forth the unique blessing of life is a fantastic undertaking. It requires extreme abilities. This I did not come upon right away. It took a lot of practical learning of skills and wisdom to know how to truly open to the essence of each woman and child and their cosmology during birth. I have witnessed women able to love with a power that exceeds words and exude a type of uncontrollable joy, a feeling that expands to everyone and into every niche of her home. It is an unexplainable satisfaction that can be felt for days.

Birth tests the fragility and strength of a family and their belief systems. Home is where families have shown me their best, their spirit, and their commitment for one another. Home is where we rediscovered the power of birth and where we have imprinted forever a type of humbling, mind-buckling happiness. We were reclaiming not only sacred birthing and conscious babies, but also healthy environments that nurture women and, in turn, the families grew not only in size but also in strength. A family supporting the notion that a woman is able to birth at home gives the woman a feeling of trust to safely birth—using her own resources—within the loving help of her family and midwives. This recognizes that birth is normal, and confirms that she has the type of home environment that she can trust to care for her and her baby during her most vulnerable and powerful moments. It requires that her extended family give of themselves to welcome the new child with plenty of love and common sense.

That type of a birth has given me hope for the future of humanity. I wanted to experience this in my own body, but then I had a tubal pregnancy that almost took my own life. In the process of healing I went to a sweat led by Archie Lame Deer. It happened in Santa Barbara where I opened my own midwifery practice after a year in Washington. I was back in the place I call my "home town." That day he asked me in a formal way to help with the healing of women. I was holding the medicine pipe of his grandfather and felt moved to the core. I began to lead sweat lodges; my journey into the women's moon lodge, now also called the "red tent" began that day. It was not an easy path to take back then. There was no one to learn from and nothing else to do but as he suggested—"you have it in you, bring it forth." He was so very right about that. It was not easy to want a pregnancy, lose a child, witness my own blood and turn it into prayer.

Yet magic was to happen in other ways. As I opened the door to possibilities, I found myself swimming with dolphins in the open ocean, and soon after that I began to attend water births. I am told that I am a "water birth pioneer" in this country. In the early years of water birth, I witnessed the ease of the laboring woman in water. It was a wonderment, and so were the babies who often swam to the surface on their own. It was from water that the American AquaNatal Program* was born. It began as a series of wellness exercises derived from my dual relationship with birth and dolphins to facilitate women's bodies for birthing and recovering after birth. I initially called my exercises AquaYoga. But now, twenty years later, American AquaNatal is a joyfully wet, sensual program. The method has spread everywhere, including North and South America, Japan, Eastern and Western Europe, Alaska and the Caribbean. Water birth, too, has taken off. It is lapping its influence on every shore and making a splash even in hospitals.

In one of my most recent adventures I developed a unique fertility awareness tool called MyMoon Cards: Understanding My Body and Monthly Cycle©. The idea was born out of a desire to teach the complex changes of women's bodies during the menstrual cycle years, one day at a time. I was working with teens in the Florida Keys and the same questions kept coming up over and over. So now, I share them in workshops, often bringing mothers and daughters together to celebrate the passage into womanhood. I mentor a magnificent group of young women to whom I have become their "Sister Mother." As I am much older now and love them as a sister and mother, they have become my "Sister Daughters."

Possibly more difficult than being a midwife has been the process of midwifing myself. It took all I had and more. From my own cycles and explorations, I have led countless circles and have helped many women who have experienced trauma concerning problems with the ovary, the womb, fertility, and sexuality. I have used prayers, songs and massage techniques to release agony, pain and pleasure all connected to being a woman. I have traveled to a place of knowing what to do for myself and many others. Women *do* have the knowledge inside themselves.

Through midwifery I have found in birth the universal truths that are cross-cultural and imperative to all living organisms, truths that require a belief in the magnificence and omnipresence of spirit manifesting again and again through an endless renewal. Birth is something that is ancient and new every time. It is something that is an unforgettable everyday act, a key to existence.

I have learned from laboring women how to welcome spirit, from the sweat lodge how to be present, from nature how to go beyond fear, from dolphins how to breathe for hours, from my grandmother how to forgive each moment, from the unborn how to be joyful, and from the heart of hearts how to function inside a miracle. My life is dedicated to bringing forth a world of peace each moment. What it takes is a belief so deeply rooted that, even if one does not know just how, one has to trust the ability of humanity to unfold the orgasmic power in body and soul. This is what I do as a spiritual practice. I midwife in gratitude for all that I have experienced and have learned and continue to learn in following my original intent of spirit-guided healer. It is all about flowing in an everlasting fertile river, midwifing life.

Again and again I saw the strength of women

RONDI ANDERSON

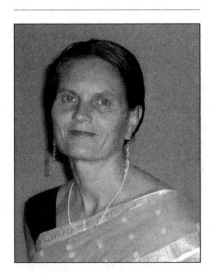

I write this as I sit here in Assam, India. My days are filled with planning and implementing reproductive health programs for some of the world's poorest people, people needing help with obstetric emergencies, antenatal care, family planning, and prevention of sexually transmitted infections and mother-to-child transmission.

I grew up in a Midwest college town. My father was a religion professor. I was the oldest; my brother was seven years younger. Between us my mother had given birth to Siamese twins that had died before I saw them, stretching my two-year-old thoughts about birth and death and humanity. In many ways we were a typical middle-class family, not challenging much of what society offered.

Then, in my early adolescence, the hippie countercultural movement arose. I was swept away by it, sitting in the streets to protest the war while my liberal father was concerned that I should be attending my eighth-grade classes instead. Filled with the wildness of youth, we attempted to cast away what we saw as wrong in our society. I left public school and joined a group of other teens to create our own school. We built shelters in the woods, experimented with mind-altering drugs and sexuality, rode bikes, studied yoga and very rarely looked at textbooks. By my late teens, I had started taking a few classes at the local community college in subjects that were interesting to me. I got involved with a man. I moved in with him on my eighteenth birthday, and six months later—after much persuasion from him—I was carrying a planned pregnancy. I was going against the wisdom and norms of the culture and felt terrified and full of possibility.

I gave birth in my home, surrounded by only a handful of friends. I was nineteen, and I had read Raven Lang's *Birth* and Ina May's *Spiritual Midwifery*, as well as *Mothering* magazine, all of which had been newly published. My labor was brutal and my body was full of the pain of the world. But the birth itself was magical ambrosia. That little wet purple girl, coming from me, coming from nowhere, connected me to all the other mothers, past and future.

With the passion that only new lovers know, my birth experience hurtled me into a new life as a midwife. In my early years I learned through watching. I was hungry for each new experience. I read everything in alternative literature, and I followed my teachers, both the midwife and the doctor who first took me to attend births. I also learned from the hundreds of women who trusted their bodies and shared with me their personal and yet elemental experiences of giving birth. In these early years we were a tribe, banded together, giving birth back to women. We were not listening to the institutions. We gathered, we chanted around fires, we told our stories, we called on each other night and day with both the unusual or the difficult. We were proud and smug of the sleepiness in our eyes and the blood on our knees; we knew we held the sacred in our hands.

But we also felt the urge to grow. We were consumed by the challenge of how to bring this awareness to the masses. We neither knew how to reach the poor and the less empowered nor how to make the powerful listen to us. Eventually we all went our separate ways, some of us holding the fort, others going off to medical and nursing school. After some internal confusion, my own desire for expansion brought me to nursing school. Five years older, with a child of my own and knowing the secrets of midwifery, I entered undergraduate nursing school. Dressed in scrubs, I attempted to share what I knew without overtly challenging my instructors or the institutions that were teaching me. I learned that I could play the game, and even though I was not always comfortable, I knew that more doors could open for me.

After I received my BSN (Bachelor of Science in Nursing) and my child was in elementary school, we loaded up our little car with bicycles and toys and drove across the country to the Navajo reservation in Arizona. I had decided that working with such an intriguing group of people would help me stomach the parts of institutionalized birth which were abrasive to me. It would be a gift to see if I could help. I spent two years on the reservation, and, in that time I became intimate with "the enemy"—an obstetrician who shared my passion of caring for women, but with almost none of my perspective. We challenged each other over IVs and inductions while amazing women pushed babies out, in spite of and because of us. I got to grapple with how to serve women within the limitations of the medical institution. In working within the hospital, I got to see if what I had learned from home births (where nature simply took its course) could also be applied to a hospital whose policies are not geared toward letting nature take its course or empowering women. Was it possible for a woman to squat on a labor bed, or could she be allowed on the floor? Could the obstetrician looking over my shoulder be persuaded to let women be in the tub? There were successes and challenges. One day a male resident physician asked me to rupture a woman's membranes. I refused because I had seen too many umbilical cords prolapsed after this type of intervention. My strong stance brought the resident to tears. It was then that I decided that my frustration with working as a nurse in a hospital was too much. I decided to become a Certified Nurse-Midwife with the hopes of having more independence and control over how I was caring for women.

So, with my now older elementary school child, and our small car again loaded with bicycles on top and a dog, we headed north for Salt Lake City to experience midwifery in a box, as it were, packaged by the college of nursing. I was to become a CNM (Certified Nurse-Midwife), fully processed. It was there that I would cut my first episiotomy and fight for women to have the choice *not* to have an epidural. I enjoyed my part-time work at a lovely birth center. And, while it wasn't quite home, it was full of freedoms for families in labor. I read about weight gain in pregnancy, menopause and female sexual response. My professors were eccentric, full of wisdom and, for the most part, affirming of me.

By the end of those two years I needed to breathe home birth again. The routine hospitalization of birthing mothers was frustrating me. I wanted to do what I knew best: sit with women while they did what only they knew how to do—give birth. I wrote to every home birth practice listed in the country. I got some replies; they were open to working with me but were not in need of new staff. Then a reply came from a midwife working in an Amish community in Lancaster County, Pennsylvania. How could I resist? I was being invited to join the most conservative to do the most radical. Those pioneer midwives before me had blazed the path and I only needed to show up. There was a home birth practice already in place that needed a midwife. So, with my daughter, who was now in junior high school, the dog and bicycles, we again headed across the country to a land where canyons were made of corn, and home births were as normal as quilting and shoo fly pie.

I spent ten amazing years there. I worked until I lay exhausted on my bed, my coat and hat still on, and sound asleep but never far from the phone. The Amish gave me everything my midwifery heart wanted. They knew that birth was normal. They let me show the world that this was a good idea. I wrote articles, I invited hundreds of midwives, doctors, nurses, students and weathered professionals to come see the work we did there. Newspapers and book authors came. I drove through ice storms and walked down lanes in the dark. I looked for husbands in barns while they milked cows. I sat with 1600 women while they shared intimate moments of their lives with me. Again and again I saw the strength of those women. I saw them make their way. In those ten years only one woman asked to go to the hospital for pain management. They walked, they did their laundry, they milked the cows, they laughed, they cried, they yelled, they held on, they pushed away, they squatted down . . . and eventually the baby came, blessing us with its cry.

Eventually I began to hear a small voice inside, asking, *What about the poorest of the world? What about those you only hear distant rumors about, those women who are dying because of lack of care?* Could I do something for them? After all, Lancaster County was only a very small corner of the universe, and I wanted to see more. I applied to Doctors Without Borders in the fall of 1997. My daughter was then away at college, and, feeling that Lancaster County was a bit too conservative, she had vowed not to come back for more than a visit. I was offered a position in the spring of 1998 but I didn't take it; I wasn't ready yet to leave the practice that I loved and that had nurtured me for so long. But my thoughts kept wandering towards Africa. A year later I came home to find two poignant messages on my answering machine, one from *Médecins Sans Frontières* (Doctors Without Borders) offering me a position in Somalia, the other from an old student wondering if I had any midwifery work for her. That's when I decided I couldn't resist. In the spring of 1999, after much mental struggle, I handed my practice over to my student and departed for Somalia, and stayed for the next thirteen months.

I felt intensely anxious about flying to Somalia. I worried about leaving the security of my practice and about missing my friends, my daughter and my parents. Yet I did not worry that I wouldn't know what to do. I figured that ten years of births by propane and kerosene light had prepared me for everything I would encounter. I was excited about exploring a new culture, but I had no idea of the totally different world I would find there.

Galcayo Somalia is a four-hour flight from Nairobi and the roads are too dangerous to drive. Like Sierra Leone, after having endured many brutal wars, Somalia is a country largely without health care infrastructure and fraught with malaria. It is also like this in Assam, India. Both Somalia and Sierra Leone are filled with people displaced from their land as their tribes struggle for existing resources. All of them tell the same story, a story that if we heard it in the West, we are sure it could have happened only once or twice, and yet this story is very real for the majority of the world's population. Death of women in childbirth is commonplace; it's one of the leading causes of death in adults. Often the chance of dying from pregnancy is more than 1 in 10. Women are poor and anemic from lack of food and malaria. They have many children from lack of access to family planning or due to cultural taboos. In some places, culture demands excision of part of the female genitals, leading to emotional and physical obstacles and pain.

The women that gather to help each other with birth have no formal education. Although they are wise when ushering in a normal birth, when problems are encountered their traditions (often arising from fear) can be quite harsh. They have no access to medical care, and if the problems are not resolved, women and infants die. The community accepts it as inevitable. It is a part of life. The clinics and hospitals I've worked in have been full of the tragic outcomes, with some small successes. Eclampsia, arm prolapse, retained twin, fetal death, sepsis, antepartum and postpartum hemorrhage, retained placenta, shoulder dystocia, prolonged labor, uterine rupture, severe anemia, newborn death—all of these medical conditions are commonplace.

Working for *Médecins Sans Frontières* (MSF), we provided assistance at government reproductive health clinics and hospital maternity wards. There we dispensed ferrous sulfate and folic acid, bednets, clean razor blades and soap, malaria prophylaxis and educational material on PMTCT (Preventing Mother-to-Child Transmission). We screened for malaria, STI/HIV and anemia. We offered family planning. We taught the communities how to recognize problems.

We tried to respond to pre-eclampsia before the seizure and to treat severe anemia before it became fatal. We responded to emergencies before the fetus or the mother died. Many were saved. And, although it was shocking to us— grounded as we were in our Western perspective—many lives were lost.

In these settings the struggle for survival often overshadowed the comforts we strive to attain in the West. When I was teaching someone how to administer magnesium sulfate to an eclamptic woman, it was often difficult to persuade that busy, minimally-educated caregiver to focus on the importance of comforting the scared laboring women lying next to her. I continued to try to hold it all, and people did learn, for example, that being upright did facilitate labor, and that drinking water was good. And soothing words and touch do feel better to every-one. But all too often these very poor women, if they received care at all, encoun-tered only an impersonal coldness rather than a welcoming embrace. Still, the sacred is there; it can be felt in the room when a baby cries, having overcome all the obstacles in the way of her survival. It can be seen when a woman, whose life has been one hardship after another, finally smiles.

In Somalia I worked in a hospital where the maternal death rate was 1 in 30. I sat with a patient who would be my first maternal death, a pregnant women who was bleeding, as I tried to convince the busy private obstetrician, one of only a handful in the country, to attend to her. The mother was poor—of a much lower class than the doctor—and so could not pay. MSF (*Médecins Sans Frontières*) had brought no surgeon to Galcayo. We were using a local surgeon when he was willing. Two international surgeons also participated in our group. So I scrambled to learn what to do. The women that came to this hospital were all sicker than most people one would find in a Western Intensive Care Unit. These women had all walked to the hospital from far away, attesting to their strength. There I was in a hospital, with no electricity, no running water, and only the very basic life-saving drugs. Luckily there was literature that could guide me. I learned about the quiet suffering of maternal mortality. I learned that the global community thought that simply giving "Traditional Birth Attendants" soap could address the issue and that clean water could prevent diarrhea. Meanwhile, I sat riveted while reading the literature written by Deborah Maine, professor of clinical population and family health at Columbia University, as she staged a largely unheard protest. She said clearly and articulately that the causes of maternal death were the same globally, that they were not predictable but that they were treatable, and that soap didn't make a difference. She said that access to emergency care could save many lives. I, who guarded the sanctity of normal birth and who firmly believed in lower cesarean section rates in the populations that I had previously worked with in the U.S., learned that the other extreme was also tragic. I went about doing my best to implement Deborah Maine's suggestions. I tried to suggest to the minimally educated hospital maternity nurses and doctors that there was hope, that is, if we provided care, then we could successfully treat the sick and most would live.

In 2006 I flew to Sierra Leone for my second mission with Doctors Without Borders. One of the poorest countries in the world, Sierra Leone is now stable but has in recent years been devastated by war. The local health administrators were often distracted by their recent rise out of poverty and had trouble focusing on seemingly unsolvable problems. In the hospitals, as many as 25% of the babies did not survive pregnancy, delivery, or the neonatal weeks. Maternal mortality was often as high as 5% of admissions and sometimes higher.

In spite of all my experience in the United States, nothing had prepared me for working in the poorest countries of the world. But the opportunity to wrestle with the problems that face the majority of poor women who give birth has been an important experience.

The problems are complex and tragic, the moments rich with the exotic. These are countries where owning a car is as rare as owning a plane in the West, and where many villages or nomadic groups must walk on footpaths for hours or even days to access health care. Here a functional hospital usually has no running water and is dependent on a generator for electricity. The majority of the staff have no professional training, yet they endeavor to take care of the most gravely ill women in the world. Here most educated people who can leave the country do leave.

The stories from these hospitals were indeed tragic. The kind friends and colleagues in the West cannot quite believe they are true, and are sure they must be isolated events. And yet, they were a daily occurrence, even two or three times a day. The problems are predictable, well-documented in the global safe motherhood literature, yet as commonly acknowledged as the problems are, it is still mind-boggling to comprehend.

In spite of the intensity and tragedy, for me it was satisfying to work with the challenges posed by such real problems and needs. I often find it less meaningful to care for people in the West, with our excessive reliance on technology. It feels embarrassing that we spend so much money to make sure one women doesn't have a problem for which she is at low risk, when that same amount of money could run a hospital in Africa for a year.

Of course, there were many rewards working in Africa—the women and babies that lived, the gratitude, and witnessing the open hearts of people who have been given so little in this lifetime. Over and over, I was presented with the opportunity to learn from the local people how to appreciate life even in the midst of hardship. For us—the privileged of the world—there was the gift of grappling with very real and very challenging issues ranging from the clinical issues to the political. It was a chance to try to be helpful in the face of extreme need.

Between Somalia and Sierra Leone I worked in the United States for five years. I knew I needed some time to settle after the experience in Somalia. Although the Somalis were overwhelmingly welcoming, calling to us enthusiastically when we walked through town, we had met with aggression, enough for me to begin seriously looking at both the intensity of the work and my own personal safety, and what risks I wanted to take.

Salem, Massachusetts is a beautiful community—the harbor is calm, a perfect respite. After returning from Africa, it was here I worked in a hospital where midwives and nurses and doctors were all friends, where we all attended the same meetings and the same parties. I shared call with a handful of wonderful midwives, and we were best friends, handing women in labor from one to the other. The nurses used birthing balls and lactation consultants, made rounds in the hospital after women gave birth. The women were interesting to me, most coming to us from the health centers we staffed. My Spanish got better. My experience there was pleasant and I had time off. I felt like the presence of midwives made people think. At the least, I felt we made people imagine that birth without an epidural could be desirable, and that rising cesarean section rates might not be necessarily good. But all too often I found that when working in the belly of the beast, I felt lulled or powerless in the face of the system. It was an okay system, one with strengths and weaknesses, but one whose values often differed deeply from my own.

So it was with sadness that I left my lovely apartment overlooking the sea, and decided to return to Sierra Leone, where the beach is beautiful and the suffering of so many pregnant women is incomparable. From there I went to Assam and Manipur India, places where reproductive health needs go largely unmet. These are places where even the organizations that support health often forget about the women laboring at home.

At face value, it might seem like home birth and Obstetric Emergency Response—the two issues I have had the most passion for in my career—are in opposition. But in truth, they are both on the same continuum. Obstetric Emergency Response within a health care system is the basic step; home birth with emergency access is a further refinement. A woman in the developing world might be facing the possibility of death as soon as she enters the passage of birth. Or a privileged woman in the United States might be lulled by the medical institutions into thinking that she can be saved, and thus she will go to the hospital to birth only to be robbed of the transformative experience to which she and her family are entitled. Though worlds apart, both women are enduring the fact that those in power often don't see or value what is important to women.

I feel good about the contributions I have made. I am proud of the research I have done and articles I have written. I know I have helped to increase the awareness of many people in these areas. Yet, there is an endless amount of work still to be done. Cesarean section rates have only increased, newborn nurseries still give breastfed babies bottles, maternal mortality in the developing world is so widespread that it cannot be counted, to say nothing of reduced. There is plenty to keep the next generation of midwives busy. I hope that they find the blissful mystery of birth and that they learn to see the silent suffering both inside and outside of our nation's borders.

The knowledge in your hands

ALICE BAILES

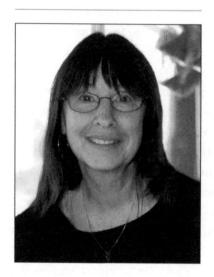

Four years ago, I built the first fire in the woodstove in my new house and wept. The self sufficient, rugged individual who was my father would have loved this place, where you can see forever across the valley to the mountains in the distance and the woods beckon you to crunch your way to the river. From the time I was two in 1948, I remember building fires with him outdoors while camping on the beach or in the woods, or inside in the living room fireplace at home. My grief at his death will forever be sweetened by the memories that inspire my life.

My mother and father worked together to design the house I grew up in. Being committed "do-it-yourselfers," they made an agreement with the builder to do the painting and finishing themselves. As a six-year-old wielding paintbrush and tools, I was welcomed to join in. They had a vision, a unique house a la Frank Lloyd Wright, different from every other house in the neighborhood, and they made it happen right in the Northern Virginia suburbs of Washington, D.C., in the1950s. They enjoyed their divergence from the surrounding landscape. It was my home throughout my school years.

Mama was a painter, puppeteer, and photojournalist. Daddy was a government accountant, auditor and investigator. His family emigrated from Romania to New York City, where Daddy was born in the Bronx. At age five, Mama left Poland with her family just before the Second World War, settling in Tennessee. Both grew up working in their families' stores from childhood through college. Education, treasured by both families, was valued for its own sake but was also regarded as the way out of poverty. They met at a Valentine's Day dance at the Knoxville Jewish Community Center. It was love at first sight and they were married four months later.

My parents filled our home with a community of friends from all over the world, people who spoke many different languages and who enjoyed international music and dance. Almost all of us were Jewish immigrants with Eastern European roots. This heritage allowed me to look at the world around me from the vantage point of an outsider, a member of a distinct minority. I noticed the workings of social constructs, and I valued my comfortable sense of difference from the mainstream. There was a keen social justice consciousness among the group. Racial segregation was very real in Virginia. From the early days of the civil rights movement in the 1950s, my mother was part of a group that created a racially integrated day camp for us kids. Living in Washington, D.C., in the 1960s, we participated in civil rights demonstrations and peace marches, putting up weekend demonstrators in sleeping bags on our living room floor. Liberal politics was a dominant theme of conversation—always focusing on what we could do to make the world a better place.

The values transmitted to me while growing up helped prepare me to become a midwife within the culture of the United States in the last half of the twentieth century. I was encouraged to look beyond the typical, beyond the usual, beyond "the way things are done." But it wasn't just a critical evaluation. There was an energy, a creativity of invention that had been woven into the fabric of my daily life, whether to beautify or to act to remediate society's ills. When I experienced the face of maternity care, these values gave me an ability to see what needed to be changed and to assume the responsibility of working to make things better.

I have said many, many times that my daughter made me into a midwife. Like many others in the field of maternity care, my birth experience was life changing. Also, like other midwives, my life experience, family background, the times, and my own identity made me more than ready to pursue this path. A vital part of that identity has always been a fascination with mind/body interaction. It has been the fulcrum around which I have made essential discoveries throughout my life. Mind/body interaction has two sides—a creative/expressive side and a technical/scientific side.

I became consciously aware of mind/body interaction in the 1950s while watching a TV special about the blood, called "Hemo the Magnificent." The grainy film showed the body's gatekeepers opening and closing capillaries in reaction to the fight-or-flight response, thus varying the rate of oxygen/carbon dioxide exchange. This was regulated by a person's state of mind. It was a potent image.

I also had the childhood experience of dancing with family friends to the uneven rhythms and complicated stepping patterns of the Balkans, and moving in the smooth flowing predictable waltz time of the Swedish *Hambo*. I felt the joy that comes from moving to music and attuning the body's movements to others. There was a special power of living and moving in your body. Dancing served as a conscious introduction to the creative, expressive side of mind/body interaction.

Another seminal event of my childhood's mind/body awareness was my mother's pregnancy and labor when I was ten. She let me read her copy of Dr. Grantly Dick-Read's *Childbirth Without Fear,* as she was preparing for a natural childbirth in 1956 for the birth of my sister. The book's introduction described a woman in labor without pain. Surprised, Dr. Dick-Read remarked on the woman's uncanny serenity. She calmly replied, "It wasn't meant to hurt, was it?" Soon after I read the book, my mother and father awakened me in the early dawn to tell me they were off to the hospital in labor and that the baby would arrive soon. I remember vividly how my mother swooped down the front steps, held onto the brick retaining wall for support during a strong contraction and then looked up at me smiling as she hustled into the car. She was joyful and confident.

So, from childhood I was fascinated with how the feedback loop from the body created emotional states in the mind, and how state of mind created physical feelings and expressions in the body. Around the age of twelve, I decided that the logical path to follow would be to examine all of this phenomena by going into psychiatry—then I would know everything, down to the last neuron about the body's feedback loop and tease out every feeling through detailed analysis. In 1965, I started out as a college freshman in pre-med. I was the only female student in a chemistry lecture hall of 399 males, and I had never taken chemistry in high school. I floated around in a sea of pedagogical confusion in a way I had never experienced before. I had always been able to "get it" the first time around at school. Clearly, I wasn't "getting it."

The professor who taught the class was also my advisor, so after the first week, I went to his office for help, thinking he'd sit down and explain things to me or at least refer me to a tutor. He opened the pencil drawer of his desk, pulled out a little pink pad, dropped it on the desktop, and said, "What's your name?" Now how many Alice's could there be in that sea of guys? So he wrote my name on the top page, tore off the note, and handed it to me without saying a word. It was a drop slip. I was stunned, confused, vulnerable, 19, a girl, and silent. I knew he was inviting me out of the program, barring me from continuing a medical education, but I didn't know what to do about it. I also didn't know that he was doing me a crucial favor. I didn't know he was redirecting me to another much broader way of thinking. I didn't know come ten years later, while my babies slept, that at every opportunity I would rush eagerly to open up my chemistry book, totally enthralled and reveling in the periodic table and the behavior of electrons.

The same year of the chemistry debacle, I had signed up for a modern dance class to fulfill my physical education requirement. From age three through junior high, I had been taking dance. My instructor, Maida Withers, was an energetic, warm woman who reawakened within me my creative/expressive side of mind-body interaction. She encouraged me to continue my dance education, so I went to New York, where I spent the next three years dancing my way to a Bachelor of Fine Arts degree. Every day I danced at least five hours in classes along with additional rehearsal time. I was living in my body and in great shape.

I could not have picked a better time in my life or in the history of the United States to move to New York. The year 1967 was a year of fervor in "youth politics" and "youth culture." It was also the year that I married the boy I met the June I graduated from high school. I was immersed in art, culture and politics all of my waking hours. It was a time bubbling with creativity and an intellectual fertile lushness. My circle of friends and I spent hours discussing draft resistance, feminism, filmmaking, union organizing, organic gardening, and how to make provocative art change society. We lived the new budding feminism described in *Our Bodies, Ourselves* first edition. We protested the Vietnam War, made our own clothes, and challenged the tyranny of experts. We were infused with the energy of youth, and our power to enrich and change our world was palpable and effective.

My dance training was a great gift. I learned the importance of relaxation, concentration and focused energy to allow myself to move with my full potential and efficient use of my body. I learned about my body as an expressive tool. I learned to read the bodies of others. I learned to perceive tension-habit patterns that give performers the ability to physically convey character and emotion. I learned about anatomy and kinesiology and the importance of the pelvis as the source of all movement. I learned about bound flow and free flow of energy and the power of each kind. I learned about and lived applied nutrition and health promotion. I had no clue how essential this knowledge would be in my future, but there was a down side to my limited focus on the creative expressive mind/body interaction. It was hard going to the studio every day while walking through the poverty of Lower East Side of New York. I wanted somehow to bridge the dissonance between the artist's ivory tower and the unmet needs in the gritty reality of the streets.

In April of my senior year, I found myself pregnant, working on a full evening of my own choreography and dancing hard. I presented my concert twelve weeks pregnant, announcing my pregnancy to the future grandparents just before the curtain rose. They had to watch as my company and I moved through the space together, running, leaping, spinning, jumping, lifting and yes—turning each other upside down. How could I have been so joyful and cruel to those poor future grandparents who watched me dance? Clearly, it did me no harm, and the little girl who was inside of me turned out to be quite a dancer herself.

My body was healthy and ready for the powerful energetic experience of labor. It was an experience that would bring together all of the elements that had touched me so deeply. As it turned out, I had a long but easy natural childbirth. The culminating transcendence and melting into the source of all energy and life that I experienced in the final two hours bringing forth my precious daughter suddenly united all elements of my being. Mind and body were one and I felt infused with a spiritual wonder. I was thrilled with the privilege of being entrusted to bring forth life and nurture this little soul. I could see clearly how the creative expressive and technical scientific sides of mind-body interaction came together. After the birth, I hungered for everything I could get my hands on to read about birth.

During my pregnancy with my daughter, I read the few available consumer-oriented books on birth. Postpartum, I happened on an ancient copy of *Williams Obstetrics* and read it from cover to cover. As I nursed my sweet baby, I took in the technical explanations about labor and delivery, getting into the rhythm of medical jargon. Before I knew it, word of my natural birth spread through my circle of acquaintances. People came knocking on my door asking me about my natural childbirth, requesting that I teach them how to do it. I did my best to share the information.

My husband and I decided to leave New York to travel for about a year. After our return, we ended up back in the metro area of Washington, D.C., where I found an amazing collection of women teaching in association with ASPO Lamaze. I was welcomed into their midst, and I began working to get certified as a childbirth educator. I read their recommended bibliography, observed passionate teachers and couples giving birth without medication; I was exposed to a radical notion—home birth.

In 1971, a growing number of families in the community endeavored to avoid hospital births altogether, especially having to take drug cocktails during birth, fighting to get fathers into the delivery room, and having to separate from their babies during the postpartum period as a result of institutional policies. Couples simply decided to stay at home to birth, and three physicians in the area were comfortable attending them. As birth educators, we realized that there was a natural and logical flow from observing the births of our students to lending a hand to the doctors at these home births. I soon found myself assisting at births several times a month, usually with my toddler in tow. It was all very informal. Those of us who assisted felt tremendous excitement and a strong desire to share our experiences with each other. In our kitchens, living rooms and dining rooms, while our babies played on the floor at our feet, we debriefed, discussed and read. And we attended more births. As there existed no formal structure for our education, we created our own. We continued to call ourselves "childbirth educators," and the families we assisted were "our couples." The doctors provided the prenatal care, and we provided the prenatal education. Eventually, the physicians felt their presence was no longer necessary at the births, and so we visited our couples in groups of two or three or sometimes more. If we had questions, the doctors were always happy to answer them. If we had problems, they would come to the home or meet their patient at the hospital. Gradually, we realized we had a name. We began calling ourselves "lay midwives."

Not long after, I was again privileged to find myself pregnant, giving birth in the warm familiar environment of my home, surrounded by eight of the most significant people in my life at that time. I needed them all—their expertise and love—as I pushed out my 9-pound posterior son. There was a profound sense of delicious peace—no conflict about defending my right to receive him and get to know him in our own time. I didn't dress him for days, savoring his soft

skin against mine, fully taking in our attachment. It was so satisfying, so different from the harsh hospital-imposed, twenty-four hours of separation from my
daughter that I experienced immediately after she emerged.

The year 1975 brought some new issues into my life. One of my lay midwife
colleagues answered her door with her five-month old nursing at her breast. The
guests at the door were police officers, and they promptly took her down to the
station, arresting her for practicing midwifery without a license. At about the
same time, a home birth nurse-midwifery practice opened in the area. It was also
the time when I became a single mom. I realized that the need for my services as
a midwife could now be taken care of by other practitioners and that the risk of
going to jail was in no way an acceptable option. Meanwhile, a nurse-midwifery
educational program had opened at Georgetown University. I made the decision
to enroll in nursing school so that I could qualify for entrance into the midwifery
program at Georgetown University.

My babies were little, and a part-time academic schedule while still continuing to teach childbirth education and assist at births, made my journey towards
attaining a Bachelor of Science in Nursing degree (BSN) a long one, taking
eleven continuous semesters, including summers. Accelerated BSN programs for
students with a previous bachelor's degree were not yet available at that time. I
loved chemistry, anatomy and physiology, microbiology, and pathophysiology,
but the rest of the nursing courses were like an endurance contest. For six long
years, from 1974 to 1980, I gritted my teeth and took my medicine.

At the Georgetown Nurse-Midwifery Program I got to take advantage of
time for study, and I made friendships that I continue to value today, for example,
with Marsha Jackson, who in 1987 became my business partner. By the time I
finished at Georgetown it was 1981, almost exactly eleven years after my flash of
integrated awareness that was ignited by birthing my daughter. In fact, I took my
certifying exam on her eleventh birthday. Three more nurse-midwifery practices
had opened to meet the demand for home birth services. One of them, Family
Birth Associates, hired me. I had been birth assisting with the owners, Joyce
Daniel and Kate Beveridge. Having already known them well, it was very easy for
me to step into their practice. I supplemented the income from my "midwifery
habit" by working full-time nights as a labor and delivery nurse at the tertiary
care hospital in the area. The contrast between practice styles was stark, but it
helped me again affirm the value I place on my midwifery work.

I settled into a new rhythm in my life as I left the structure of formal education.
The women and their families proved to be my best teachers. I reaped the benefits

by learning how to provide what was called full scope midwifery care. Twice a week at office hours, I met families full of hopes, dreams, worries and anticipation of the moment when they would welcome a new person into their lives. I was able to watch them consider how they would make the delicate shifts in their family constellation and take on their new role as parents. By the time labor began, I knew them well. I was able to provide a presence that could instill confidence—the reassurance that all was proceeding normally—and to serve as a vigilant lifeguard who watches from the sidelines. I was able to see them open their eyes and work with the ebb and flow of the wide range of possibilities that is called "normal labor." I loved being there as they navigated from each totally present moment evolving into the next totally present moment. I was awestruck by their profound efforts filled with the salt of sweat, blood and amniotic fluid, the juicy, unpredictable intensity. These moments prepared them to open their arms and their hearts as their baby emerged to fill their hearts with the passion and tenderness of attachment to this sweet, pink, soft, vulnerable yet powerful being.

I loved living in this rarified world where my focus was undistracted and protected. There was sanctity in the separation from the disruptions of daily life. I could devote my entire concentration to the energy of labor, how the mother could use it to its maximum, how to conserve it, how to replenish it. Sometimes just my presence in another room was all that was needed. Other times a word, a touch, changing the lighting, straightening up the environment, or simply opening a window brought support. Sometimes I needed to be very directive to reduce the numbers of well-meaning guests who unintentionally diverted the mother's hormones away from making labor proceed at its own pace. It was often the simplest things that would make the labor proceed as it should. I remember one mother of three whose body labored erratically, unproductively with baby number four. Then her mother-in-law arrived. Grandma's home cooking was the trigger that put those labor hormones in gear. When Grandma turned on the oven, the aroma of familiar, plain, wholesome food wafted its way upstairs into the bedroom. The laboring mama then knew she and her household were taken care of. The baby arrived shortly thereafter.

With each day I learned to step back to give the families more and more space to bring their own creativity to their labor process. This work that they did together, depending on and leaning on each other, was a kind of glue. After all, I was a temporary figure who would go home after a few hours postpartum. With visits lessening from days, then weeks, then months after the birth, we experienced a gradual weaning from one another. But the birthing mother and her partner would continue to be there for each other day after day, living their lives. Sharing the intimacy and work of birthing helped the family to build a solid foundation for taking on the act of parenting together.

As time passed, I finally began to attain the financial means and cognitive capacity to broaden my horizons from my little family and my practice. A midwife friend invited me to join her at the American College of Nurse-Midwives (ACNM) conference and annual meeting. The conference brochure piqued my interest with educational offerings, and I looked forward to finding out more about the concerns shared by other midwives throughout the country. However, when I arrived at the conference, I was surprised to discover that I was in a very tiny minority of those interested in home birth. I sensed an overt hostility toward home birth, and in fact, the organization had officially endorsed an anti-home birth policy. This attitude was something I had never encountered from other midwives in the Washington, D.C. area, and something I hadn't come across in the ACNM's *Journal of Midwifery & Women's Health* or other publications.

Not too long after my attendance at the ACNM conference in the mid-1980s, I received a flyer for a "Midwifery Today" conference where some amazing speakers would be giving presentations. I was very excited about listening to so many notable speakers in the same conference program. The educational sessions proved inspiring. It was so reassuring to hear what I believed in coming right off the speaker's podium. But it wasn't all roses at the conference. Again I encountered a strange reception from some of the other conference attendees. Some clearly did not appreciate my Certified Nurse-Midwife (CNM) credentials, and some hostility was specifically directed toward me because I sullied my work accepting money for attending the sacred and holy moment of birth.

I was lured into going to the next ACNM conference program, which included a session about the transition of lay midwives to CNMs. Fran Ventre, Kate Bowland, and Peggy Garland-Spindel gave presentations at the session. I found great comfort in their company. Fran suggested forming something she called the "Bridge Club" for outcast midwives who had experienced harassment from both sides. She created a logo and published a newsletter called *View from the Bridge*. To add my support, I vowed to do something to assure that home birth would not remain an ACNM stepchild.

Back home in Washington, the 1985 national malpractice insurance crisis reared its ugly head. When I first started practicing as a CNM in 1982, I purchased my malpractice insurance policy for $15. The premium went up to $35, then $150 without us paying much attention. Then our premium shot up to $850, and we read about obstetricians in Florida and New York getting charged $100,000 for their insurance. The rise in insurance costs made no sense but certainly caught our attention when the ACNM insurer couldn't find a carrier at any price. Because the ACNM national office was close by, I chose to become involved in ACNM's negotiating work. With the help of the national staff and other D.C. area midwives, we worked hard to assure that whatever policy we could negotiate would include home birth.

In 1987, the Family Birth midwives made a decision to slow down and reduce their workload. However, as I was not at all interested in slowing down, I decided to open my own new home birth service. I called the practice BirthCare and Women's Health and worked with a designer to create a logo. My father, a CPA, delighted with my entrepreneurial spirit by helping me set up the books. I started seeing prenatal clients in my home, enjoying a very relaxed affair with long prenatal visits over glasses of iced tea on my back deck. I knew I needed a staff to help me, so in May I went to the ACNM convention looking. There I ran into Marsha Jackson, my former classmate from Georgetown and handed her the ad I was passing out to everyone at every opportunity. She was the director of an adolescent pregnancy program attending births in the hospital, but she also had a few private home birth clients. We agreed to become business partners, continued seeing clients in our homes, and by August had enough money to rent an office and hire a part-time office manager. In 2010, we celebrated our twenty-third anniversary.

Gathering information about home birth safety came very naturally to us, and more articles began to appear in both the international and domestic literature. We prepared written material for the ACNM staff to use when questions about home birth came to the attention of the national office. We worked to resurrect ACNM's Ad Hoc Committee on Home Birth, Marsha serving as chair and working to make it a standing committee. I succeeded as chair when her term expired. We were both deeply committed to rehabilitating and legitimizing home birth within the ACNM. With the help of other home birth midwives across the country, we strived to ensure having at least one home birth educational session presented at the annual convention. We were asked to write an article and coordinate an entire issue on home birth for the *Journal of Nurse-Midwifery*. We co-edited ACNM's *Home Birth Practice Handbook*, helped to launch a national prospective study that was published in the OB/GYN journal, and were invited to write the chapter called "Birth in the Home and Birth Center" published in *Varney's Midwifery, 4th edition*. The evolution of ACNM's acceptance of home birth was acutely apparent at ACNM's 50th Anniversary Conference gala opening celebration. A film, proudly illustrating the roots of nurse-midwifery in the United States and showing a home birth, was met with cheers and a warm reception. As Marsha and I sat at the gala together, we felt very gratified to see the shift towards a positive attitude regarding the value of home birth.

From the beginning of my involvement with birth, my focus has been on the process of taking birth back. We women have been fortunate to be the actors in this awesome and totally creative event. By now, the dark and hazardous clouds of poor public health, poor nutrition, infection and postpartum hemorrhage have largely been lifted. What remains is an opportunity in the United States for birth to be safer than it ever could be in the past, provided that technology is kept in the background and brought out only when necessary. What has happened instead? Birth, this elegant, simple, yet intricate process has had unnecessary, complex, expensive technology superimposed onto it, creating a dangerous environment for birthing women. Powerful economic interests have created an "obstetrical-industrial complex" of convenience that has intruded into the birthing suite. The coordinated décor in hospital rooms houses machines that replace the presence of human touch. Starting the "cascade of interventions" is made all too easy by implementing packaged surgical solutions paid for by skyrocketing insurance premiums. And somehow, women have been made to feel that they do not have the ability to birth safely without all of this. I feel that my natural birth with my daughter was easy to accomplish in the unsophisticated obstetrical world of that time in 1970. Even though the hospital staff was unfamiliar with natural birth, they didn't stand in my way. Back then, fetal monitors and epidurals were not available, IVs were not standard procedure, and the birth environment was not permeated with the fear of horrible complications emanating from inappropriate application of technology and ensuing lawsuits. I labored unhampered by equipment, unsupported by staff, but hospital rules allowed my husband to remain with me. Today, rather than receiving the support a woman needs as she takes on the work her body knows to bring forth life and claim her baby, she must instead waste energy in defending her rights to move unencumbered by machinery, fighting for peace and an expectation of healthy outcomes, and advocating for undisturbed contact with her baby. Too often her desires are foiled. It is our responsibility as midwives to be the guardians of the normal, to hold the space for the woman to do what her body knows how to do—bring forth and nurture life.

No big money supports home birth simply because there's no big money to be made from home birth. Birth is simple, and birthing at home keeps it simple.

Home birth promotes those labor hormones to increase the likelihood of normal. And not a lot of money gets spent as long as everything stays normal. Authority, centrality and privacy are the bulwarks that support the free flowing of labor hormones, and these hormones are what make labor go. Our job is to assure that families labor in an environment where they have authority to run their own lives and labors, where the woman is central and every action we take emanates from *her* needs, and where she has the privacy she needs to relax and feel uninhibited. I believe that we should banish the words "allow" and "permission" from our vocabulary when we are working with families. No woman in labor should have to move over for someone else's needs. I don't know how families in labor can take in the names and intentions of all of those people on staff in a strange place. It is an unnecessary and unwise waste of precious labor energy.

As midwives, being our own bosses is at the root of being able to practice the way we want and may be the essential element of the survival of our midwifery practices. We cannot set up practices whose existences are at the mercy of outside forces. Rather, we are more likely to be able to practice according to what we think is clinically appropriate when we are setting up the rules and writing the protocols *ourselves*. Then we are not vulnerable to the whims of an obstetrician, a hospital or the board of an HMO. There were two cases in which the midwifery staff was fired from obstetrical practices in the D.C. metro area. As a result, the midwifery option was no longer available to many women. In both cases these midwifery services had operated for years, and the clients felt satisfied with the care they received there. In one case, the OBs held onto a grudge for twelve years, and when they found the opportunity, they saw to it that twenty midwives were fired and hence closed the midwifery service. In the other case, there was a change in the practice ownership personnel, causing a thriving service of twenty years to suddenly close. So we must be bold, and like my parents we must be "do-it-yourselfers."

I have long been a believer that if we get information out to the masses, things will change. In the mid 1990s, I contributed to the design and data gathering of a prospective study on home birth published in *OBGYN Journal* by Patricia Murphy and Judith Fullerton. The study described great outcomes for home birth families in a sample size of over 1000. At the time, I truly believed that the study, with two respected PhD epidemiologist-midwife-authors published in the most prestigious OB journal in the United States would make a difference. I believed that its publication would be greeted with celebrations across the country and even around the world. I expected home birth practices to open everywhere and flourish. As it was, hardly anyone noticed. And to top it all off, the American College of Obstetricians and Gynecologists (ACOG) reissued their anti-home birth statement without a stitch of evidence, while complaining about the quality of our research. It is said that the definition of insanity is continuing to do the same thing over and over again and expecting a different outcome. So perhaps I am insane. But I believe that we need to continue to keep collecting data, and that eventually more data will enable us to reach the tipping point. There is a hospital in the D.C. metro area where the cesarean rate reached 70% in 2007, while BirthCare's c-section rate was only just over 3% the same year. Is the physiology of our clients so different from the ones who go to that hospital? I plan to maintain my "insanity," because someday women will notice and we will reach the tipping point. Women will advocate for themselves and for their rights to appropriate support to labor physiologically, to birth normally and to use technology only when it is truly necessary.

I have reaped the benefits of the longevity of the consumer movement to change childbirth. I have been blessed with a growing number of clients who were born at home themselves or were present when siblings were born at home, or whose mothers have had natural births. This is one of the advantages of living in the same community for a long time. The daughters and sons of clients have benefited from experiential learning, so there is so much less that has to be taught regarding attitude and expectation. When working with a first-time mom whose mother has had a natural birth, there is also less worry and less pressure from those grandparents. They understand when patience is working.

One case I remember vividly. A beautiful young man lifted his baby out of his wife's vagina and placed this new, wet little life on his wife's breast, saying tenderly to his baby, "Here baby—here—this is the best place in the world." His was not an action motivated from learning from a book. No one had to teach him about the benefits of breastfeeding. He knew from his own experience at his mother's breast. There was not a dry eye in the room.

I am grateful that my work as a midwife offers me learning opportunities daily. These lessons are often not in the clinical realm. I may learn about honoring some aspect of human relations because I am dealing with people daily. The lesson may be about the intricacies of family dynamics. I may learn about some ethical system that helps with decision-making. I may learn about some spiritual practice that guides life's path. I may learn about some new business system that makes the practice work better and smoother. And of course, touch puts many lessons into my hands. My hands possess their own wisdom that they have gained from feeling many, many babies inside their mothers. The direct line from my hands to my brain and vice versa has opened up a quick path to knowledge. Without thinking, I can make the leap to understanding. I am not a fan of "intuition" but rather of sensitivity, of heightened perception. Whether that knowledge in your hands is there, or whether you see a look revealing attitude, or watch the way a touch is given, or how an expression floats across someone's face, or the tensions of muscle groups—all of these things tell you what is going on. It is also important to cultivate humility and to keep an open mind to surprises—to expect that anything may change at any moment. In the world of labor, progress is often not what you expect it to be. Any conclusion you draw must be ready to be altered. It is essential to always be mindful that perceptions may not be accurate and that suggestions for change may not be effective. I've learned that I must always be ready, paying attention with my heart, my head and my hands.

I will always be a birth junkie

MAGGIE BENNETT

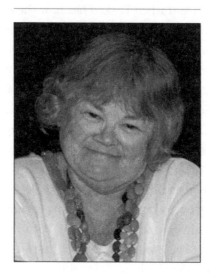

The births of my children changed the course of my life. It was as though I was traveling along a highway headed for a specific destination, only to meet a detour sign and be diverted so drastically that I ended up in a completely different destination and a different life. I feel that my son Johnny made an adult of me. In choosing to have him, I chose to become an adult, to care for another's well-being more than my own, and to plan a life that is conscious, productive, and family centered.

In 1964, during my last semester of college, I became pregnant, decided that I was thrilled and happy to be becoming a mother and absolutely clear that I was not going to marry the father of my child. I finished student teaching. To my parents' dismay, I turned down a position at the University High School in Champaign, Illinois, and admission to graduate school at the University of Illinois. Instead, in January of 1965 I boarded a train bound for California. The first thing that I did on the train was go into the restroom and remove the girdle that I had been wearing to hide my pregnancy from my friends and parents. I was five months along. In 1965 girls who were pregnant and unmarried either went to a home for unmarried women where they birthed and gave up their babies or they left town for either coast. My sister lived in San Francisco, so that is where I headed.

I gave birth in June of 1965 in Walnut Creek, California. I must say that I did not have expectations going into my birth experience. My own mother had had seven children, and when I asked her how she handled childbirth, she calmly answered "With fortitude. Women can do this." So, I innocently trusted my doctor and childbirth and simply expected things to go well and to end up with a baby in my arms. Years later, looking back, I became angry about many things—unwanted drugs, rectal exams, women on scopolamine screaming down the hall, being strapped down in the delivery room, and my son being routinely circumcised without choice. Yet at the time, my son's birth seemed more than wonderful to me. In spite of my own lack of knowledge and the mechanized system of the day, I managed to have a simply beautiful birth experience. Flat on my back, wrists strapped down, legs in stirrups, and appalled at the lack of dignity, I was suddenly overtaken by the amazing feeling of pushing! I tried to get the doctor to adjust the mirror so that I could see the birth, but he said he was too busy. He was trying to give me a saddle block (the newest hot anesthesia), but I couldn't stop pushing. Then I felt my baby sliding through my vagina, creating the most incredible throbbing, orgasmic sensation! I was totally unprepared for such a thing! I wanted to say something, but there were no words. Surely this was not a feeling that had been mentioned in any of the childbirth books I had read. I remember staring at my skinny little baby boy draped over the doctor's hands while trying to take in the sensation of birth as my body experienced it and the emotions that I felt at seeing my very own baby boy! I felt very sorry for everyone in that delivery room, because they had not just had a baby. And I felt especially sorry for the doctor and the male nurse because they never could! My child was whisked away, but I had a million questions for the doctor, who finally got around to adjusting the mirror. He pointed out my cervix, explained what he was doing while he stitched up my episiotomy and apologized for not being fast enough to get the anesthesia in place before the birth.

I waited for ten years to have another baby, not only because I loved being a mother and wanted more children, but because I wanted to experience the moment of birth. It was really not until I was a midwife that I began to hear of other women experiencing orgasms as they birthed. I think it is rare, but would be more common if women knew it was a possibility. I was so unprepared, so unconscious, and so very lucky!

Ten years passed before I was in a committed relationship. We soon owned our own home in Monterey, had a business, and Ralph was a wonderful father to my son. We were also pregnant. It was then that I began to reflect upon my first birth—the good parts and the bad parts. Meanwhile, my sister had her second child in a teepee in Big Sur. In attendance were her husband, their five-year-old daughter, and my husband. Ralph was committed to home birth. I was not so sure about home birth, but mostly I just didn't want to be told what to do. I studied a lot, including reading Sheila Kitzinger, Grantly Dick-Reed, and Marjorie Carmel, *whose Thank You, Dr. Lamaze* became a pivotal book. In the book, Carmel describes the doctors who she encounters on her path to finding Dr. Lamaze and the perfect natural birth. I felt that she was describing every jerk with a medical license that had ever abused my body or insulted my intelligence. It was clear that the only thing to do was to have a home birth and avoid the hospital altogether.

Nevertheless, there were no midwives in Monterey. Most of the women I knew who had home births did it on their own, receiving prenatal care from an obstetrician and birthing with sisters or husbands, much as my sister Kathleen had done. There was a fledgling midwifery community in nearby Santa Cruz, but the midwives often missed the births because they were too far away. So Ralph and I borrowed tapes from the Santa Cruz Birthcenter and began to study up. We learned that there was a support group for homebirthers in our town. It was called the Birthcenter comprised of folks who met weekly to share their home birth experiences and advice with expectant parents. We knew it was a bunch of hippies, so I bought a long skirt at the Goodwill (Ralph already wore torn jeans), and we set off for our first meeting in a funky, little Victorian house in Pacific Grove. And there the magic took place! We arrived at the end of a long summer day and walked into the living room. Everyone was seated in a circle on the floor. Backlit by the setting sun were four or five beautifully pregnant women. They were wearing long diaphanous dresses that were sheer and which revealed the shapes of their bodies. The sunlight made halos of their hair and outlined their shapes with gold. To me these women were a vision of goddesses of birth. I always consider this singular moment as my calling to midwifery. I knew in a flash that I longed to sit at the feet of these women and to serve them. I knew my life had changed. I was twelve weeks pregnant myself, and these women became my first teachers.

In one of those inevitable curves that life throws us, my second birth was a disaster. After attending Birthcenter meetings for six months, reading *Williams Obstetrics* from cover to cover, even the yucky parts, and assembling the perfect team, the right candles and best meditative tapes ever, I ended up with a scheduled cesarean! Here's what happened. I decided to go to my obstetrician one more time to make sure that everything was lined up just right. Going on my less than perfect LMP (last menstrual period) date, he decided that I was more than two weeks late and that my baby was too big to be born. I have always suspected that the X-ray pelvimetry they performed on me was one of the last done in our local hospital. It suggested to my doctor a cephalopelvic disproportion. He called me up and said that I needed to have a c-section that afternoon. I was frantic. I called my mother who said she was relieved that I would be in the hospital. I called my brother, a doctor. He said to believe the technicians. I called my friends at the Birthcenter. They came over, and we put our arms around each other and cried. My husband was devastated, but what could we do? I asked my doctor about a second opinion, and he said, "Go ahead, but don't come back to me." It was all too much. I refused sedatives and a drug called Atropine. A nurse ran out of the room yelling, "Are you trying to kill your baby?" I remember lying on the gurney all alone waiting for surgery. I was tempted to just get up and walk away. But I was also afraid that the doctor and his X-rays might be right. What if my baby couldn't get out and I did kill it? I went into surgery so freaked out that the epidural anesthesia didn't work. I thought I could feel them cutting into me. The doctor, showing a truly humane side of himself, stopped the surgery and came around to my side. He touched me and assured me that he would never do anything to harm my baby or me. Then they gave me general anesthesia. I was awakened by a male nurse who was slapping my cheek and saying, "Wake up . . . you have a son." When I did finally see my baby, it was an effort to care. I knew that I must hold him and nurse him, but any motherly feeling was stifled by my anger and disappointment at the loss of my birth dream and the violation of my body. He was only 10 ounces bigger than my first baby and less than 7 pounds. When I asked the doctor how a cephalopelvic disproportion could have happened, he dropped a total bombshell when he answered, "Childbirth is a mystery. Sometimes this sort of thing happens on a first birth." I said, "But I have given birth before!" He just looked at me with a blank face and left the room.

It took a year for me to recover emotionally from that birth. I was definitely a little crazy as I tried to align my love for my beautiful baby boy with the feeling that my body had been violated. The birth of Shayne was one of the worst experiences of my life. However, if the goddesses in the sunlight had called me to birth, my son's birth made me into a warrior with a mission. Bearing a child should not require a choice between the ecstasy of birth and sacrificing your body unnecessarily. I spent the first five years of my midwifery training learning to understand what happened to me. The rest of my career I grew more and more committed to helping women find some of the same joy I experienced in my first birth and avoiding the unnecessary and harmful surgery that dominated my second birth. I also began to go to births as a "Lady of the Birthcenter," primarily to help the father.

For the next ten years, being a member of the Birthcenter dominated my life. I continued to attend meetings and began attending births within a month of Shayne's birth. This organization was now my life, my spiritual path, and my connection with the other women who were to form the most influential relationships on my path to becoming a midwife. In the beginning, those of us who continued to come to meetings after our babies were born organized a set of ten classes that covered topics for parents like us who wanted to birth at home without professional attendants. The classes that we taught covered all aspects of prenatal care and labor management, both normal and complicated. We taught couples how to encourage labor with herbs and homeopathy. We taught mothers how to deliver babies in a variety of positions. We taught fathers how to unwrap a cord and what to do if the baby had trouble breathing. We taught third stage management and breastfeeding and discussed circumcision, sex, immunization, and the politics of home birth. We had no time to waste on Lamaze breathing. Frankly, we thought making noise was more useful. As we taught our classes, we learned to be midwives. We graduated ourselves as Certified Birthcenter Instructors. Unlike every other childbirth education program, CBIs had to have attended at least ten births, only one of which could be their own. So we knew of which we spoke. The other thing that was important about us as birth attendants is that we came to the work totally untrained. The Ladies of the Birthcenter only attended births as invited guests. Birthcenter was an educational organization, and everyone was welcome to be at our classes, either as a student or as a person available to help at births. Many women were interested in being present at births, and so there were often many "helpers." However, over time only a small number of us were repeatedly chosen. Ultimately, four of us became the community-called midwives, meaning, the community identified us as their chosen midwives. We studied together every week for years and shared our experiences with each other. It was as though our working knowledge of birth was multiplied by knowing everyone who came to Birthcenter functions and the stories we told each other of the births we attended. It was a very different paradigm for learning and sharing. Because there were no confidentiality issues in those early days, we were free to teach and learn through sharing stories about each other. In fact, in those days the stories were far more valuable than any information in the books that were available. At the heart of every Birthcenter class were the stories that people returned to tell. Sharing our stories and learning from them was how our knowledge of the business of home birth was created and honed.

It was about three years before I began to call myself a midwife. We were proud to be lay midwives as opposed to institutionally trained. I have always felt that an important factor in those early days was that we attended births out of passion. I felt so thrilled to be present when a birth occurred! I felt that I was in the presence of a divine event and that the woman was a transcendent being giving birth to a holy child. Indeed, I needed those mothers as much as they needed me. This reciprocity of choice and need was a basic component of the "New Midwifery" movement of the '70s. It was very personal, very one-on-one. It was the basis for the magic and, unfortunately, is probably very much at risk of being lost as direct-entry midwifery becomes more and more professionalized, both in education and standardization of practice.

Nonetheless, we did not oppose the notion of becoming more professional. The goal was always to proliferate home birth and to present it as the very best way to bring children into the world. We needed credibility to grow the movement, and once we acknowledged that we were midwives, we needed to earn money in order to be able to continue to offer our services. At one time or another, many a good midwife stopped attending births because she needed to get a job that earned money for her family. And many of us who continued to be midwives have gone through life exchanging passion for poverty, lack of health insurance, lack of retirement funds and, worst of all, lack of money to fight legal battles that are often part of practicing in an illegal state.

I remember well the time when my friend Teri and I decided to charge for our services for the first time. We had just finished interviewing a potential "client" over tea at my kitchen table. With much nervousness we had announced that our fee for services would be $300.00. At that very moment a recent father arrived with the gift of a lemon tree for our help at his child's recent birth. With true Birthcenter passion, he raved about how wonderful we all were in helping his wife have their baby, how committed and tireless, and so on. And then he closed his soliloquy by saying, "And the best part was that it was completely free!" Fortunately, the story had a happy ending for us because the couple told us later that if we had charged nothing, they would not have seen us as good midwives at all.

Once I became involved in my state organization, I quickly realized that the evolution of midwifery that we experienced in the Monterey area was not an isolated case. Such stories had occurred simultaneously all over California and, by extension, throughout the country. The circle of women who had gathered in Monterey living rooms was part of a greater community of women willing to risk a great deal to make home birth available to women and their babies.

Before I became a midwife, I was an art teacher. I taught in the inner city school in Los Angeles and in a district in Wisconsin where I traveled from school to school. When Johnny was in high school and Shayne was about seven, I was offered a job teaching art at Briarcliff, a small, very enlightened private school. I was part of the original faculty that helped define the direction and mission of the school. When hired, I made it very clear that I was a midwife and that midwifery was my primary role in the world. For some amazing reason, they accepted that. For seven years I taught art four days a week to kindergarten through eighth grade students. Not only was art curriculum an integral part of the whole educational plan, my midwifery was completely supported by the administration and faculty. Over this period of time, life handed me an amazing experiment. My midwifery practice never slowed down a bit during my career at Briarcliff. If anything it grew. However, I was adamant with the pregnant mothers that I could never leave a classroom of children unattended. Therefore, I was available on weekends and on Fridays. All other days, they had to call me before 6 A.M., so that I could arrange a substitute teacher. If labor began during the day, I would have to wait in my classroom until I could send the children back to their classroom teachers or a substitute arrived. It seems that this would have been off-putting and that clients would have gone elsewhere for care. However, this proved not to be the case. Sometimes the principal would come to take my classes or cancel them for the day. While these remedies did happen with very little grumbling, it was the birthing women themselves that really controlled the situation. Over seven years and over 150 births, I missed only one birth, and in that instance I was merely the assisting midwife. In spite of all the media drama about taxicab births and unexpected deliveries, it has been my experience that women will not let go of their babies until all the component parts of their birth plan are in place. A woman will rarely have her baby when her husband is out of town (unless she is mad at him). She won't have her baby until she gets in the hospital door if that's where she means to go, and she won't have her baby without her midwife unless she really doesn't need her for the birth. Of course, all this is contingent upon the mother knowing well in advance what are her limitations and choices. The psyches of women are very powerful. If a woman visualizes that she will birth at dawn for long enough, she probably will! The value of having a woman write a fantasy birth story is that she will plant that vision in her subconscious and be more likely to achieve it. Every experienced midwife knows that if she wants to go on a vacation, attend a conference, or attend her kid's graduation, she has to let her clients know—probably when they hire us. We think of the fight or flight mechanism in terms of fear or danger. However, my experience at Briarcliff and in the years since is that this control mechanism is also available to the mother well in advance so that she designs her own best birthing situation.

In 1987, our lovely little school was given away to a local prep school, which changed the format of the program. I consequently found myself out of a job. I also found myself brokenhearted and without a husband. I also knew that I could never go back to public school education. These events made life looked pretty bleak, but as so often happens, were the catalysts for the best thing that could have ever happened to me. I decided that after fifteen years, I could take the leap and create a solo midwifery practice and depend upon it completely for my family income. No more juggling multiple careers, no more split loyalties. I was simply and completely a midwife. I learned many things from the poverty of my first couple of years of business unaided by any other income. First and foremost, I had to give up the fantasy of providing midwifery services solely for the love of birth. Of course, I will always be a birth junkie, but in those days while I was still getting a kid through high school and another through college, there had to be more than love. I had to learn what my services were really worth in light of the expenses I had for food, rent and a car in which to get to births.

I recall this as a difficult transition in my community. The tradition that birthed me into midwifery was community service, self-reliance, and most importantly, non-professional. But now I had somehow bridged a gap and was forced to look at myself and what I did in a different light. Once while teaching a class in our old ten-class Birthcenter format, three couples announced that they would be having their babies on their own. To my surprise, my gut turned over, and in my heart I felt concern for them. From my own early years in the home birth world I couldn't help but remember how often we went to the hospital for what, in retrospect, I consider poor reasons—prodromal labor and unexplained pain, anxiety that can accompany transition, and fear of a new and unknown process. It was in this instance that I realized that I had crossed over into being a professional. I knew suddenly what I, as a midwife, was doing at births. I was there to keep the faith, to know the difference between painful early labor and the real thing. It was my job to keep that "flight" instinct at bay when the transitional mother thinks she can't do it after all. I knew that at least two of these couples would end up going to the hospital if they had no midwife or experienced person with them during labor. At the very least, a midwife's presence creates harmony at the time of birth so that its sacred nature doesn't get lost in quick moving, unfamiliar events.

So, I had to rebirth myself into another care provider who, in spite of charging a fee, possessed love, compassion, courage, common sense, and an awesome secret bag of tricks to offer. I had to convince myself that I was making a living to make it possible for midwifery to survive in the neighborhood. I experimented with fee schedules, partnerships, apprenticeships and marketing schemes. I learned how to manage my passion as a business owner. A friend and client, seeing my disarray, offered herself to me as a bookkeeper as her service to the goddess. And even though I now pay her for her services, she continues to be the silent partner of my business, doing the billing and the taxes and paying all those bills that I find odious. Eventually, I created a website and advertised with brochures and a Yellow Pages ad. All these endeavors changed my life as a midwife and expanded my services to the women in the community. I consider my efforts to become a good businesswoman a major accomplishment in securing the means to provide midwife services.

One of the greatest joys of my life has been working with midwives in training. I have always had a student midwife. That is the midwifery way! Midwifery is a path, which women follow for love of birth and reasons of their own. Students stay with their teacher for a period of time that may or may not lead to actually becoming a midwife. To be on the midwife path is to seek the meaning of womanhood. Women find answers to their own birth puzzles (as I did following my c-section) and then go on into other avenues of endeavor, enriched by what they learned about the Divine Woman within themselves.

Each of my apprentices has been remarkable for bringing to midwifery a unique perspective and a beautiful way of working with women. In return, I love passing on my knowledge to them. I am happy that these women have been able to learn to be midwives in the shelter of a practice. As proud as I am of being largely self-taught, apprenticeship is better than experimental midwifery. It is also better than schools and clinic training. Apprenticeship is slow, methodical and confidence-building. True apprenticeship is a total way of learning; it is not the same as a preceptorship, which is separate from book studies. The five women I trained are all better midwives than I was at that same stage of learning. They have gone forth into the profession with great confidence and the long tradition of women's learning.

I have accomplished far more as a midwife than I ever set out to do. Originally, it was my goal to attend fifty births. I wanted to feel that I could help a woman—a neighbor, a stranger, a friend, any sister in need to give birth outside of a hospital. I did that within the first couple of years that I was involved with birth. If that had been all that ever happened to me, I would have been amazed, thrilled and satisfied. After all, how many of us in these modern times see a baby be born, let alone touch one as he or she make entry into the extra-uterine world? As far as my life is concerned, even as a very small girl I meant to change the world. Midwifery has been a vehicle for fulfilling that desire. It is not what I did or didn't do as much as my *willingness to act* in the role of midwife that has made the difference for hundreds of women. Women need a person to be with them in childbirth. Although we can do it alone, I don't believe that we are meant to birth alone. But we are also not meant to submit our bodies to an external force in order to get the child within us out into the world. A midwife plays a role, which is different for every woman she serves. Sometimes I hear women describe how I served at their birth and I wonder whom they are talking about! Sometimes we are shadows on the wall, sometimes kind of bossy in a motherly sort of way, sometimes we step in and make decisions . . . and a lot of the time we just guess until the woman takes a suggestion that is right for her. Years ago, I coached women like mad; I went early and snuggled into bed with them. Nowadays, I encourage mothers to be alone with their partners, and when I'm with them, I hardly do anything at all. Everyone has a picture of me sleeping at their births. Yet, women still see that there is a midwife there with them and they hear and see what they need to make them feel comfortable and confident. I see the confidence that they have and mirror it back. So, I have changed the world for every woman who has seen in me a midwife whom she could trust. I have helped to change the lives and fortunes of every gently born baby whose mother I helped. I have, by being willing and present, helped dozens of women avoid cesarean births and assisted others in having VBACs (vaginal birth after cesarean). I have, by my presence and not a great deal else, made it possible for a few sets of twins to be born vaginally, a breech or two to be born without interference. Previously there had been no midwife service in my community, and so women did not have any choice but to birth in the hospital. My presence in the community has made it possible for women who knew of me to be able to choose between home and hospital. These are accomplishments indeed.

For the greater world out there, I would mention only one other thing of importance to me. In 1993 the Midwifery Act passed in the California State Legislature. I was the Chairwoman of the California Association of Midwives (CAM) during the fifth attempt by midwifery activists to get a law passed that would license direct-entry midwives. Frustrated by a struggle that lasted years, the California Association of Midwives adopted a certification process that was the brainchild of the Bay Area Guild of Midwives. This process involved documenting a certain number of births, submitting charts for review, and passing a didactic test of obstetric knowledge. It was our strategy at the time to certify as many midwives as possible and to offer this certification tool as a potential template for utilization by the state. The Wall Street Journal found out about our self-certification and labeled us the "Brazen Women" of California. Achieving CAM Certification was a personal high point in my career. I count it as a great privilege to have been a part the sisterhood that worked so hard to get this bill written, sponsored and passed into law. There are two lessons that I learned in 1993. One is the truth of a famous quote by Margaret Mead: "Never underestimate the power of a small group of committed individuals to make a difference. Indeed, that's the only thing that ever has." We were a small group– probably fewer than ten really front line players involved in this effort. The other lesson was that even in our admittedly flawed nation whose government draws deserved criticism and cynicism, democracy does work. A small group of very committed women with a clear vision of a better future changed the law in a very large state against the very powerful lobby of the AMA. Because the legislative process did work, there are more midwives in the world, more access to midwifery care and better, safer births for hundreds of babies. Being one of those "Brazen Women" of California will always be a big achievement for me.

Becoming involved in the home birth movement helped me find my particular path as an activist for social change. From childhood, I had had an inkling of the importance of standing for certain principles of human justice and for consciously striving to make a difference in the lives of human beings. As a young woman, I was involved in civil rights activities, including interracial communications, inner city education, and at one point even considered missionary work in Africa. I was involved in early feminist activities, the ERA movement and welfare rights for single mothers. But none of these areas of activity grasped me with such a white-hot passion as midwifery did. I needed to be with birthing women, and the home birth movement needed me! I felt that I could and must be an agent of change in my community. Here was a feminist movement so new that demonstrated that the activities of a small group of women could change lives. We could stand up, one woman at a time, against hospital policy. We could teach couples what they needed to know to have a home birth. We could attend those births and bring a measure of confidence and safety that would ensure success at home. We could be with women who had had cesareans, were pregnant with twins or breech babies. We could, simply by being willing to be present, empower mothers to birth naturally and on their own terms.

It was, after all, the '70s and civil disobedience was in! The first twenty years of my career, I was a "felon" waiting to be caught. I was charged with practicing medicine without a license, and it was not uncommon for California midwives to be faced with that charge. One of my dearest midwife friends was prosecuted, and the trauma of her experience affected us all for many years. I remember well discussing civil disobedience with my children. Looking back, I would not have been surprised if I had had to face prosecution or even jail. Nonetheless, I was willing to risk my personal freedom because I believed in a woman's autonomy over her body, and I understood that such a right was threatened by the prevailing obstetric customs and the laws of the state.

Having said this, I would not like to give the impression that my early career was fraught with fear. It was not! It was a fact of midwifery life in California (and many other states) that if something unfortunate happened at a birth, that the midwife would be prosecuted, often over the parent's objections. But I seldom thought of that sort of thing. Bucking the system was a by-product of attending home births, not the reason for the activity. It is inspiring to know the kind of people who choose home birth. They are hardy and strong in their beliefs. They are self-reliant and responsible. Women in labor are indeed beautiful, and the man who joins the dance of birth with his loved one is heart-melting in his tenderness. There are moments of intimacy between partners that are so sensual that one feels almost like a voyeur. And the moment of birth, whether it is easy and flowing or hard won, is a transcendent experience. To be a midwife is to hold a sacred space and be part of it as well. I have always felt humbled and honored to be at a birth. The power of the birth experience has always transcended any of the scariest moments of labor.

For me, one of the greatest challenges of midwifery has been in dealing with my feelings of inadequacy. I have spent far too many hours worrying about not knowing enough to do my job. There has been a long standing argument between the logical part of my brain, which can never be satisfied no matter how many births I attend or books I read or skills I acquire, and the intuitive part of me that believes that women were born to birth and that my only task is to hold the space in which an individual mother can believe in herself to connect to the quintessential Great Mother. I suspect that this is not a bad situation. On the one hand, learning new things is deeply satisfying. I'm pleased with how responsive midwifery is to new ideas—we are quick to learn from each other and the mothers we serve. On the other hand, I know that I can never know enough to cover every situation that comes up. And it is just not possible in a small solo home birth practice to have gained enough experience in advance to be able to handle complicated situations like breeches or twins. You just have to have common sense and realize that you must give in to a higher source of knowing. It is truly a challenge to face a situation for which you may not be prepared. In those moments, when I realize that my conscious mind must give way, I have experienced a phenomenon that occurs in no other part of my life. I have experienced a tangible feeling as though an energy is moving down through my head, through my body and out my hands, seeming to act independently to make the change, move the hand or body of the baby or do what is necessary to affect the ability of the baby to be born. I know that this can be explained as a shift from the logical right brain to the intuitive left brain. But I also know that it can happen only when I trust completely in birth and in my heritage as a midwife rather than as my trained self. It is the occasional stress of a complex birth that creates the only seriously important challenges for me as a midwife, while at the same time is the source of my most amazing experiences and the foundation for my confidence.

I have been a midwife for a long time. I have participated in midwifery politics on local, state and national boards. I helped to bring about legislation in my state, and I have been honored with my share of awards. I have helped change midwifery into a more visible and legitimate profession. There are many more stories still to tell in another time and place. But right now, what I am most proud of is my work as a community-called midwife. When I meet clients on the street, they want to introduce me to their kids, who are understandably reluctant. I like to rub the back of their heads and tell them that it is the part of them that I knew first and that I knew they would turn out good by the way their hair grew.

It is enormously satisfying to know that, because there was a midwife in this community, these children were born gently, usually at home, and surrounded by all of us who felt thrilled at their arrivals. It seems enormously lucky that I have been that midwife. As much as I loved being an artist, a teacher, a mother, and knowing my children as adults, nothing can touch what it has meant to me to be a midwife. If I had not encountered this spiritual path…ah, but I did! I was meant to be exactly what I am. I made a million tiny and large choices that led me to midwifery, and I am what I am, heart and soul.

Women give birth in all sorts of ways

PATRICE BOBIER

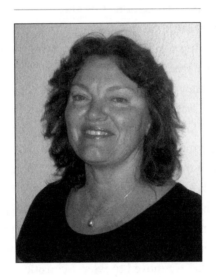

*M*y *parents were both still in college when I was conceived.* My dad was in medical school in Atlanta, and my mom was in nursing school in St. Petersburg, Florida. Although married and twenty-one, my mother was the first student allowed to graduate pregnant. I was born on September 29, 1951, in Tampa, Florida, and my mom went back to school and dorm life just four weeks after my birth. My dad had taken summer classes so that he could take fall term off to care for me, along with my grandparents, and still graduate with his class. We moved to Atlanta when I was about four months old and lived in married-student housing in a decrepit settlement called "Mudville," a group of clapboard wooden shacks on red Georgia clay roads. My mom worked as an obstetrical nurse to help put my dad through school. I grew up hearing stories about me playing with cadaver bones that my dad had brought home and telling him, "Come visit again sometime," as I didn't understand his role in my life when he was caught up in the frenzied schedule of internship and residency.

When I was five years old, we moved into a real house in a real neighborhood. Kindergarten wasn't available in much of the South in the 1950s, so I started first grade in 1957. I remember loving school and mistakenly thinking I got to go to second grade after my birthday in late September because I had already learned everything in first grade.

In the fall of 1957 we moved to Burlington, Vermont, because my dad had been drafted into the Air Force as soon as he graduated. I loved Vermont—snow, family trips to the mountains, camping, a huge backyard. It was the only time I remember my dad having regular work hours, being home for uninterrupted dinners and able to have weekends off.

I have an early memory of my grade school teacher being pregnant, though I didn't know what that was. Soon I learned where babies came from and played "having babies" with the Lutheran minister's daughters who lived next door. I recall riding in a car with my mom while she talked about women laboring alone and how it wasn't right. The things she told me, and TV, books and magazines, too, made me imagine wards of wailing women separated by curtains and all alone. My dad's medical books always fascinated me. I looked at the pictures from an early age, read the texts and read all I could find about the human body. I loved biology studies in school and did reports on bacteria, antibiotics, and crib death.

In the spring of 1960 we moved to what I consider my hometown, Haines City, Florida, where I lived until leaving for college. It was a small town in central Florida in the 1960s. I skipped sixth grade after only six weeks and graduated from high school when I was sixteen in 1968. My adolescence was turbulent. Many girlfriends dropped out of high school pregnant. I also was involved in alcohol and drugs. I got involved in some very dysfunctional relationships and so was in a hurry to leave.

I attended an alternative three-year, small, private liberal arts college where I was exposed to people from all over the country and many foreign countries. It certainly broadened my horizons! I read, talked, experienced many new things, but did not concentrate on studies, and so I dropped out after just two semesters. I remained living on campus for about another year or so. In the summer of 1969 I hopped on a VW bus full of friends and drove north to attend the Woodstock

Music Festival in New York State. I remember being awed hearing a baby had been born on the festival grounds. I wondered, *is it really that simple?*

It was having my own babies that sparked my interest in pregnancy and childbirth. Birth control was sporadically available during my teen years. I had an IUD and then went on "the Pill" off and on. In the fall of 1969 I met my future husband and father of my children. At that time there was a lot of press about complications from birth control pills. We were starting to learn more about healthy eating and living a natural lifestyle, and so I stopped taking the pill. A few weeks later I was pregnant. Having always had irregular menstrual cycles, I didn't realize I was pregnant until twelve to fourteen weeks when I saw a doctor for what I imagined might be a serious problem related to consequences from using various birth control methods. But it wasn't that there was a problem; I was pregnant. I was only eighteen years old. At that time there were very few books out about pregnancy. I read about birth in the *Whole Earth Catalogue* and discovered that women were having babies at home. I liked the idea! I found a copy of Grantly Dick-Read's *Childbirth Without Fear*, whose premise was, "If I am not afraid, it won't hurt." But that was not my experience. My husband and I moved to Michigan, his home state, when I was about seven months pregnant. I made my second prenatal visit to his family-friend obstetrician (OB) who had delivered him in 1950. He was a very kind man who told me I had a great pelvis. His partner, who was from India, told me I could squat or stand or whatever I wanted to do in labor.

My naïveté led me to believe giving birth would be a breeze. I went into labor three weeks past my due date (about a week past when I thought I was due) and I went into the hospital in a state of excitement. I was dilated all of one centimeter at about 11 P.M. By 3 A.M. contractions came hard and fast, so I took the Demerol that was offered. My husband was one of the first fathers allowed into the labor and delivery rooms, but since he knew even less about what was happening than I did, he wasn't a big help. I remember being very tired and it hurt! I remember laboring on the toilet for a while and looking at myself in the mirror. It all seemed so surreal. Medical staff took only a few fetal heart tones with the fetoscope. I did not have an IV, they would not allow me to have any food or fluids, and we were pretty much left alone. I was given some pain medication via pudendal and paracervical injections, and the physician cut a huge medio-lateral episiotomy. I quickly progressed and gave birth to our first child—a son—before 6 A.M. I was draped, but when I refused to have my hands tied down, I was scolded for reaching out for my baby and contaminating the sterile field. It was a typical birth in

1970, except for the fact that my bewildered husband was by my side. Our baby was nestled in my arms for the brief gurney ride back to my four-bed ward. That was it. I didn't see my baby for hours after that, and I didn't really get to care for him until three and a half days later when we were dressing him to go home.

My only experience with breastfeeding was as an early teen when my mother and I visited a German woman who very nonchalantly nursed her newborn baby in front of us. Now, it seems impossible to think that I had briefly seen only one nursing baby before attempting to nurse my own. Our son was born with a cleft lip and soft palate, and we weren't successful at nursing. Knowing what I know now, I think breastfeeding would have been possible with more knowledge and support. Nonetheless, my husband and I bought a goat and devised our own baby formula. Author Adele Davis' advice guided me through these early months of feeding a new baby.

Soon my pregnant friends came to me with questions, because, I suppose, I had had a baby and the fact that there was so little information available—no Internet, no good books, no childbirth classes, no real information from doctors. I got my hands on an early copy of *Our Bodies, Ourselves* and a few mass-market books, sharing the information, as well as my personal experience, with as many women friends as possible.

My husband, our six month-old, and I moved to impoverished rural Western Michigan in 1971, landing on a farming commune as part of the first wave of back-to-the-landers. We still reside on part of that farm, though the original commune is long gone.

In 1974 we had our second baby, a daughter. I knew I was in labor early in the day, again weeks after the original due date. I waited till early afternoon to walk to a friend's house to get a ride to where my husband was working. It still seemed too early to go to the hospital—I didn't want to be one centimeter again—so we drove to a friend's house about fifteen minutes from the hospital and hung out there for a short while. I can remember distinctly the change from hanging out, laughing and talking with everyone, to sitting on the toilet and feeling the baby suddenly descend, with the immediate strengthening of contractions. I thought, *OK, now I'm ready to go in.* The bumpy truck ride was awful in hard labor. I was four centimeters at the time of hospital admission, and I remember shouting, "Is that all?" They shaved me and gave me an enema and then I hit the shower. Two girlfriends had come with us, who were briefly allowed to take turns sitting with me in labor. Less than an hour after arriving at the hospital, I felt like pushing! My doctor couldn't be located, so one of his partners came in at the last moment.

I have vivid memories of being perched on the delivery table, feet in stirrups, and so afraid I was going to push and my baby would fall on the floor. As it was, no one but my husband was in the room, and he was told to stay by my head. The doctor finally arrived, washed his hands, gloved up, cut and caught. In trying to be a compliant patient, I didn't reach for our daughter who had been placed on my belly. But the doctor and nurse encouraged me to touch her, and it was so wonderful to feel her bare soft skin! My girlfriends had been able to stand outside the delivery room door and hear the birth. We all got to be together briefly in my hospital room before they were told they had to leave, my husband included. All I had wanted for my second birth was to have been spared staying up all night in labor. She was born about 7 P.M., and there I was—alone and wide awake for hours that first night. Eventually, I was able to get her from the nursery for a little while and undress her to look at her and touch her. And she nursed! We left the hospital AMA (Against Medical Advice) about forty hours after she was born. The discharge staff didn't know we had to ride in a trailer pulled by a tractor from the road back to our little cabin in the woods, as it was a muddy springtime season. This second birth was a much better experience than my first, but it still felt like the wrong way to bring babies into the world.

A year after my daughter was born, acquaintances who were pregnant with their first child were planning to have a home birth. They invited three women friends who had given birth to about eighteen babies between them to attend. I took food and a few supplies over in the afternoon, but I didn't stay. Hours later I got the word the baby was stillborn and that the mother was in the hospital. A friend and I walked the half-mile back to the little cabin in the woods in the middle of the night and cleaned by lamplight. It was my first smell of home birth. . . and home death. Would it have been preventable with a skilled attendant? This experience, too, did not feel like how babies were supposed to be born.

Two years later, in 1977, new friends in the community became pregnant. They had had their first baby on The Farm in Tennessee and planned to have a home birth again. They asked me to come. The thought of another baby dying was ever present in my mind, but I was drawn to be there. A nurse friend who had seen a home birth was going to be the attendant. The birth took place on a snowy, cold November day, the same day that also happened to be my son's seventh birthday. The natural light reflecting off the snow glowed in this quiet home while the woman labored silently. It was an amazing experience to watch the baby crown and ease out onto the bed, then cry and be soothed by her mother and nurse for the first time. She was tiny—we estimated her to weigh in the

5-pound range, and perfect. I loved it! I raved about it! I relived every little part of it! This baby—the very first I ever saw be born—is now thirty years old. She has given birth three times at home into my waiting hands.

The same birth team assembled about nine months later to attend another friend's second birth. I helped out more with labor comfort and was more observant about what was actually taking place. It was another easy emergence of a sweet baby girl. We all were blessed. I was this woman's midwife for two more babies in later years. A pregnant friend decided to attend this second birth in preparation for her own first birth. The nurse friend refused to attend a primip (first time mother), but the family was able to find midwives who lived more than an hour away who agreed to attend. I accepted the invitation to attend and had my first exposure to midwifery care in what turned out to be a simple, run-down farmhouse without running water or adequate heat. The baby was born in the kitchen, as that room was the warmest. None of that mattered, however. I thought, *Ah, this is what birth can be like.* It was a more complicated and longer birth with a larger baby, longer pushing, and a nuchal arm. But the minimally-trained midwife team knew how to check the baby's heart tones with a fetoscope, assist the mother with labor and pushing, untangle the arms and shoulders, and stimulate the baby boy when he was born. The birth happened back in the fall of 1978. By the spring of 2008, thirty years later, I had helped deliver two babies for that "boy" who had grown into a man.

Midwife—the word resonated with me. It was what I wanted to be. I wanted to know how to do what that midwife team knew how to do. In my pursuit to becoming a midwife, my life changed in all sorts of ways.

I spent about a year or so traveling, many times in borrowed cars, to Grand Rapids, 70 miles away, to attend workshops for pregnant women and families. I volunteered to labor-sit with friends planning hospital births. I recruited pregnant families in my community to plan home births. I was trained to do postpartum care for the midwives' clients. We were emulating the European system of multiple follow-up visits after the birth, so I made the time to go and do the perfunctory checks, and then the dishes, laundry, bring the older children home with me for the afternoon—anything I could do to assist the mom and family afterwards. I was invited to a few of these births and got to see more midwifery care in action, basic though it was in those days. I read everything I could find about midwifery care—journals, English texts, obstetric books, the first crude newsletters from a budding national midwives organization. Everything to do with midwifery held intense fascination for me.

Around that time, some midwives, with all of 50 to 75 births between them and with an expanding practice, invited another woman and me to train and assist them at births. About six months later we became apprentices, a new concept that was gaining favor as a way to train more midwives. I committed to making the two and a half hour round trip two days every week for two and a half years. I got a phone so I could be on call. In 1980, we attended a gathering of other midwives from around the state of Michigan. There were perhaps fifteen of us present at that first meeting. I was in awe and quite shy, not yet knowing where I fit in, as I was one of the first apprentices in Michigan. It was inspiring to be in the same room with these women telling their stories and sharing information.

Learning midwifery through the apprenticeship route was unique in providing me with first-hand experience with women and families from all sorts of backgrounds. One of my senior midwives was an RN who was married to a doctor. I thus gained access to medical texts and journals, of which I read profusely, taking the time to study the texts at home and learning a lot about body physiology in general, as well as how it related to the maternity year. I was very inquisitive and asked only some relevant questions so as not to be bothersome. I learned to think things out for myself, to observe and qualify what I was seeing.

It was hard to make time to study and give up two days each week for appointments and training, besides attending births. In reflecting back, it was a very stressful time in my home life. I had two children under age ten, a bustling small farm business, with both family and farm depending on my daily involvement. We were very poor and had unreliable automobiles. What's more, my husband was not supportive, as he expected me to be a full-time partner and thought the timing was wrong, that I should wait a few years. Regardless, I was determined to become a midwife.

Observing hundreds of prenatal visits, I learned to palpate a baby's position, to answer clients' questions, and provide assurance for their safety and health through the process. My senior midwives were getting busier and covering a larger area. I attended births, and due to the vast territory the midwives were covering, I sometimes was the only one arriving in time for the birth, the midwives getting there soon afterwards. My rudimentary studies were put to good use, generating more and more questions and building my confidence and knowledge base. Almost two years into the apprenticeship, my senior midwives split their practice, and I took a more responsible role in providing care. I had attended about forty births at this point. The midwife with whom I remained working began plans to go back to school to become a Physician's Assistant. Then I was notified that my apprenticeship would be coming to a close.

In the spring of 1982 I opened my own practice—Full Circle Midwifery. I had attended between 60 to 70 home births, hundreds of prenatal and postpartum visits, and dozens of workshops to broaden my knowledge, and I had voraciously read everything I could get my hands on. Though I still didn't feel ready for the responsibility, I was thrust out of the nest and into my own hotbed of life experience, and not quite sure I was yet a midwife. In order to ease more slowly into primary practice, I kept in close contact with the other former apprentice midwives, and as a team we attempted to attend as many births as possible. Having worked together, we trusted each other, so it made for an easier and safer transition, despite longer driving times from living one and a half to two hours apart.

My early midwifery practice was quite different than it is today. Back then I was not as trusting of birth or myself. Growing and changing and evolving into a better person and midwife is a lifelong process. I let my passion for this work light the fire in me to be a good midwife. I'm still growing, changing and striving to become better at what I do.

Living in a rural area and working in counties with a high poverty rate used to bring many lower and middle income people with no insurance to midwifery care and home birth in order to save money. Medicaid now pays for a larger percentage of births in Michigan, so the niche of people who pay for their own maternity care is smaller. Most low-income families now choose a "free" birth in the hospital even if it isn't their preferred choice, rather than pay out of pocket. I get inquiries from a dozen or so women each year who are interested in having a home birth until they find out Medicaid doesn't cover the cost.

I began attending births with Amish families in 1982. Their simple lifestyle settled me more as a midwife, simplified how I thought of birth, and changed how I taught childbirth classes. I learned to accept "what is" without needing to explain or blame. What's more, I learned to have respect for families with very different lifestyles.

Hearing speakers, such as Nancy Wainer Cohen and Michel Odent, and reading their books, added to my trust of birth. Attending midwifery and other allied professional conferences, subscribing to midwifery journals, especially from other countries where birth is treated more as a natural process, has also helped shape my midwifery practice. The first VBAC (vaginal birth after cesarean) I attended was in 1983. That woman's knowledge of the safety of VBAC and unwavering trust of her body aided and spurred my rethinking many of the dictums about birth in this country. I have always been pushed more with VBAC clients. They had so little choice from medical providers in the 1980s. And after a brief period in which VBAC was on the rise, choices have again become limited for women who want this option.

I have been a board member of my state organization—the Michigan Midwives Association (MMA)—since 1983. We took some first steps toward licensing in the early 1980s without success, so we set up our own credentialing program and standards of care. We continue to hold educational conferences two to four times a year and have sponsored regional and national conferences. It's been a real support system for me all these years.

The Midwives Alliance of North America (MANA) has succeeded in professionalizing midwifery with standards and guidelines for practice. I have been challenged even more to learn new ways of practicing that are safer and have better outcomes. As an early supporter, I took part in the surveys about direct-entry midwifery practice and statistics gathering, including the CPM 2000 research project on outcomes of out-of-hospital births. I earned the Certified Professional Midwife (CPM) credential in 1997 and trained to be a Qualified Evaluator of CPM candidates. I have made it a priority to attend many MANA national conferences in order to improve my practice and skills.

I have had a job most of my adult life, beginning at age fourteen or fifteen as a Nurse's Aide in nursing homes, and then as a clerk in a small upscale jewelry store. In college I briefly worked in food service and started a little catering business cooking brown rice and vegetables for students who didn't want to eat in the cafeteria. After we moved to Michigan, I worked as a waitress and bartender in a couple of local taverns, as a woodworker with a successful small cooperative woodshop business, and manager of our own firewood business for a few winters. I have always worked some other part-time or full-time job while being a midwife, as the income from midwifery wasn't enough to adequately support my family, even though we chose to live simply.

Today, a very important part of my life is my work as a farmer. My husband and I have always grown our own food. We have a 200-acre farm, raising vegetables, beef, pork, chickens, and hardwood timber. We operate a Community Supported Agriculture (CSA). Our land is a great place to have my office, and families are welcome to come when the women have their prenatal and postpartum visits. In the spring we have new calves, early lettuce, and flowering bulbs. In mid-summer we have red ripe tomatoes, acres of sweet corn, and hay cutting. And in the fall we have squashes, pumpkins and autumn-hued woods. It makes it easy to provide good examples of how to eat. My clients have become CSA members and purchased eggs and meats from us. Food customers have been exposed to midwifery and have subsequently chosen to hire me as their midwife. Midwifery and farming have been completely intertwined in my life.

In 1990 my husband, Bill, decided to run for State Representative, after being involved in local politics for ten years. He was elected and served in the legislature for eight years before being term-limited in 1998. Our lives changed dramatically from the simple alternative lifestyle of farmers and homesteaders, to more mainstream. We both discovered our messages were better heard if we looked and acted more like our audiences. My practice grew from about 30 to 40 home births per year to 40 to 55 births per year. We have been able to expose many people in his expanded legislative work arena to the ideas of midwifery and home birth. With his new income, I could afford to build an office onto my home and upgrade my equipment and library. It also enabled me to not raise my fees out of the range of lower income people. We have always considered some of the reduced–fee care I provide as direct tithing.

Trust is at the very core of the midwife-woman partnership, and my aim is to have the same trust flow to the mother-baby relationship. I know I have helped women keep healthier through their pregnancies and attain safe, family-centered birth experiences. I have learned so much from watching women in labor who were truly in tune with the process: their reactions to pain and discomfort; their ability to find measures of tolerance; their physical movements and subconscious and conscious acts that allowed labor to progress; the ways their bodies pushed the babies out. I have also learned from the women who didn't like being pregnant, who fought their labors and clenched their legs together, and didn't want to push. Women give birth in all sorts of ways and most of them work. I have experienced many moments of being fully present in the process and paying close attention to what I was observing. That has always been a huge learning experience, molding and shaping me to calmly and quietly assist in the natural process when needed, but mostly to trust how the birth was progressing and to provide simple comfort and encouragement to the birthing woman.

I love watching babies' responses too, taking their first breaths, stretching and unfolding, nuzzling and nursing for the first time. It amazes me that babies who haven't breathed spontaneously, even ones who have needed positive pressure ventilation, come around, and are almost always okay after a little more time to recover. Babies are filled with a strong life force and are very resilient.

It has been hard work to pay attention to my intuitive self. Yet, many times I acted and spoke with no clue as to why, just a knowing it was right. Many times I ignored gut feelings of discomfort but later regretted making those choices as both a person and a midwife. Within the past six or eight years, I have had a clearer idea of how I feel when making the right choices.

Being a midwife has changed how I interact with everyone—my family, husband, children, and community. Always being on call affects everything. I have had to be responsible twenty-four hours a day, seven days a week most of my adult life. I have had to be organized and able to plan for sudden change. My family struggled to adapt, and we worked hard to compromise how best to integrate a full-time profession into full-time family responsibilities. We bought better cars; we stayed close to phones before the days of reliable pagers and cell phones. My equipment had to always be packed and ready, and we always made backup plans. Such a lifestyle is quite disruptive to the normal flow of home life, allowing for very little spontaneity. The phone calls from women in labor are the spontaneous inserts into my daily life, affecting me and everyone around me.

Interrupted sleep is another hard issue. In a typical week I receive five phone calls between 2 A.M. and 7 A.M., and yet no baby was born! Women and their families and other sister midwives simply needed support and so I made myself available. Naturally, it's draining on me and hard on my husband to deal with the disturbances to normal sleep patterns.

I'm still surprised at my adaptability to what life throws at me. I'm smart and know how to think things through to find solutions that usually work. I have developed resilience and strength. My knowledge base is constantly expanding from all sorts of sources. I trust body processes. I am a more patient person in all sorts of ways. I think in nine-month cycles.

I have faced fear and it has changed me. I have been arrested for practicing medicine without a license. I have had babies die and a mother die, and yet I grew stronger, busier and became a better midwife. I have made mistakes but kept on learning. There were times when I did everything right and still suffered with sad consequences.

One of the toughest challenges in midwifery has been in assisting families with the death of a much loved baby, whether from a miscarriage at 13 weeks gestation, a stillbirth at 34 weeks, or the death of a week-old baby with a lethal congenital defect. You cannot expect to be continually intimate with the miracle and joy of life coming into the world without experiencing some sadness. I know I have changed peoples' lives profoundly with love and support at a crucial time of growth and change for them. Helping families to bond strongly with each other and their new babies makes all the hard work, sacrifice, and sadness worthwhile.

I love the way a dawning day feels when a new baby is just born! I have personally attended over 1200 births. I love knowing babies are born drug-free, never being separated long from their mothers, able to cuddle and nurse to their contentment, be loved and cared for. I have assisted my daughter with the births of my three grandchildren. I have delivered as many as eleven babies for one family. I have really enjoyed my work. It is a pleasure to assist families at such a special time in their lives. I am now catching the babies of babies I have helped deliver, and catching grandbabies for some of the parents I worked with thirty years ago! Many of them have become dear friends.

I became a midwife before I knew midwives are the safest birth attendants for low-risk women. It is a global fact. The United States ranks pitifully poor among developed nations—about thirtieth in the world for infant mortality—meaning twenty-nine other developed countries have better infant outcomes. Those countries with the best outcomes have midwives providing most of the care for childbearing women. Obstetricians in this country need to pay attention to World Health Organization recommendations for good maternity care and tell the truth about outcomes in America compared to other countries. The medical system in this country is ingrained with one of the most hierarchical power structures in our society. I yearn for the day when our health care system isn't so deeply wrought with turf issues. There's more than enough work to keep all providers busy. Specialists should keep to their areas of expertise and quit trying to make a natural process so complicated. Pregnant women and women in labor should not be treated for the "what ifs," and medical practitioners should use their knowledge and intuition to distinguish who really needs intervention. It is possible to lower risk factors, cesarean, and intervention rates while still providing positive outcomes. For over twenty years, the cesarean rate in my practice has remained at 3% while the national c-section rate is currently ten times higher at 32%. Granted, I work with exceptionally motivated women, but all women deserve the education and support to make good choices about their care. It saddens me that the medical profession has done such a sales job for epidurals and inductions. It also amazes me to be asked if I do cesareans at home. People think it's just another way to have a baby! How has this happened? How can we all work to stop the tide against natural childbirth?

I am always thinking about how best to train new midwives. Some great steps in the right direction have been taken in the past two decades. These include the process developed by the North American Registry of Midwives (NARM) that documents midwifery skills obtained through apprenticeship (the Portfolio Evaluation Process, or PEP); the creation and implementation of the Certified Professional Midwife (CPM), a credential that requires knowledge and experience in out-of-hospital birth; and the growth in new midwifery schools. My vision is a maternity care system based on the CPM in which the textbook and laboratory learning would be integrated in the community college system. Coupled with a two to three year apprenticeship in one or two midwifery practices, such a module would be followed by internships with a half dozen other midwifery practices in order to round out education and expose midwifery students to many styles of practice. I think the required number of births that family practice doctors and midwives must attend before certification is too few; the number of births should be doubled or tripled, with at least a third of those encompassing continuity of care.

I can offer some advice to new midwives. First, it is important to set your boundaries and respect them. Understand they will change over time as you gain more experience and confidence, but know what is outside your comfort level and don't be forced to compromise your standards. Next, start out being more conservative; let responsible and educated clients push you when you are ready. Third, take care of yourself. Eat healthy, get regular exercise, and sleep well. Do the things that work to refresh and renew you. I garden and spend time outdoors. I know other midwives who walk daily, or get their recharge from their spiritual affiliations, or make time for self-improvement and centering work. Schedule vacations with family and friends. Take occasional time off call. Fourth, be truthful and consistent. Treat all clients fairly. We all have our favorites, but every client deserves to think she's special. And finally, it has always been important to me to have peers I can count on for support and advice. Don't hesitate to consult with other trusted practitioners for a myriad of reasons. Spend time with seasoned midwives you admire. Learn from them. Let them mentor you.

Remember that as midwives, listening to women and their partners is a large part of the service we provide and an important aspect of the care. It is something that can't be "fudged." Listening deeply, observing that actions match words, providing simple reassurance, being kind and respectful, referring to other professionals if indicated, are all as important as taking a blood pressure or catching a baby.

Most important, trust a woman's body and its cycles. Believe in the ability to give birth naturally. If you ever lose your passion for midwifery, take a break. Find something else to do. This work of building strong families is too important for half-hearted attention.

I never intended to be an outlaw

KATE BOWLAND

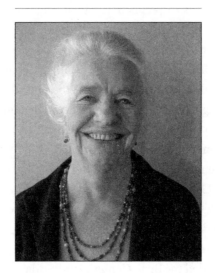

I never intended to be an outlaw, but I was born into a time when the midwifery profession had been nearly eliminated and was illegal in many states. Future generations of midwives will wonder why we risked going to jail and our freedom to do midwifery. It was and remains our hope that our grandchildren and great grandchildren can be born without fear, safely and surrounded by love, into the hands of midwives.

I began my midwifery profession in February of 1972 after earning a degree in art from the San Francisco Art Institute in1968. It was the time of the civil rights movement. When laws are unjust or immoral, it is our responsibility to disobey. I made the conscious choice to disobey the law. For me, midwifery was an act of civil disobedience. I fought for what I believed to be my constitutional right to be a midwife, all the way to the California Supreme Court. My sister midwives all over the United States revived a profession that had almost been eliminated. I have been a midwife for thirty-six years, long enough to see some of the laws play catch-up with the will of the people.

Often I am asked why I became a midwife. It was an accident, I say. In 1972 I left my home in Oregon to visit my friend from art school, Raven Lang. When I arrived, she was leaving to go to a birth and invited me to come along. I climbed into her old Volvo, and so as she drove the redwood-lined back roads, my life as a midwife began. On the way to the birth Raven explained that the mother had contracted toxoplasmosis in pregnancy, which might have damaged the baby. The woman in labor lay in a candle-lit room with music drifting in from the living room where her husband played the flute and piano. I stayed up all night applying pressure on her back to relieve her pain, all the while I felt awed by the magic of the energy that surrounded her. In the end, the baby was born with extreme head molding from its posterior presentation, and I thought that he was deformed. But I fell in love with him anyway. I saw him as perfect.

Raven had written to me about having started "The Birth Center," a collective of women giving prenatal care and attending home births in the small coastal town of Santa Cruz, California. She was also writing a book about those births. She shared her black and white photos of naked women squatting, standing, kneeling, and on hands and knees as they gave birth. The photos were stark and graphic, shocking to my Midwestern sensibilities, yet absolutely intriguing. The following week I attended the Birth Center's Wednesday clinic and began attending prenatal visits.

For a long time I have said that I became a midwife because I was a feminist and wanted to empower women. The fact was that birth in the early 1970s was a culturally warped ritual of isolation, humiliation and disempowerment for most women in the United States. I said then that I did it for the women, to give them the choice of a natural birth and to protect the natural process and help make it safe and empowering. Now I understand that there is a deeper reason. I do it for the babies . . . and for the baby I once was.

My mother conceived me in the summer of 1944, during WWII. Protein was in short supply, so my parents opened their house to another family with three young children and shared their rationed food supply. My mother loved being pregnant, and in her journal she wrote that she felt closer to God in pregnancy and giving birth than at any other time in her life. She had read *Childbirth Without Fear* and given birth to all four of her children naturally, having breastfed all of us. She also wrote, "I think that weaning is more about weaning the mother than the baby."

I was born in Detroit Michigan in Henry Ford Hospital in April of 1945. My mother told me that Henry Ford visited me in "his nursery." He was very proud of the hospital, designed on his assembly-line model. This model involved bringing in the "ore" or the raw material (that would be my pregnant mother) and separating the father from the mother, and the mother from the baby. The mother went along the conveyer belt from labor room to delivery room to postpartum room and then out the door to home. "The product," that was me, was taken to the nursery for ten days and put on a strict four-hour schedule for feeding.

I was weaned abruptly at ten weeks when my mother got pneumonia and was hospitalized for months. This was prior to the development of antibiotics, and when one of her lungs collapsed, she nearly died. She wanted to die, wanted the nuns who prayed over her to leave her in the arms of God where she felt peace. My father begged her to want to live. "You have three children at home who need you," he said. "You have a little baby." In that moment, she willed herself to live and to work for each breath.

I thank my mother for giving me positive messages about pregnancy, birth and breastfeeding and for unique opportunities to experience life fully. As an artist she taught me love and respect for the human body. She gifted me with the confidence that birth works.

She also gave me what I call "mother deprivation syndrome." Because she was mostly absent my first year, I asked her, "Who took care of me?" She said she arranged for a wet nurse to breastfeed me. I clung to that story, liked to think that someone held me to her sweet breast. However my father reported that it was "anyone who we could find." It was the separation from my mother at birth and during that first year that has been one of my primary motives and inspired me to work so hard to keep a mother and baby together after birth. Each time I slip a baby into the mother's eager hands, each time I witness an outpouring of unconditional mother love, with the cries of wonder and joy and declarations of love to this new being, I am healed. Midwifery became my passion, a calling and a healing journey.

As a child I spent long summer days watching frog eggs hatch and tadpoles turn into frogs. Cats had kittens on my bed, and under my bed puppies popped out. When I was nine, my mother pulled me out of school in the early spring and arranged for me to ride along with Miss Wells, a public health nurse for

Sweetwater County. She drove to the remote ranches in southwestern Wyoming and northern Utah in the foothills of the Uintah Mountains.

On my first trip I gripped the door of the Jeep as Miss Wells carefully worked its wheels to keep them on the top of the icy tracks beside the Henry's Fork River. We passed a work crew with a bulldozer clearing snow and gravel from the edge of the ford where the road crossed the frozen river. She turned the Jeep south and slowly moved out on to the sheet of ice. The edge was thin and cracked under the tires. My stomach was full of butterflies. Ice groans under weight, ice is used to moving slowly, and slowly it does. The ice gave a long groan, then a loud crack like a firecracker, or more like ten firecrackers. I gripped the seat with both hands as the back wheels dropped down from under us; all four wheels were spinning on an ice slab slanted ever so slightly uphill. The Jeep's back bumper dipped into the water, and rested against the gravel bottom. My heart was pounding. The workers laughed as the driver of the D 9 Cat hooked the Jeep and pulled it to safety on the other side of the river. They all treated the event like a sport. We visited four ranches that day. Each time we arrived at a house Miss Wells opened her black bag and did basic health care, including vaccinating children, testing for anemia, and checking blood pressure and urine for sugar. She also checked the cistern water and sanitation systems. I was allowed to accompany her except when there was a pregnant woman to examine, and then they would retreat to a bedroom. Miss Wells, it turns out, was a nurse-midwife trained at the Frontier School in Kentucky in midwifery and public health. I credit her with giving me a vision of home care, a taste for adventure, and an understanding that the journey is much of the story.

I moved from Wyoming with my family to the San Francisco of the mid-Sixties, rented an apartment in the Haight-Ashbury, enrolled in the San Francisco Art Institute and found myself in the midst of a cultural revolution. My generation was questioning every value, everything we had been raised to believe in the post-World War II era. Our fathers were war heroes; our mothers were back in the kitchen. We wanted to stop the war in Vietnam, and give peace and love a chance. Our generation was optimistic, believing that we could make the world a better place if we would just "do it." We went back to the land to grow our own food and raise our animals; it was our dream to live a self-reliant, self-sustaining organic, environmentally sensitive lifestyle. It was the "do it yourself" American way, the help-your-neighbor-raise-the-barn spirit. In the city we opened free clinics, free shelters for the homeless, and centers for free food distribution. Swept up in the joy of the Beatles music, peace marches and the introduction of eastern religions and spiritual practices, we were determined to change the world.

My generation of women re-launched the feminist movement, demanding equality with men in work, in equal wages, in childcare and in our reproductive rights, including birth control and abortions. While our great-grandmothers had marched for an end to slavery and for women's emancipation and our grand-mothers had marched out of the Victorian era for women's right to vote, they also marched for pain-free childbirth. Childbirth had been moved from home to hospital. Women were told that they couldn't bear the pain of labor or breast-feed. Medicated births and bottle-feeding on a schedule became the norm. The feminist movement did not include the right to give birth where, with whom, and how you pleased, or the right to breastfeed in public. Feminists did not fight for maternity leave; instead they fought for "disability leave."

A small subset of women who wanted to breastfeed their babies realized that in order to do so, they had to have more control over their births and they wanted their babies with them continuously after giving birth. These women had moved back to the land and valued a natural life style. They realized they could not get their needs met in a hospital. They trusted themselves to give birth naturally at home with a little help from their friends, thus creating a need for home birth midwives.

After college in 1968, my husband and I combed the west in a VW Camper Van looking for land, and with two other couples we bought forty acres at an end of a road in southern Oregon. One of my land partners, Ruth, was pregnant with her first child and decided to tour the local hospital. After the tour, she felt in her gut that she could not give birth in such a sterile environment. In early labor she called her family doctor and asked him to come to their home. He had attended numerous home births in his practice over the past three decades. Doc came over and sipped whiskey with her father-in-law until she was ready to push. She was the first home birth mom I knew, and she told me she was ecstatic with the results of her birth.

In 1971 Raven Lang opened the Santa Cruz Birth Center in that small coastal California town, with a group of women in response to the refusal of local doctors to provide prenatal care for women planning home births. Raven wrote to me in Oregon about the Birth Center. In 1972 I visited her and attended my first birth with her. I decided to stay. The Birth Center midwives quickly learned the basics of birthing from a handful of supportive nurses and doctors willing to share their knowledge. The women met in a large Victorian house where the housemates opened their bedrooms to become examination rooms once a week. The living room became a center for pregnant women and their families to exchange infor-mation and create community. The Birth Center quickly grew by word of mouth, with the midwives soon attending ten to twenty births a month. It wasn't long before the Birth Center was in need of a new location, and so I offered my house for the Wednesday clinics. I became immersed in birth and the midwifery movement.

Raven's philosophy of non-intervention became the foundation of the midwifery model of care. We held clandestine meetings with other home birth midwives in northern California where we "talked story" and invited guest speakers to teach. In the beginning we only shared our first names. Later, as our trust grew, we started a newsletter, and out of this "school without walls" grew the California Association of Midwives. After approaching the state's Maternal Health Department and legislators, we proposed new laws to legalize midwifery. At this time there was a concerted effort by the California Medical Association to suppress other alternative health care givers, including acupuncturists, massage therapists and herbalists. Law enforcement officers arrested practitioners, charging them with practicing medicine without a license. Little did we know that midwives were included in their investigation.

The second birth I attended took place six miles up a winding redwood-lined road in the mountains. Valerie lived in a small tourist cabin in an old resort by the river under giant redwoods. I was the first to arrive and I found her on her bed laboring quietly with her man by her side. Valerie's red hair curled around her head, spreading out like seaweed floating back and forth between waves. After each contraction she fell back onto the bed and into a deep sleep. Her husband sat beside her in silence. Out of her endorphin-induced haze, she would rise, feet flat on the bed, and support herself with her arms behind her, and brought the baby into sight, then fell back again and snored for a few minutes. As this was only my second birth, I felt I was not yet a midwife. And I still felt unsure about becoming one.

We were waiting for the midwives to arrive. On the table was my new copy of *Myles Midwifery* to study while I waited. Even at the crowning we could tell this was a redheaded baby. As the baby crowned, Valerie's partner, Jeff, moved into a position between her legs to receive the baby. He flew into Jeff's cupped hands with a flood of clear fluid and a loud cry. Our laughter burst the air as the baby settled into quiet breathing. I covered him with warm blankets from the oven. Valerie sat up, placed him between her breasts and he bobbed his head while we admired his strength. I turned for a second blanket and heard the distinct sound of sucking as he latched onto her breast. We all laughed again in surprise and celebrated.

Fifteen minutes later she looked up at me and asked, "Would you hold the baby?"

I said, "Sure."

She said, "I don't feel well." Then she pitched backward in a full faint and fell into unconsciousness. I quickly cut the cord and handed the baby to Jeff, kneeled on the bed, placed her flat and shook her shoulder.

"Are you OK?" I asked. No response. Beneath her bottom was a large pool of blood. I jumped up to look up hemorrhage in *Myles*; I really did not know what to do. The English spell it differently than we do, so it took me some time to find it. I treated her for shock by putting her legs up on my shoulders. Color returned to her cheeks and she opened her eyes.

"What happened?" she asked.

"You fainted. You have to stop bleeding." I placed my hand on her stomach and tried to rub up the uterus. Everything felt soft, and I could not find a hard grapefruit size uterus to make contract. Suddenly, the sound of a car's tires crunching the gravel outside the house announced the arrival of the midwives. Kitty and Dora swept through the door, and with one glance Kitty, also a cardiac nurse, quickly assessed the situation. Without any hesitation she said, "We have to get her to the hospital. I'll get my car ready." When I carried her to the car she passed out again, and as the car drove away I wondered if she was going to live. There I was—left alone with a newborn baby boy in my arms. In that moment I promised him that if women were going to choose home birth, then they needed to have midwives who knew how to help them to make it safe. I decided I would learn what to do. I would become a midwife. It was a simple decision: there was a need, and I knew that I wanted something to do that required all of me. Valerie arrived at the hospital where the doctor removed her placenta with his hand and gave her two units of blood. She was reunited with her baby a few hours later.

A few days later, Kitty called me at dawn from her home in the mountains and asked me to go to Linda's house just a block away from my own. As this was Linda's first baby, Kitty was sure there would be plenty of time before the birth. Carrying my mini-birth kit, containing a blood pressure cuff, gauze pads, dental floss to tie the cord, sterile scissors, and hemostats, I walked down the alley to her house. The house was warm and quiet; candles were burning in her bedroom where she lay on her left side grunting like a weight lifter. Her husband was on a futon on the opposite side of the room with his back to her, groaning with her and complaining of his back pain. When I pulled back the blanket, I saw the baby's black hair surge forward into a full crown. I knelt down and the next surge delivered the head. A shiny cord was wrapped twice around his neck. Carefully, I unwrapped it, and he plopped out, wide-eyed, very blue and crying.

After the birth, the first person I called was my father.

"Daddy!' I said, "Daddy! I just delivered my first baby!"

He said, "Well . . . weren't you scared?"

"No," I said, "and there were two loops of cord around his neck, and I just unlooped them. He's fine and he's nursing."

"Well, I guess it's all right. I was born at home on the farm in Ohio and I'm OK. I guess it's all right. You know, it cost my mother five dollars for the doctor to come out in his horse and buggy to deliver me on the kitchen table. You know that my mother helped women have their babies, don't you?"

I said, "No, really? My Grandma Ona was a midwife?"

"Yeah, I guess so. She was the one they called when someone was being born or dying. They would give her a piglet or a chicken or potatoes." After Linda's birth, I attended births as the senior midwife. I came from the see-one-do-one-teach-one school. About a year and a half later a pivotal event in my life occurred.

At the Birth Center's weekly chart review meeting in my bedroom, I threw Terry Johnson's chart down on the floor in the middle of the circle of the Santa Cruz midwives.

"Look at this chart!" I said. "Terry has not brought in her blood work or signed up for a childbirth class; she has missed prenatal visits, and her baby seems too small for her due date. I get a weird vibe from her. I don't think she is taking responsibility. Who wants to go to her birth?" No one spoke up. So we decided to confront Terry at her next prenatal visit the following day.

Later during that meeting I said, "What we are doing here? Giving free prenatal care and doing home births is radical, and we are all in danger of being arrested for practicing medicine without a license." The very next morning, on March 6, 1974, during the Birth Center's prenatal clinic day, the phone rang. It was Terry's alleged husband. He spoke hurriedly.

"Terry is in labor. Come quick and bring all of your midwives and all the equipment you can." I took down the address and turned to the other midwives; no one wanted to go, much less go alone. We talked about how weird he sounded; we knew that the baby was too small for a home birth, and we were afraid that he was preventing her from going to the hospital. We decided to send two midwives to get her to the hospital. Linda Bennett and Jeanine Walker drove to the cabin in Ben Lomond.

Thirty minutes later I looked out the window over the shoulder of the woman I was examining to see two cars pull up across the street. Six men in suits got out and ran between my house and the neighbor's. I knew immediately that they were plainclothes police. I heard loud knocks on the front and back doors of my house, the knocking accompanied by "OPEN UP. IT'S THE POLICE!" I sprang to my feet, grabbed the medical contents of my birth kit, Pitocin, syringes, sutures and Xylocaine and plunged them deep into the pocket of my mother's black velvet coat in my closet. Carol opened the front door to see holstered guns underneath their suit coats while I fled to the back of the house and into the bathroom with a sudden need to defecate. Just as I flushed the results, a police-woman opened the door and ordered me out of the way and plunged her hand into the swirling mess, thinking I was flushing some evidence. I enjoyed a little satisfaction seeing her disgust.

The house was searched and some things were confiscated—my birth kit, diapers, stethoscope, sterile gloves, and only a few of our charts. Dr. Lewis Mehl was reviewing the other charts, about 300 charts of them, at Stanford University for research on home birth. Terry Johnson and her alleged husband turned out to be undercover police officers who had been investigating the Birth Center for months to set up the sting. I was arrested and marched off to jail to be booked along with Jeanine Walker and Linda Bennett who had been arrested in Ben Lomond. We were released an hour later on our own recognizance. At the time, I was early pregnant with my first son Shane. Over the next three years I would attend more court dates than prenatal visits, and I would go through two pregnancies and two home births with the lay midwife of my choice, Carol Brendsel. The case went to the Appellate court twice before the Supreme Court ruled on it.

The women's movement was at a high point. We had the support of a large birth community and women's groups all around the world. The money they donated paid our legal fees. Our arguments in the case were that midwifery and home birth were legal actions for mother and midwife, that, in fact, constitutional law protected these rights. We demurred (a demurrer is a response in a court proceeding that admits the facts of the opponent's arguments but claims it is not sufficient grounds to justify legal action), asserting that we were midwives, and that midwifery was not the practice of medicine. In other words, what we were charged with was not a crime. I felt proud of my actions as a midwife defendant, confident in our cause. Ignoring the advice of my attorney Ann Flower Cummings to remain silent about the case, I was very outspoken in public and to the media. I was arrogant and very defiant of the male authority in the medical-legal complex. Meanwhile, I was term pregnant with my second son when I stood before the Supreme Court of California and listened to nine old men in black robes, most of whom were born at home, rule that while I did have the right to give birth at home, I did not have the right to choose my unlicensed friend as an attendant.

The California Supreme Court wrote a very confusing thirty-six-page decision in response to our constitutional augments. The Court ruled that it was legal for a woman to give birth at home, but stated that "pregnancy was a physical condition, and that during the course of pregnancy or labor, a person holding them self out to be a midwife, or undertaking to render skilled material assistance in the birth process, or to be able to recognize the development of certain problems that may occur, or to cut the cord or engage in acts that involved the assumption of responsibility for delivery of the child could be guilty of the practice of midwifery or medicine without a license. Midwifery is characterized by legislation as a 'healing art' because a midwife is consulted for her expertise or as an advisor and or an assistant."

The Court further stated that the State recognizes an interest in the life and well-being of the unborn child, and, quoting from *Roe v. Wade*, said, "for the same reasons for which legislature may prohibit the abortion of unborn children who have reached the point of viability, it may require those who assist in childbirth to have a valid license." The court further stated, " . . . because women rely on those with qualifications, which they cannot personally verify."

It is noteworthy that the fetus was referred to as the "unborn child," and that the rights of the unborn superseded the rights of the mother, thus pitting the rights and welfare of the mother against the rights of her own child.

The court referred us back to the municipal court for trial and added that we should address the legislature to change the laws. Three years later, in 1977, the local district attorney dismissed the charges against us for lack of evidence. There was a rumor that his wife threatened him with divorce if he prosecuted us, but the fact is that the medical-legal complex had what they wanted, and they began arresting midwives in California and all over the country any time there was a "sad outcome" such as a stillbirth.

I often summarized the story of the new wave of midwifery in the following words: At first we got arrested. Then we had to write new laws and get them passed, and then create schools and go to them. We were then tested, certified, and licensed.

After exploring my options for licensure, I decided to return to school for midwifery. Though the Nurse-Midwifery Practice Act had passed in December of 1974, I knew that it would be many years before the Licensed Midwifery Act would be passed (in fact, not until October 1993). I wanted to be in bedrooms, not courtrooms. In December of 1983 I stood talking to the program director of the University of California San Francisco nurse-midwifery program, Susan Libel. I had just graduated. She handed me the current California Association of

Midwives newsletter that listed all the midwifery arrests in California, beginning with the Birth Center Bust. It filled nine pages. I looked at her with tears in my eyes. "This is why I went to nurse-midwifery school."

Earning my Certified Nurse-Midwife (CNM) license propelled me into an unanticipated crisis of identity. I was no longer an outlaw, for I had a signed contract with four OB/GYNs who had agreed to back me up. I could draw blood, order labs on my own, and administer medications legally. As I was no longer a lay midwife, the earth-mama hippies now considered me too much in the medical establishment while the more mainstream families choosing home birth with nurse midwives in town found me too much of a hippie. It was a difficult transition. I felt like a mule—neither horse nor donkey—and in making my way through this transition I began talking with other CNMs with lay midwifery roots. Fran Ventre, Peggy Spindel and I did a survey and wrote a paper about these hybrid midwives. Later we created a home birth committee within the American College of Nurse-Midwives to advocate for home birth. We wrote a handbook for CNMs, and in 1995 an entire issue of the *Journal of Nurse-Midwifery* was dedicated to home birth. We had the vision of unity for the two major streams of midwifery with the creation of the Bridge Club to bridge the gap between the nurse-midwives and the direct-entry midwives.

For twenty years now I have been fortunate in being in partnership with Roxanne Cummings. We have shared the responsibility and passed the "on call" baton back and forth. I am grateful for the twenty years that we have had as partners and friends. We have midwifed each other through the various family joys and crises that make up life, including births, marriages, and the departure of loved ones. I treasure our deep friendship and am proud to be in one of the longest professional home birth midwifery partnerships in the nation. As I write this story, I have been in home birth practice for thirty-six years.

We cannot predict or control birth. As a midwife I can only show up and meet the challenge of the moment. I have learned to be eclectic and open to change in the ways that I practice, as new information or research is gathered. As a naturalist, I have learned that I am conservative in the sense of conserving energy and using as little technology as possible or necessary. I have learned to balance the principle and value of non-intervention and undisturbed birth with the need to incorporate actions and interventions to preserve the health of baby and mother. I have learned to listen to women and my gut and be decisive. I have learned to transport women to the hospital earlier rather than later and without regret.

Looking back, the hardest part has been the conflict between my family's needs and the needs of my clients. My poet friend Greg Keith summed up the conflict when he wrote, ". . . the strands of the family gone slack without her. Laundry piled, love unmade, dishes undone." But I made the simple decision to put the woman in labor first, to avoid the conflict of feelings between my work and any other life event. I missed birthdays, Christmas, Thanksgiving, school plays, play dates, celebrations with friends, and dental appointments. Because of my exhaustion, I sometimes had little energy to give to my family.

Actually, fatigue is the easy part. Early on, I learned that being tired is not the worst thing. A nap of twenty minutes or a few hours of sleep would allow me to go safely on to the next birth. My advice to young midwives is to learn to nap and to ask for help from your midwife friends.

I have written several stories under the heading "The Times I Quit Midwifery." They are the stories of births where I was faced with a life or death situation that I had to handle alone. The fear of being arrested or sued for a sad outcome proved harder than the hard stuff of the emergencies. To this day, every time I see a police car or hear a siren I feel anxious, knowing full well that I can be arrested and taken away even if I am innocent. Or if sued, I could lose everything I have worked for all of my life.

The wolves of the medical-legal insurance complex are constantly nipping at our heels, making it harder to practice the midwifery model of care at home or even in the hospital. Laws related to the practice of midwifery make it difficult to practice. Barriers limit the scope of our practice to an extremely narrow window. They include the requirement that midwives have physician supervision, while malpractice insurance companies deny coverage not only to midwives but also to the doctors who are willing to supervise them. Many HMOs and so-called health insurance companies refuse to pay midwives for their care at home. Furthermore, the social movement of natural birth and breastfeeding that gave birth to the midwifery movement has been replaced by an epidemic of epidurals and cesarean sections and a culture of fear around birth.

Here is my vision: Pregnant women would have maternity leave beginning at twenty-eight weeks and stipends to stay home for the first two years. Their first pregnancy contact would be a midwife who would refer to doctors as needed. We would have a health care system with "mal-occurrence insurance" instead of malpractice insurance. There would be a fund to take care of women and their babies who are injured by giving birth or being born. Midwives would be well educated, autonomous, legal, and licensed. They would be supported culturally, politically, economically and socially. This would include the integration of modern medicine with ancient wisdom and holistic health practices. Midwifery education would be for direct-entry midwifery, from an apprenticeship model to bachelor's and/or master's degree education. Community-based midwifery education would available at local community colleges, universities and remote learning programs. Every midwifery practice would be a training site where student midwives would have a practicing midwife as a mentor/preceptor. The health care system would support practice in all settings according to the desires and needs of women, their babies and their midwives.

My story is a simple one. My friend Raven took me to a birth and birth spoke to me. I felt that God had grabbed me by the scruff of my neck and set me down and said, "This is your work." I had found my calling, a clear path to service to which I have devoted my life. I have sustained a home birth practice since 1972 and attended more than 1700 births. I have kept driving through the days and the nights, the full moon, the dark of the moon, star-studded nights, the big wave nights, the fog-shrouded nights, storm-pounding rainy nights and clear calm nights. I have left my bed and, in my somnambulant state, have gone out to the woman in labor. It seems as if it is always 3 o'clock—3 P.M. or 3 A.M. I warm the blankets, offer a drink through the bendable straw and chant to the woman "This is normal, this is normal . . . you are doing well," and at the crowning of the head I chant "Beautiful, beautiful, beautiful."

In my culture, woman is the first environment

KATSI COOK

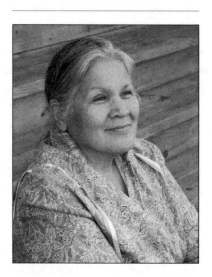

*M*y belly button is buried in Mohawk territory at Akwesasne, an indigenous kinship nation of about 12,000 Mohawk people. Our lands
and waters straddle the United States-Canada border where the St. Lawrence
River first meets the St. Regis and Grasse Rivers in Northern New York. My
Reservation is unique in North American Indian Country in that it has the
political complication of being tri-sected by three governmental jurisdictions:
Quebec, Ontario and New York State. Over the twenty-five years of my traditional Aboriginal midwifery practice, I have worked in all three jurisdictions at
one time or another.

My paternal grandmother, Elizabeth Kanatires Herne Cook, delivered many children in my generation, including me. She and her mother—my great grandmother, Millie Garreau Herne—served the many extended families of Akwesasne as midwives from the mid-1930s and the Great Depression to the post World War II industrial boom of the 1950s that brought the St. Lawrence Seaway development to our territory. My grandmothers raised their large families and served many others at a time when rural communities, especially Indian reservations, pretty much had to take care of themselves. There was no money for the few and far away hospitals that there were at the time.

Sometime in the 1930s and 1940s, my grandmothers made the downstairs bedroom of their large farmhouse into a birthing room, or "baby room" as it was called. I was born in that room—into the hands of my paternal grandmother in her big white iron bed in mid-winter of 1952. I have been told that my grandmother bundled me up and put me aside in a basket while she tended to my mother. When she later circled back to me, she found that I was bleeding from the cord stump. Using her common sense, Grandma took a needle and thread, sterilized it and sewed up my belly button. Growing up in her care, my cousins and siblings would tease me, saying "You better not make grandma mad or she'll take her thread back!" As a young girl I used to sit on my little bed, a chintz curtain away from my grandma's big white iron bed where I was born, and search my belly button for that thread. When I carried my first child in 1975 at the age of 23, Grandma's long lost ligature became the connection and continuity that led me along the path of midwifery.

My mother, Evelyn Kawennaien Montour Cook, was integral to my intellectual development. She was a Kanawakeh Mohawk who, when I was eleven years old, succumbed to the effects of mitral valve stenosis that developed secondary to childhood rheumatic fever at a time when antibiotics did not yet exist. I will never forget what she told me when I came home crying from Catholic school in second grade. I was the only Mohawk attending the off-reservation elementary school besides my older sister. Sister Mary Patrick had picked me to read aloud in class from a chapter in our history book about the martyrdom of missionary Isaac Jogues at the hands of the Mohawks. I hung my head in my hands as I read the page, embarrassment burning my cheeks. I was only seven years old. I hadn't known that Mohawks had ever been that cruel. At home, my mother took me in her arms, looked me squarely in the eyes and said in a revelatory tone: "Just remember who wrote that book." Ever since then, I have increasingly grown to understand the power of the one who controls the metaphor.

Along with other communities that are part of the Six Nations Iroquois Confederacy, Akwesasne was a leader in the struggle for sovereignty and self-determination throughout Indian Country. I became involved in the traditionalist movement of my *Kanienke:haka* (Mohawk) longhouse as a youth, as well as in "Akwesasne Notes" and "White Roots of Peace," our international communications outreach. Throughout the 1960s and 1970s, the voice of Native sovereignty was being raised throughout the hemisphere. The national grassroots Indian Unity Caravans of the 1960s later evolved into the hemispheric International Indigenous Movement that culminated in the historic Geneva Convention of 1977 in Geneva, Switzerland, where indigenous nations of the hemisphere met together for the first time.

Back home in the Six Nations communities, my generation of activists organized action around five key issue areas of sovereignty: control of our land base, control of jurisdiction within that land base, control of education, control of psycho-religious life, and control of production and reproduction. Within each of these areas are issues in need of decolonizing strategies that indigenous peoples must develop and implement for ourselves. Women could be productive leaders in any of the five areas, but control of production and reproduction is the women's domain. This area captured my attention early on, involving as it does the powers of reproduction and performing the work of procreation—not just biological reproduction of Six Nations' babies and bodies, but also the reproduction of our society and culture, of clanship, kinship and language.

As a young woman in the longhouse, I asked my wolf clan mothers, "How do we teach the young about birth?" "Begin with the story of the first birth," they said, referring to our Iroquois creation story.

Pregnancy is a re-enactment of creation. The power of the birth story is that each birth is a re-weaving and re-creation of the world, encoding patterns and knowledge that inform the growth and development of the individual as well as the culture.

Sky Woman of our Iroquois creation story carried seeds and bits of sacred things embedded under her fingernails from the uprooted celestial tree of the Sky World to be used in the creation of this world on turtle's back, a renewal in fulfillment of a dream. Midwives also carry sacred knowledge of reproductive processes of birth necessary for the transformation of women and society. The mother-infant bond, for example, is so central to the aims of healing and social transformation that for me, midwifery occupies all of that space. It's not just about delivering babies. It's about the power of women to transform life.

A memorable character in my childhood growing up at Akwesasne was an elder Mohawk midwife named *Karati:the* (*She wears a hat*). Dressed in work overalls and a French beret, drawing on the stem of an old corncob pipe, she strolled the dirt roads of Saint Regis Village where she lived not far from the Mission Church. *Karati:the* was in her early seventies when I asked her to deliver my first baby at home in Saint Regis, Quebec, where I lived at that time not far from her house. I was twenty-three years old.

"I can't see anymore, I'm blind," *Karati:the* told me. "I can't even find my way across a room, let alone deliver a baby. But if you come to see me in your last two weeks of pregnancy, I'll give you Indian medicine for your delivery so you'll have an easy time."

There were many influences around me in my early days that created the currents that would carry me through many years of struggle to train, to practice and then to become a place holder in midwifery between my grandmother's generation and the generations coming towards us. Would these future generations be able to speak with our ancestors on their tongues?

I was determined to birth at home within the power of my own beliefs and knowledge. At that time in the 1970s, lay midwifery was emerging in the alternative world. During my first two pregnancies I spoke with elders and read books like Ina May Gaskin's *Spiritual Midwifery*, Maggie Myles' *Textbook for Midwives* and even *Williams Obstetrics*. My interest in pursuing midwifery began growing exponentially.

In 1977, with two young children under the age of five years and a fearlessness borne of my determination, I traveled to The Farm in Tennessee to study in a direct-entry apprenticeship model with Plenty International Midwifery Training Program. I initially spent three months at The Farm, learning hands-on in the pre-natal clinic and attending births with the birthing crew described in *Spiritual Midwifery*. Over the years, I visited The Farm in Tennessee again for month-long periods of time, as well as The Farm outposts in Washington, D.C. and in Lanark, Ontario. My family hosted a number of The Farm delegations to Akwesasne, whose members came to help train an ambulance crew and provide assistance in various other nation-building projects of the late 1970s and early 1980s.

Through the valuable assistance and generosity of friend and mentor Dr. Ann Boyer, OB/GYN, I was privileged to attend the University of New Mexico's Women's Health Training Program in 1978, funded by Planned Parenthood of North America. It was one of a class of only six students in a six-month clinical training program led by clinician and researcher Dr. John Slocumb, OB/GYN with Medical Director Dr. Sharon Phelan, OB/GYN. I was trained as a Women's Health Specialist, learning the SOAP (Subjective, Objective, Assessment and Plan) model of health data collection, taking and documenting medical histories, conducting complete physical exams and working in a variety of clinics providing a full range of primary health care to women who lived in areas without doctors. I attended complicated hospital births with Dr. Ann Boyer and lived in her home throughout my training. The strength of my preparation for midwifery practice was the recognition of the normal woman and infant and knowing when to consult and/or transfer care to a physician. In every sort of clinic that served women and their reproductive health needs—Planned Parenthood, VD clinics, maternal and child health clinics, surgery clinics, well-woman clinics—I provided primary care for Planned Parenthood clients, including a number of Native Americans from several of the many communities of the region's Pueblo and Navajo Nations. I was surprised by my clients' apparent lack of knowledge regarding their birthing experiences, seemingly deprived of their own agency. These observations were of great concern to me, because at that time, in the late 1970s, sterilization abuse of Native American women throughout the hemisphere was an emerging issue.

Having gained the clinical and counseling skills I felt necessary for a safe lay-midwifery practice, I decided to travel to spend time with my brother, Tom Kanatakeniate Cook, and my sister-in-law, Loretta Afraid of Bear Cook, in the Slim Buttes District of the Pine Ridge Reservation in South Dakota. My wonderful sister-in-law had shared with me the amusing story of her own mother's birthing at home for her youngest brother Aloysius Weasel Bear during a peyote meeting. Loretta's mom, Beatrice Weasel Bear, had served many years as a community midwife on the Pine Ridge Reservation. I wanted to learn "traditional" midwifery from her. Beatrice generously indicated to me: "Daughter-in-Law, if you want to learn about that, you have to go into that ceremony," directing me in 1978 to the relationship between ceremonial practice and birth.

While in South Dakota I attended the founding conference of Women of All Red Nations at the Mother Butler Center in Rapid City, South Dakota. From there I spent eighteen months in Minneapolis-St. Paul working out of the Red School House Survival School Clinic, training an Anishnawbe birthing crew, working to prevent reproductive abuses of Native American women. I returned to Akwesasne in 1980 where I continued my midwifery practice, assisting in the development of the Akwesasne Freedom School. I also organized an Akwesasne Mother's Milk Project, which later evolved into the First Environment Project.

I worked with Health Departments at Akwesasne to generate multi-disciplin-ary, multi-generational, human health research studies funded by a variety of government agencies, most notably CDC (Centers for Disease Control), ATSDR (Agency for Toxic Substances and Disease Registry) and NIEHS (National Institute of Environmental Health Sciences). From 1987 to 2002 I served as a research associate, co-investigator and principal investigator for a variety of human health research projects which sought to characterize impacts to human health from exposure to Akwesasne's local food chain that had been contami-nated by industrial chemicals, including heavy metals and organo-chlorines. As a founding member of the Akwesasne Task Force on the Environment and the Haudenosaunee Environmental Task Force, I helped develop research protocols in a framework of respect, equity and empowerment. I have conducted a number of research projects in compliance with the Institutional Review Board's process for human health research. Since I am not a Certified Nurse-Midwife, I have always chosen to initiate professional work that was congruent to my traditional Aboriginal midwifery practice.

Was midwifery a "calling" for me? The word "calling" implies belief. When one is "called," there is an understanding of a difficult journey ahead fraught with obstacles that must be overcome and sacrifices to be made. Associated with an understanding that ritual connection and thanksgiving is involved, a calling to the art of midwifery requires tasks of intense preparation and the responsi-bilities of proper communication and reciprocity. As art, midwifery is sacred performance at the confluence of a clear set of biomedical clinical (procedural) competencies, compassion, and women's ways of knowing involving our intuitive capacities. Midwifery is a way to make a living as well as a way to live a life.

It wasn't until June 9, 1984 that I actually received my "calling" from the spirits in a dream. Oddly enough it was in a moment of doubt, when I thought that the movement towards midwifery as a regulated profession would close the door to a culture and community-based practice. My dream revealed a magnifi-cent turtle constellation in the midnight sky. Like a bursting pod of milkweed seeds the stars that produced the Great Turtle's pattern unfurled into a continu-ous line of Iroquois women dancing across the sky towards me carrying their babies on cradleboards. Weaving in unison, like slender tendrils of bean plants climbing their way up a stalk of maize, they were singing the fertility songs of the women planters' society.

Ten years later, a remarkable door of opportunity opened in the province of Ontario, Canada, due to the hard work and political organizing of lay midwives in that jurisdiction. After attending the Michener Institute Pre-Registration Program for previously practicing lay midwives that was sponsored by the government to bring us "up to standards," seventy-four of my colleagues and I became eligible to become the first Registered Midwives in that province. We had been broken into three separate, consecutive classes of twenty-five midwives each. We lived in dormitory style together for one month in downtown Toronto in the winter of 1992-1993. My peers selected me as their class representative to the midwifery faculty that came from New Zealand, Sweden and England. I will never forget the diversity of women I was privileged to study with and continue to relate to as a member in what is now known as the Canadian Association of Midwives (CAM).

As a professional member of the Transitional Council of the College of Midwives of Ontario in 1993 and 1994, I helped write and review the standards under which Registered Midwives in Ontario practice their profession. In so doing, I guarded indigenous rights in the interpretation of jurisdictional issues recognized in the 1992 Ontario Midwifery Act and Regulated Health Professions Act that exempts traditional Aboriginal healers and traditional Aboriginal midwives from any regulation by the government. "If we don't use our rights, we lose our rights," I told my colleagues when I chose not to become registered as a midwife in the province of Ontario after the Midwifery Act was proclaimed by Parliament in 1994. From this ground, I was the founding Aboriginal Midwife of the Six Nations Birthing Center—*Tsinonwe:ionakeratstha/Onagrahstha*—at Six Nations, Ontario, where traditions of matrilineal clan knowledge are again honored and valued in strengthening the woman and her family. I recall our first day of prenatal clinic in our beautiful new building, entirely staffed by Six Nations women. At last we experienced the feeling of a having a creative space of our own. For a generation, Six Nations babies had been delivered into the world at a facility called Lady Wellington, long since closed.

Births that arise from the ground of an indigenous identity and the processes of social and cultural memory underpin the reproduction of our Aboriginal midwifery knowledge. Birth is a ceremony. Its transformative power lies in the expansion of relationships, increasing depth of identity and in the possibility of purification. Of many extraordinary births that I have been privileged to assist, a particularly memorable one enfolds the congruency of birth, dream and ceremony. It illustrates the potency of dream as a vehicle for empowerment and connection at the "threshold," a psychological space of the Iroquois ceremonial complex.

About 16 years ago, during an initial prenatal visit, Tewakierakwa recalled the words of her maternal uncle who had passed away several years before. Clearly, he was the most significant male in her early development. She said: "When I was 15 years old my Uncle Moises, a great man and a wise bear clan chief in the Oka longhouse, said: 'Our people die at birth for they are no longer born the way Mother Nature had intended. The birth is always hurried and women's stomachs are cut open. Drugs are used that make babies born half asleep. The first words they hear are the tongue of a foreign man. Then he's tossed from nurse to nurse, washed and measured on some Apgar test. Then he is placed at his mother's breast if he is lucky. That's why our ways are dying. There is no respect in the pain women feel at childbirth, the only time that the pain of life can be associated with joy.' "

The following spring, on the night when she went into labor, Tewakierakwa had conducted a full moon ceremony near the driveway outside her kitchen door. Sacred tobacco, water, and song were offered to the fire, Earth and moon, while her clan relatives and friends expressed their sincerest words in our Mohawk language for a safe journey for her and her coming child.

Afterwards, sitting at her kitchen table finishing up the ceremonial feast, a fierce storm suddenly kicked up outside. I was sitting in front of an open kitchen window when a great gust of wind came blasting past me and down into the hallway to the room where she planned to give birth. Just as people quickly ran back outside to close car windows, I heard someone shout, "Watch that fire, it might catch the cars!" The wind was so powerful that the big drops of rain could not extinguish it. Upon entering her bedroom to catch the flailing curtains and close the open windows, I could see the fire outside dancing in the wind. The wind was so strong I couldn't even leave the windows open a slight crack. I closed them completely as people jumped in their cars and took off for the refuge of their homes.

In the middle of the chaos, Tewakierakwa was feeling uncomfortable with contractions, so I sent her into a warm shower with just a night-light on in the washroom to promote her relaxation. A while later, after calm was restored to the household, she came out and settled into her bed. She was in active labor and soon began to push. It was a lovely scene. The woman's mother was beside me, waiting to receive the baby in a new deerskin. The room was darkened and we kept quiet. During an especially hard contraction, Tewakierakwa grasped a small turtle shell rattle of the kind used in the seed blessing rite of the Tonwisas Society of our Mohawk longhouse. With each swell of the heavy contractions, she shook the small turtle shell rattle grasped in her hand. The gourd rattle or small turtle rattle that is used in the germinal rite of the march of the women planters in the spring finds symbolic significance in women's ovaries, fluid, and rain necessary for growth and ritual performance. The privileged cultural knowledge and ritual praxis of the Tonwisas Society is part of a larger constellation of procreative practices of our longhouse women, tied to the maintenance of the gardens and the matrilineal group. Entering through the logic of ceremonial practice, the seed itself is singing to the singer of the song in a dance of reciprocal consciousness, complexly interwoven in indigenous concepts of reproductive power. The root language of the expressions within the song evokes seeds of consciousness pertaining to fertility, procreation and the *orenda*, or sacred power, of women. Here, Tewakierakwa applied her experience of ritual performativity to call her baby to its birth.

Upon my day one postpartum visit, I found Tewakierakwa in a state of euphoria. After she had given birth to a healthy boy, she had fallen asleep and had a compelling dream. Elated, she told me: "I had forgotten what I had experienced in the intensity of my birth, but when I fell asleep everything came back to me in a dream. Do you remember when you sent me into the shower? I was standing in that shower having a hard time, thinking, *I can't do this*. Standing there, I remembered that when I was only a couple of months pregnant I went to a seer. I was told my baby was going to be born in a thunderstorm. Everyone waited so long for me to actually go into labor that I kept thinking, *When is this thunderstorm going to come?* In the shower, I began to feel the whole house shaking. I thought, maybe it was my husband and brother-in-law shaking the house to make me think there's a thunderstorm so I'll go into labor. Then I realized that you couldn't shake a house that easy. It occurred to me that when the False Faces come into your home after mid-winter ceremony, they come in with their big turtle shell rattles, pounding the floor and dancing, and the whole house shakes. For a minute, I thought it must be them, the grandfathers. Then just when I thought I couldn't do this anymore, I turned in my shower. Standing there, I saw my Uncle Moises face. He was standing in a field of green grass against a blue sky with white puffy clouds. There was a light around his eyes and forehead. He spoke to me in Mohawk, encouraging me and giving me the strength I needed to know that I could do this. Just then I felt my baby move down through my bones. When I came out of the bathroom in my dream, I walked into my bedroom and saw a wall of fire burning outside where our tobacco fire had been. The wind picked the fire up out of the earth. It was very powerful. When I was in my bed pushing my baby out, do you remember that moment when I yelled?"

I remembered her yell. It rose from her depths as she lifted her buttocks off the bed letting loose energy from her throat like the great gust of wind that had blown through the window the night before. She continued: "When my breath left my mouth, it went out into the room. It circled the room and came back into me through my ear and went down into my body where my baby was. You know how they say when you die there's a light at the end of a tunnel? Well that's what I saw—a light at the end of a tunnel."

"That must have been my flashlight," I said. "A life before birth experience."

"You know how you can hear underwater when you're swimming?" she asked. "Well, that's what I heard. I could hear people talking like we were talking underwater. I could hear everything my baby heard, and I could see everything my baby saw. I felt a great peace. I knew my baby was OK. And when he was born, I was born!" She exclaimed excitedly, "I'm never going to be the same. For so long I have let the White man tell me who I am. I now know we can do this. I'm not going to go one more day without speaking my language. I'm not going to go one more day letting the White man define who I am . . . and who we are as a people."

When a birthing mother awakens to her personal power, when her mind, body and spirit converge in an elegant display of her personal *orenda*, or enspiritedness, this is the moment when life grasps hold of purpose.

The National Aboriginal Council of Midwives (NACM) was established under the umbrella of the Canadian Association of Midwives at the 8th Annual General Meeting, November 12-14, 2008. NACM exists to restore birth to our communities and to the core of our healing path from intergenerational trauma. Our primary objectives are to preserve, develop and share Aboriginal midwifery knowledge, education and practice by strengthening and amplifying the voice of Aboriginal midwifery. The ranks of Aboriginal midwifery in the Canadian provinces are steadily growing, nourished by provincial and federal support of midwifery education models. With increased organizational and leadership support, pathways to midwifery practice are increasing. In 2003 a cross-border partnership was established under a Memorandum of Understanding (MOU) and was signed by Canadian Minister of Health, A. Anne McLellan, and Secretary of the U.S. Department of Health and Human Services (DHHS), Tommy G. Thompson. The purpose of the MOU was to stimulate collaborative action on improving the health status of mothers and infants. Other such partnerships are gathering momentum. In May 2008, under this MOU, the Indian Health Service Maternal and Child Health Office and First Nations and Inuit Health Board brought together an Invitational Gathering of North American Indigenous Birthing and Midwifery in Rockville, Maryland. Unfortunately, there exists only a handful of American Indian Certified Nurse-Midwives currently in practice in the United States. Under the shadows of the overarching health care crisis—in particular, the maternity care crisis in both countries—there is a pressing need for Native American women to commit to restoring this vitally important piece to our community life and family realities so that we might once again be whole.

One of my deepest concerns is the trend towards the industrial production of babies and reproductive technologies that remove women from the mind-body-spirit continuum approach to childbearing that an earth-centric culture supports. Native American families continue to suffer the intergenerational effects of the "civilization regulations" era, with its associated movement towards detribalization and disintegration through the residential school era, relocation programs, and undermining of our languages, governance and spiritual traditions. The blow that paralyzed Native people was so brutal that nineteenth century Cuban prophet José Martí observed that it was going to take "mountains of love" for Native peoples to recover from it. I think that at the heart of this healing journey and recovery of our Nations is the continuous flow of life protected by the spirit of the mother and midwifery. Midwifery is itself a cultural intervention with great capacity to heal with its holistic and woman-centered approach. A new generation of Native American women must come forward to receive the call to midwifery. We continue to prepare the ground so that this is possible.

My current work is as Program Director for Woman in the First Environment Collaborative, an initiative that brings the voices of indigenous women into a growing visionary movement to connect the fields of environmental justice and reproductive justice. Its overarching goal is to promote Native American women's epistemologies—births, dreams and ceremonies—as key aspects in restoring reproductive health and well-being.

In my culture, an original sacred instruction is that *woman is the first environment*. In pregnancy, women's bodies sustain life. Their unborn see through the mother's eyes and hear through her ears. Everything the mother feels, the baby feels, too. At the breast of women, the generations are nourished. From the bodies of women flows the relationship of those generations both to society and to the natural world. My lifelong message is that, as the ancestors said, the Earth is our mother, and in this way, women are Earth.

The foundational idea of the First Environment Project is that society must consider the community-based and culturally-defined models in which the health of girls and women is protected at the same time that healthful cultural practices—which have long been the key to individual and community health—are maintained and restored. These concepts are vital when considering the socio-cultural risk in closing the gap in health disparities of American Indian and Alaska Native peoples. The restoration of culture-sustaining practitioners, such

as midwives and doulas, have always been included with strategies for the restoration of the holism of women's environment, in the protection of women's health
over their life span. Promoting Native women's epistemologies and ceremonies is
at the center of such health development. Women's bodies, minds and spirits are
indeed the doorways through which one must pass to enter into this world. For
example, by resourcing generative visionary epistemes of the Mohawk Creation
Story (*Tsie tsi tsie koia tehn ah tsi karon iateh—She Who Fell From the Sky*) and
Thanksgiving Address (*Ohenton Kariwah:tekwen—The Words that Come Before
All Else*), the First Environment Project aims to prepare a new generation of girls
and women to think critically in making choices about the realities of their lives.

Putting my clearest thoughts, sincerest prayers and greatest hopes together
for future generations of mothers and midwives; acknowledging the grandmothers among us—past, present and future; greeting sister midwives throughout the
world with my fondest and highest regards; I throw down the tobacco into which
I place these words into the fireplace of the generations so that our generations
may continue. *Neh toh.*

The connection between this world and another

IDA DARRAGH

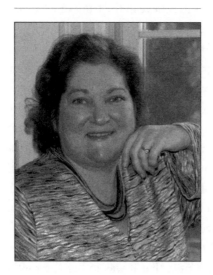

I have spent all of my life in Little Rock, Arkansas, one of the few urban areas in a very rural state. I was born in a hospital in 1948, just about the time that all the community midwives who had been issued permits during the previous thirty years were sent thank you letters with instructions to retire immediately. My parents were among the many urban families who considered the move to Little Rock to be a form of escape from the poverty of the small towns where they grew up. They placed a great deal of stock in the notion that money could buy better things, including medical care. A hospital birth for their children was something they were proud to afford, unlike the home births that they and their siblings had—not by choice but by necessity. My mother did breastfeed both of her children—something that was still encouraged in those days.

Growing up in the biggest city in a small state provided a perspective on life that was both small-town and urban. Our town was too big to know everyone in town, but small enough that anything you did was bound to get back to your parents. We had two high schools by the time I was that age, with lots of accompanying rivalry and school spirit. My interests were not really with the school crowd, though. I spent one summer as a candy striper at the medical school hospital, an experience that cured me of an interest in medicine or nursing. I ventured instead into the community theater, developing a love of performing that later translated into teaching childbirth education. Teaching always seemed to be a lot like performing—the audience needs to believe in the truth of what you say.

My interest in theater led me to join a performing group sponsored by a local church. We composed and sang "Life of Christ in Folksong," traveling on weekends during the school year, and around the world in the summers for seven years. I was no singer, but I contributed as a speaker in the program and as a treasurer in the organization. I spent my high school years with this group, and went to a local university in order to remain in town to continue to participate. The most important thing I learned during those years was the value of relationships and the work that it takes to sustain them. I met my husband during those years and formed friendships that still hold a place in my life forty years later. I learned a sense of what it means to "be in it for the long run," which pretty much characterizes the relationships that followed me throughout the next four decades.

After marriage, I tried several jobs. I was looking for my real calling in life, only to find, four years later, that it was in being a mother. I never expected to take to motherhood the way I did; I had always assumed I would be a professional something. The powerful impact of birth and the profound relationships of mother, child, and family, became the focus of my entire being for another thirty years.

First and foremost, my children were the major influence in my path to becoming a midwife. Before giving birth, I had never even remotely thought about midwifery. Their births, and my relationship with them as babies, were life-changing experiences for me, and I knew immediately that I would be involved with birth in a significant way.

During my first pregnancy, I knew neither midwives nor any women who had given birth at home, so we prepared for a hospital birth. I had taken childbirth classes almost reluctantly, more out of fear than a desire for natural birth.

My childbirth educator, Beth Cravens, imparted a sense of peace and calm about anticipating birth (as well as a bag of tools, including focal points, tennis balls, and socks), and we found ourselves in the hospital four weeks early—in labor—with a charge nurse who had the authority to "allow" or "not allow" fathers in the labor room. That night she did "not allow." When my physician arrived, I told him that my husband and I had taken Lamaze classes and hoped to be together for labor. Since that wasn't currently allowed, my doc rolled my bed out of labor and delivery (L & D) and onto the labor floor where we could labor together in a private room. That turned out to be an unanticipated critical event, for we were alone for hours without the constant interruption (and intervention) of hospital procedures. There was no choice but to use what we had learned about breathing and relaxation to get through the labor. Of course, there were several times when I thought I couldn't do it, and if we had been in L & D I probably would have agreed to the epidural in a moment of vulnerability. But those moments passed without the offer of meds, and I found that I could, indeed, work "with" the pain. My doc checked on us periodically, and when I was completely dilated we went to the delivery room, leaving my husband, Kramer, out in the hall since he wasn't "allowed" in delivery. That was a disappointment, but it was overshadowed by the intensity of the birth. I pushed out my firstborn, and when I held him and looked into his newborn eyes, my life changed forever. I have never felt a deeper emotion than that first look into my children's eyes as they came from the womb and were cradled in my arms. Within a week of that birth, we were back in childbirth class to tell the story of the most magnificent experience in the world. A month later, I was volunteering to help with the monthly film showings and talk-backs. A year later, I was training to be a childbirth educator. This became my new vocation and calling. I joined a group of four childbirth educators—which grew to twelve in the next few years—to help other women prepare for the experience and to change the hospital policies that interfered with the natural flow of birthing energy. I taught classes for many years, benefiting from the invitation to accompany many women and their partners through their birth experience.

My second child was born four years later. By then, I was a true activist having demanded to labor and birth in the same room without routine hospital procedures. My doc, again as supportive as he had been with the first, came in quietly to stand in the corner as I lifted my first daughter from my womb into my arms, with my husband rubbing the top of my head as he didn't know what else to do at the moment! That birth taught me how powerful birth can be without interventions and interference. I had still only seen hospital births, but I was learning to make it an intensely personal and private experience. Our third child, born almost two years later, again taught me how little we are in control of the whole thing but how unique and powerful the experience can be. She was breech throughout the pregnancy. We did the tilt-boards and pelvic rocks to no avail. She stayed breech. My doc, an older experienced OB, was willing to deliver a breech birth for a multip (a woman who has already given birth), but the younger doc in the practice said it would be a cesarean section if he were on call. I sought out older docs from other practices who would agree to help if my own doc wasn't available. Fortunately, that wasn't necessary. Her birth was the easiest of all three, though the minute from the birth of the body to the birth of the head seemed to take a lifetime. Her little feet rose up by her ears for a week, mimicking her fetal position, as we waited for her body to resume a more newborn posture!

I've used this opportunity to tell my birth stories, but they are each such important parts of who and what led me to midwifery. All were hospital births, but all were very unique and powerful in my understanding of birth.

It was about a year later that I met the woman who had the most direct influence on my path to midwifery. There was a couple in my childbirth class who were planning a home birth with a midwife. All participants in my classes had planned hospital births, so I was surprised that there were any home births in the community. I had known Sheila and Joe years ago in college, but we had lost touch until she showed up in class. I was really interested in what was going on with her that she would be thinking about a home birth, and wanted to know more about her plans. She invited me to meet her midwife and to attend her home birth. Their midwife was Mary Alexander. Mary had her own baby at home about twelve years earlier and in another state where she could not find a midwife but where she did find a friend who had had a home birth. Mary had her baby at home with a small group of friends, none of whom was a midwife. After that, other women called her to come to their births as a friend. She began to read and study about birth and continued to go when called. By the time she came back to Arkansas, she had been to fifty or more home births and continued to go when invited. By the time we met, she had been to close to a hundred births and was beginning to call herself a midwife. She had evolved into this profession as a friend and helper, and had not really thought much about record-keeping and childbirth classes and such. My route had been through credentialing as a certified childbirth educator, complete with syllabus and extreme paperwork, and I had a notebook listing of every client, their class dates, their birth dates, their baby's name and weight, and all my interaction prenatally, intrapartum, and postpartum! Mary and I came to birth from opposite ends of the spectrum, and yet our knowledge and experience complemented each other's and our personalities meshed well. I attended Sheila's home birth as an observer and helper and began a lifelong relationship with Mary. Sheila's first birth was my first home birth to attend, and then I began assisting Mary at other births. Sheila's second home birth two years later was my first catch. I still stay in touch with Sheila through a local women's group, and both of her daughters are now grown and out of college.

I continued to teach hospital classes because there was such a need, but my heart was growing towards home birth as I began to work with Mary. I worked to organize the home birth classes and our birth charts, and Mary began to teach me about midwifery. We taught classes together, did prenatals together, and went to births together. In 1983, we created a practice called "Birth Works." We met together with other midwives in the state for discussions.

One of the midwives in our state had opened a birthing center in her community that attracted the attention of the local physicians, some of whom objected to the number of clients who were coming to see her. Soon, a complaint was filed, and she was issued a cease and desist order to close her birth center and stop practicing medicine. She obtained the support of a local attorney whose uncle was a prominent legislator, and so the first effort toward licensure began. Mary and I lived in the capital city, so we were naturally drawn into the lobbying effort. There were several other midwives working on the issue, both for and against, and that legislative year also taught us about the conflict that grows among strong-willed women who disagree on the best way to get things done. It was a stressful year, but we eventually put aside most of the conflict and worked together for a licensure bill. The medical opposition to the licensure of direct-entry midwives was strong even then, and our bill was eventually gutted so that licensure would be available, but only to midwives in counties with at least 33% of their population living below the poverty level. This was an introduction to politics: midwifery could be legal, but only for poor people. And it was not enough to be poor; you also had to live in a poor county. So, even though our county had higher numbers of people living below the poverty level, the percentage was not high enough. Midwives could only be licensed in six counties in the southeast part of the state. The Health Department was assigned the task of overseeing the licensure program, and Mary and I were on the committee to write the rules and regulations. An entire book could be written about that experience alone.

By that time, four other states had licensure for direct-entry midwives (South Carolina, Arizona, New Mexico, and Washington), but we had no Internet back then and no way of knowing what was going on in other states. We were learning midwifery and grassroots politics by the seat of our pants. My early years as a midwife were inextricably entwined with the political issues—which would come to be a big part of my life's work, though I didn't know it then.

Even though I did not live in one of the six poorest counties of the state, I applied for the license, passed the test, and received the first license in the state. That piece of paper said I could practice in six counties about two hundred miles from where I lived. But, I did have a license! The next year, when the license expired, I was told it could not be renewed because I did not live in one of those counties.

About that time, two midwives in another part of the state had a precautionary hospital transport for an unborn baby with slightly irregular heart tones. Mother and baby were fine at delivery, but the local obstetrician was very annoyed at having to attend this birth. He had turned the mother away early in her pregnancy because she did not have insurance or the total fee up-front. So, the mother had gone to the local midwives. Because the midwives decided to transport, the doctor ended up taking care of this uninsured woman anyway. He filed a complaint with the local prosecuting attorney. These midwives did not live or practice in the six poor, legal counties so they did not have a license. That case went to trial, and Mary and I, along with most of the state's midwives, attended the trial. I had always believed in my heart of hearts that if the average person really had a chance to understand midwifery they would surely be supportive. This was another one of those turning points in my development as a midwife. Eleven people on that jury thought that catching babies was the practice of medicine. Only one person held out for acquittal at the end of the two-day trial. Fortunately, she held her ground and the judge declared a hung jury. The state had one year to re-try the case. We went back to the legislature that year and lobbied successfully to have licensure expanded to cover the entire state. Now we were legal and highly regulated.

I continued to teach classes for hospital birthers for many years after becoming a midwife, primarily because there was such a need in the community but also because I loved teaching. As a midwife, I also taught classes for home birthers, eventually dropping out of the hospital venue altogether. Many years later, I organized a non-profit called Arkansas Childbirth Institute, which sponsored classes for both home and hospital births, as well as doula and midwifery training.

I had done other work before becoming a childbirth educator and midwife, from cocktail waitress to psychological examiner, but combining the intellectual aspects of teaching with the spiritual aspects of nurturing and birthing seemed to suit my particular talents as well as allowing a strong commitment to family priorities. I did not want a career that kept me away from the family all day, every day, but I enjoyed the sporadic and intense nature of being called away to births. The support of my husband and children, and the help from other family members and neighborhood carpool mothers, seemed essential to making it all work. But, I also saw my friend Mary manage single parenting, midwifing, and sometimes second jobs to make it all work. All the midwives I ever met were remarkable in their ability to juggle multiple tasks, take care of their families, and meet the needs of their clients. That's not to say there weren't times of melt-down and burnout for all of us; but somewhere deep inside was a strong sense of the importance of what we were doing, and a sense of being privy to witness life's most extraordinary passage.

At the moment of birth, there is a rare and brief glimpse of the connection between this world and another, of before and after, of mortal and immortal, of spiritual and physical, of known and unknown. That brief glimpse happens at the moment of death, too, but is much more visible at birth, and infused with joy rather than clouded with grief. We make those passages ourselves only twice. As midwives, we stand in awe each and every time we are invited to witness that intimate journey taken by another. It is said that when midwives retire, they sometimes become hospice workers because "midwifing" happens at that end, too. I have had very limited experience on that end, but it makes sense. We are drawn to the work of birthing because it speaks to something inside of us. This is the part that is the "calling" that so many midwives use to describe how they got into this work. It's a feeling that we were meant to do this; it's beyond what we can be taught or what we can learn, it's something that we are. The learning part is important, too, but it builds from a place where we know we must do this— we just cannot turn away from it. I think that is why the apprenticeship model works so well for midwives. We can learn from someone, but they can't teach us. Looking at that statement, it seems a strange one for an educator to make. But, it's true. Nobody can teach you to be a midwife; you have to learn it. We can learn it from teachers, whether they know they are teaching or not. We might learn more from one teacher than another. We learn from every birth, no matter how many births we have been to. If we stop learning, we've stopped listening to the birth.

Midwives often say they don't want to get involved in politics; they just want to go to births. They say that, usually, when they find themselves in the middle of the politics. I can hardly remember a time when politics didn't go hand-in-hand with midwifery. Maybe that's because I got licensed so early in my career as a midwife, and licensure keeps the politics in sight all the time. There were "Rules and Regs" meetings and Advisory Board meetings, and state association meetings, and eventually Midwives Alliance of North America (MANA) conferences, which were part educational sessions, part networking, and part politics. Because of my work with state licensure, I joined the Legislative Committee at a MANA conference in 1986 and shared with the committee the notes that we had made on getting legislation passed in Arkansas. Computers were just beginning to become household items (does anyone remember the DOS operating system and 8-pin dot-matrix printers?), but there was no Internet. We made occasional conference calls, mailed packets of information around, and tried to meet every year at the MANA conference. I was only able to attend every two to three years, so my contributions were limited. Licensure for direct-entry midwives was still very controversial, but we could see it coming. Seven states had licensure by 1986, but investigations and cease and desist orders seemed to be increasing, and we weren't winning many of those battles. Midwives didn't seem to mind working underground, but no one relished the idea of being the poster child for illegal midwifery. The extreme cost, both financially and emotionally, of defending oneself against charges of practicing medicine without a license, was not an easy burden to bear. We saw the toll it took on our sisters, and we saw the effect it was having on the number of midwives willing to stay in practice. We needed to find better solutions.

The Midwives Alliance of North America held regional task force meetings across the country to discuss the development of a direct-entry midwifery credential. The leaders of MANA and ACNM (American College of Nurse-Midwives) met as the Inter-Organizational Workgroup in 1991 to discuss midwifery core competencies and to find common ground in our divergent backgrounds. I read about these events in the *MANA News* while participating at home as chair of the state Midwives Advisory Board. At that time, still without the Internet, state midwifery organizations mailed their newsletters to each other. As newsletter editor for the Arkansas Association of Midwives, I relished reading news from many state midwifery organizations. The politics of midwifery, while being the polar opposite of attending births, was also exciting and challenging. We sensed that change was going to happen, and we could either get involved and have a say in what those changes would be or withdraw from it and see what would be done about that pesky "midwife problem."

MANA had created the Interim Registry Board (IRB) to develop an exam to measure midwifery knowledge. The idea was that midwives could voluntarily take the exam, and those who passed would be listed on a Registry. Being listed on the Registry would prove that a midwife had attained significant midwifery knowledge. The Interim Registry Board would be a first step in proving that we neither posed any danger to the public nor needed to be "managed" by the medical system or the judicial system. Later, the IRB became the North American Registry of Midwives (NARM) and, with the advice of testing consultants, developed and administered the first NARM exam in 1991. NARM was looking for midwives to take the test who were already credentialed or who had already passed a state midwifery exam. Several other midwives and I, who had taken the Arkansas midwifery exam (an absurd document written by health department nurses from maternity nursing textbooks), volunteered to take the exam administered by the North American Registry of Midwives. We who passed were listed on the national Registry.

The next few years were filled with raising children, going to births, and working at the local level on our licensing program. We adopted the NARM exam as our state licensure exam. Although the NARM exam was a much longer and harder exam than our state exam, it was much more relevant to midwifery practice. NARM had also added an experience component that documented attainment of skills learned through apprenticeship, as well as supervised clinical experience, which would lead to a credential called the Certified Professional Midwife (CPM). The midwives who had already passed the written exam could document their extensive experience and receive this credential. Three of us who were licensed in Arkansas and who had passed the NARM exam applied for and received the CPM credential in 1995. Since we were already licensed, the credential was not required for us, but we believed strongly that this was an important step in the support of the profession of midwifery nationwide.

Mary and I continued to work together in our practice, Birth Works, training a few apprentices, some of whom continued to work with us or in other parts of the state. We were both members of MANA and CPMs through NARM, and we felt a commitment to the goals of these two organizations. In the summer of 1997 the CPM newsletter solicited volunteers to join the NARM board. Mary suggested that I apply. It took a bit of urging, but I eventually let her put my name forward. She may have regretted this later, as it turned out to be a pivotal change in the direction of my energies! The first step in my application was a phone interview with the NARM Board. Still being awfully provincial (and not yet with daughters living in other time zones), I misunderstood the time of the call and was not home when they called! I came in forty-five minutes later, thinking I had fifteen minutes before the call, only to find out that I had missed it. They were on my answering machine, wondering why I wasn't there. Not a good beginning, but a huge step forward in my education. I called back to make amends and was given another chance. After the phone interview, I had an in-person interview at the 1997 MANA conference in Seattle. At that interview, I learned that each NARM board member had a specific job in the running of the program. The woman who had been answering the toll-free phone line was leaving the board shortly to move to another country, so someone was needed to take her place. By the time the MANA conference was over, I was accepted as a member of the board and would be taking over the incoming phone calls. Wow. My first job with NARM would be to answer questions! Being a talker, I was excited about the task, but being new on the board I wasn't sure I would know any answers!

The first thing I learned about the NARM board was that we all work together to make things work. I joined an incredible group of women who were making things happen: Ruth Walsh, Sharon Wells, Alice Sammon, Shannon Anton, Pam Weaver, Sharon Evans, Carol Nelson, Robbie Davis-Floyd, and Debbie Pulley. Some were on the NARM board already, and some were MANA committee chairs who worked closely with NARM and would join the NARM board in the next few years. All were very dedicated women who were committed to the future of midwifery and to the role of the CPM credential in that future. It was a steep learning curve to join these women, and I spent countless hours on the phone with Sharon Wells learning what I needed to know to answer the 1-800-line. We had (and still have) a weekly conference call for three hours on Friday morning to discuss the work of each board member and to make the decisions that keep NARM functioning. All of these women work as volunteers, with heavy personal responsibilities as midwives, mothers, wives, and community leaders, to carry the workload to keep NARM going. At one time, NARM had hired a company to manage the applications and testing duties, but it soon became apparent that only midwives could really understand the process that is involved in becoming a midwife. NARM board members have taken on those responsibilities, relying on a professional testing consultant only for certain aspects of scoring and evaluation of the exam.

After a year as the phone person, I relinquished those duties to Debbie Pulley and took the helm as Director of Testing, replacing the irreplaceable Alice Sammon as she left the board to pursue midwifery in the northeast. After surviving prosecution in New York, Alice moved to Maine where the climate may be colder in temperature but is warmer to midwifery. As Director of Testing, I became an apprentice to NARM's testing vendor, Jerry Rosen, who oversees the development of our exams and the statistical evaluation of our test scores.

In college, I had taken courses in educational psychology and statistics, never knowing how those courses would influence my future work with NARM. I learned the role of psychometrics (psycho = mind, metrics = measurement) in testing. I loved learning how each test question performed on the NARM exam; how many respondents chose each answer and whether those who chose each answer passed or failed the exam; how to write effective test questions; and how to set the passing score. This work merged with my undergraduate degree in psychology, with my universal education in midwifery, and with my belief that we can measure what midwives need to know. I believe we can maintain control over the criteria state legislatures want to set regarding who can be a licensed midwife or a CPM.

In my role as NARM's Director of Testing, I have overseen the application and maintenance of our accreditation with the National Commission of Certifying Agencies (NCCA). We achieved that accreditation in 2002, after an extensive application process that involved writing and rewriting many policies and procedures to document that we met the standards for accreditation. Though we *did* meet these standards, our accreditation hinged on documenting *how* we met the standards. Getting NCCA accreditation was not difficult once we put into writing precisely what we were doing. Ironically, I realized that this is exactly the same process that we require of the CPM candidates—to document how they meet established standards.

In 2003, Ruth Walsh left the position of Chair of the NARM Board of Directors to follow her career with West Virginia University, and I assumed the duties as Chair of the Board. The NARM board works as a cohesive unit with all members contributing to the leadership. My role is to facilitate the weekly board calls and the twice-yearly board meetings. I do this with great delight, as all members of the board are a joy to work with. We have had some changes in board membership over the past few years, with some leaving and some joining. Working on the board is not everyone's cup of tea, so we hope to nurture those who find their calling with NARM and to graciously excuse those who need to move on for personal or professional reasons. My role, both before and after becoming the board's chair, has increased to include teaching workshops and speaking on behalf of NARM to legislators and legislative committees. Our most significant workshop, "Preparing for Legislation," was based on the experience of the prime leaders in recent successful (and unsuccessful, but progressive) state legislative efforts. It is offered in collaboration with the MANA Legislative Chair and the entire NARM board. The workshop has been presented in every state that is seeking (or recently obtained) licensure or legal status for direct-entry midwives. As of 2010, that number stands at twenty-six states, and we hope to see many more added in upcoming years. Our goal is to promote midwifery as a viable and effective maternity care option for all states. We hope the CPM will contribute to that effort.

My role has changed in the past few years. I am no longer in private practice, having been replaced by competent and caring midwives who work with Mary. I stay involved with the state organization and with the state-licensing agency. I travel a lot with NARM, presenting workshops or speaking on behalf of the CPM credential, and I coordinate the work of the NARM Test Department. The Internet has become a huge element in our communication, and I am on what seems to be hundreds of lists, national, international, and state-based, for discussion of midwifery practice or state political work. I speak regularly about midwifery and the CPM credential and continue to work with state groups who are seeking licensure.

I truly believe that if we keep the licensure mechanism based on direct-entry midwifery, and if we keep the national credential as a respected and accredited credential, we will attain legal status in all states for direct-entry midwives. We hope the legal status will be based on the CPM credential because the CPM credential was created and is maintained by and for direct-entry midwives. It is my pleasure to work with so many dynamic and soulful sisters (and brothers) in this process.

In my travels for NARM, I have been pleased to see many young women interested in becoming midwives and many of the older, experienced midwives taking apprentices. As midwives, it is our responsibility to see that our knowledge and our "midwives' model of care" are passed down to the next generation. It is also our responsibility to see that midwifery is legal and economically viable for the next generation. To keep this flame alive, more people need to know about midwifery. Even women who are not choosing midwifery care should know about it. Women who are past the childbearing years should know about it. Men who never gave much thought to childbirth options should know about it. Midwifery care should be available in homes, birth centers, and hospitals. Midwives should be able to attain their education through apprenticeship, midwifery schools, and universities. It's going to take cooperation and mutual respect among all midwives, and between midwives and other healthcare providers for families to have the best possible care. We have been working on this for a long time, and we still have a long way to go. We can do it.

We were a survival experiment and we survived

INA MAY GASKIN

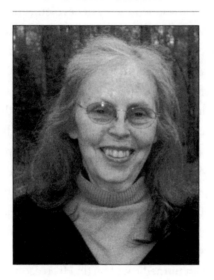

I didn't know what a midwife was until I went to my grandmother's house in rural Iowa and saw a duck casserole dish. The bottom part of the dish was an oval nest and the duck sat on the nest full of eggs, so you would lift off the duck and you've got a casserole dish. It had been given to my great-grandmother, who had been the local midwife, for helping at a birth. There are family stories about my great-grandmother going out into the Iowa winter and sometimes not coming back for ten days or two weeks because the mother needed rest and care before she could safely take up her usual household responsibilities again. Knowing what Iowa winters can be like, I'm sure that the snow sometimes made it hard for her to travel home in her buggy or sleigh after a birth.

Another trickle of my knowledge of midwives came through eighteenth or nineteenth century novels that I read while working on my Bachelor's Degree in English at the University of Iowa. From these novels I learned that a forceps delivery was something to avoid if possible. And then apart from my reading, I think I remember every birth story I was ever told. As a sixteen-year-old, I read Grantly Dick-Read's *Childbirth Without Fear* and asked my mother if childbirth was something to be afraid of. She said "No" and added that a lot of people would scream but that it really wasn't necessary, leaving me with the impression I could do it, that it was nothing to worry about and that my body was capable. She didn't say all of those words, she was just reassuring. I remember leaving the church with my mother and her making sure that I was introduced to the doctor who had attended my birth. He seemed totally benevolent, and from him I formed an idea of what a doctor was. I imagined that all doctors must be like him.

Two visiting nurses who lived next door provided my mother with enough practical in-home health care and education to get my three siblings and me through childhood without need for hospital care or visits to a doctor—other than a tonsillectomy for my brother. Growing up with those two women next door gave me the idea of the benefits and conveniences that ensue when people in the neighborhood can and will take care of you when you are ill or injured.

My first birth provided me with a powerful experience in how women should *not* be treated during pregnancy and birth. My obstetrician (I had taken a friend's advice to hire an obstetrician rather than a family doctor) prescribed diuretics for me during pregnancy to keep me from gaining more than 12 pounds, and then he made sure that I had a mandatory forceps delivery, even though I had already told him that I wanted an unmedicated birth. His reasoning was that he believed in the DeLee "prophylactic forceps delivery," which called for spinal anesthesia, a big episiotomy, and forceps for every first baby in order to protect the baby from brain damage due to the battering on the "iron-hard perineum." This sounded like nonsense to me, but I had no idea then how to deal with a doctor who seemed to have no common sense. I decided to follow my usual strategy for getting my way by quietly doing my thing and not attracting attention to myself in order to avoid the anesthesia. I did actually have many hours of labor without medication. I know now that I did really well, but when I was almost fully dilated, they ganged up on me and pulled my daughter out with forceps. They didn't show me my daughter before rushing her off to the nursery, and I was warned that I had to keep my head down for at least 12 hours to avoid a spinal headache. When they finally brought her to me, I didn't feel the emotions of joy and relief that I thought I'd feel. I felt some guilt for my lack of an appropriate emotional response to my new baby. I recognize now that what I had was a kind of post-traumatic stress disorder. We didn't use terms like that back then, but I knew that what had happened to me wasn't right. During the five days in hospital, we were allowed to be together for only three or four hours. She was in the nursery the rest of the time, even though she was perfectly healthy. After that experience, I was sure of one thing: there had to be a better way to have a baby.

We moved to San Francisco in the summer of 1967, where I began hearing home birth stories. So many of the women who told me their birth stories had had similar experiences to mine, but they found the inner strength to devise a better way—even though there were no midwives attending home births in those days. The typical home birth story was that the mother was assisted by a labor and delivery nurse acting as a midwife. If the mother developed a complication that required medical attention, the nurse would recognize it and take her to the hospital. Each of these birth stories impressed me greatly, and I knew that I wanted a home birth if I became pregnant again. I also knew that I wanted to be a midwife someday. I was called to be a midwife, and I chose it, but at that time I didn't know that there was any training available.

While living in San Francisco in the late 1960s, I witnessed a whole cultural movement sweeping the world, the "love generation," the Beatles, all of it. Hippies have come in for a lot of mockery over the years since then, but I have to say that we were right about many things, including environmentalism, making bonds with indigenous people, learning from them, and giving respect to those peoples, finding nonviolent ways to solve problems, the superiority of organic food, the safety of being a vegetarian, and about living more closely aligned with nature. We were also right about childbirth and breastfeeding. Nobody has any idea how many women and couples rebelled, how many either didn't go into the hospital or went into the hospital under their own terms between 1968 and 1971. One couple had a big impact on hospital birth in San Francisco. The hospital absolutely refused to let the baby's father be present at the birth, so when labor began, the couple went in handcuffed together. That birth ended the policy of keeping fathers out of the maternity ward. Meanwhile, home birth stories spread like wildfire, and the word got out that some hospitals even had nurse-midwives working in them. Almost overnight, it seemed, their roles were enlarged, as hospitals began to change their policies as a way of continuing to attract women to give birth there. So women started telling their home birth stories, and the word got out that there were people emerging who were now being called midwives and that some of them actually had training as nurses. There were nurse-midwives at some of the hospitals in San Francisco who now saw that they didn't have to fight to attend births; they were being *invited*. And they were being hired by hospital after hospital because the physicians weren't as present. Women assumed that when they hired a doctor to attend a birth that they would actually see him more than just for the last five minutes. They were confused by the fact that he would just be there for the time the baby came out and that the rest of the time they were under the care of the nurses.

Those first really brave couples opened the doors for midwives to start working in hospitals. Those were the halcyon years, when hospitals listened to midwives and put locks on the doors so that the mother's privacy could be insured. They didn't want to risk people bursting into the room because they knew that that type of curiosity and lack of privacy could negatively affect the process of labor. We knew things then that have been lost along the way. For a while that was the heyday of hospital midwifery. It was a time when midwifery schools were being established—and we got up to where we had fifty—which was an average of one per state, although not every state had one. Now we are down below forty nurse-midwifery programs, and that's a sad thing because I want to see the day when we have more midwives than we have obstetricians. That's not to put down obstetricians; it's just to recognize the nature of birth. The best demographic for mothers and babies is the one that has been proven over many years and in many different countries—the demographic of midwives outnumbering obstetricians. Since birth is a physiological process and not pathology, I'd like to see that ratio be about 7 to 1. Then you don't have as many surgical births for low-risk women, but you are able to have surgical births when you need them. And those physicians should be well distributed so that they are able to give expert obstetrical care, whether they are obstetricians or family physicians trained in obstetrics. Hopefully there is a growing number of these people, but most family physicians don't provide obstetrical care anymore. It was once a requirement that they had to have the skills, whether or not they used them.

I finally had my first chance to observe a birth in the fall of 1970, when I was one of nearly 300 people traveling in a caravan of school buses and vans converted into campers on a five-month lecture tour of forty-two cities with my husband, Stephen Gaskin. Stephen had been persuaded to make the tour by a group of clergymen who had heard him speak at a San Francisco conference about the phenomenon of the hippie culture that was spreading across the country in 1970. Stephen was about to give a lecture at the university when there was a knock on the door. A fellow traveler—who was pregnant and determined not to give birth in a hospital—was in labor. Her husband wanted to know if Stephen could help his laboring wife. Because Stephen was the leader of the caravan and a veteran of the Korean War, the husband figured that he would have the courage and knowledge to get them through the birth. I, who had had my first child four years earlier, knew something about how women shouldn't be treated in childbirth. It was my dream to become a midwife. But at that time I didn't know of a way to get the necessary training. I thought that a good beginning might be to at least see a birth (something I had never seen before, not so much as a photo or drawing of birth). Seeing that the laboring woman's husband was satisfied with my offer to come, I grabbed my friend Pamela Hunt, and together we went to the school bus where the woman was laboring. We simply gave the woman love and respect and, in turn, were lucky enough to witness a perfect birth.

We were all lucky that the woman's birth happened quickly and perfectly, making this the best possible birth for a first experience. And that is really profound, because you would have a really hard time finding a medical student or a doctor alive today in this country who has witnessed a beautiful birth for their first time. I think more often they see something that is really bloody and really frightening, and it marks them in a certain and different way that I was not marked. Altogether, eleven babies were born while we were traveling, most of them first babies. Along the way, a friendly obstetrician gave me a quick course in emergency childbirth, an obstetrics textbook and some medical supplies. The eleven births during the caravan period gave all the women of our group a great and growing confidence in their ability to give birth with the care of a midwife.

In 1971 our group bought 1000 acres in southern middle Tennessee, and soon after that we bought the adjoining 750 acres. We continued living in the school buses and campers we had arrived in but then began to move into larger quarters—tents left over from the Korean War, warmed in winter only with woodstoves. We faced multiple challenges. We had to keep from pissing off the neighbors; we had to deal with all of our pregnant women and new babies; and we had to learn how not to get sick. To say we were living in the "wilderness" may be going too far, but it wasn't as well set up as your average national park. There was certainly no outhouse waiting for us. And we didn't have camping sites, so we had to learn how to deal with all of these things simultaneously. But we were a survival experiment and we survived. Fortunately, we met a local family doctor who was not afraid of home births, having served an Old Order Amish community for the previous sixteen years. It was a matter of fantastically good luck that we settled ten miles away from his home. His help was invaluable. He taught us, as he put it, some "country medicine" that we would have to have in order to survive. He became my mentor after my first introduction to breech birth. I brought a woman into the hospital, recognizing that she had a breech presentation and because she labored so well, I was allowed to stay with her throughout her time in the delivery room. That was the first breech birth I witnessed. It was also the first episiotomy that I had seen because I hadn't been taught to take great big long cuts in the perineum. Now we have an interest among doctors in medical school—especially those in which midwives are a strong part of the faculty—in learning how to preserve the perineum. They used to think that the way to preserve the perineum was to cut it and then sew it; now there is a desire to do it differently. This all comes from contact with midwifery knowledge.

Thankfully, we were able to document these things. In building our community, which we called The Farm, people were free to choose the type of work that they wanted to do. Some were interested in organic food growing, some in teaching children, repairing vehicles, construction, and many other occupations. As soon as we could get a video camera that could be supported on the camera person's shoulder, we began to video births. Some members of our community went to medical school. Naturally, they told their stories of The Farm, and so it wasn't long before some of their professors began to invite me to speak to their Introduction to Medicine class, or to the Family Practice faculty, or to the obstetricians. I usually began these sessions by showing some of our statistics and videos of home births. Since there were virtually no such videos available in the early '70s, the viewing of home birth provided most of the students with their very first chance to witness a woman giving birth without damaging her perineum, without bleeding—a joyful and triumphant experience. These teaching experiences taught me how fortunate I'd been to learn in the way I had learned. I remember that once I was at a well-respected medical school, and one of the residents had just come in after the first so-called "catch." He had dropped the baby in the bucket because he hadn't been prepared for how slippery it would be. He was devastated. I thought that harsh incident must have really marked that person deeply (even though the baby was fine), but that it would have taken only a few seconds for his instructors to say to him, "The baby is going to be slippery . . . so be careful."

We midwives took a very strong part in the way our community was organized. We actually had the idea that if you make a community in which the mothers and the babies both flourish, then the men will flourish too, that it doesn't come at the expense of men. When I look back on it now, I think it's remarkable that a bunch of amateurs who had no prior training were able to get some training on the fly. I think that the most important thing that we accomplished was that we learned our bodies still work, and that we can take care of ourselves safely in a way that is intellectually, emotionally and spiritually satisfying. After I had witnessed three births, I was fortunate that an obstetrician gave me and two other women a seminar on prenatal care and common obstetric emergencies. He also equipped us with medications and tools, including syringes, hemostats and scissors, blood pressure cuffs, urine testing sticks, and that type of thing. He prepared us for what was to come, and with his help and that of an obstetric handbook that he also gave me, we got through 186 vaginal births before we needed to have the first c-section. No lives were lost as a result of our learning, so I think that was pretty good. The other thing we learned was that every mother could breastfeed. This was important because we had put ourselves into a situation where we were living in a forest with no running water, no electricity, and no cash.

I'm lucky to have been able to work in this community. From the beginning I have been able to pick out women who I thought would be great candidates as midwives, and they became my partners. Together we would choose from among several hundred other women, and we'd say "That one, she'd be a great midwife," and we would reach consensus and invite her in. We've had a long relationship, working together for three decades, so we really know each other well and we work well as a team. I think that is why we've been able to keep from suffering burnout; rather we've succeeded in continuing to build our experience and helping each other. That's why we've been able to attain such a low c-section rate because we didn't have to get so exhausted. We've been at this for a long time and we've seen a lot of changes. We've had a lot of relationships with different people in the medical field who have come to visit us, and many of our own community members have gone into medicine. So it has given us a view on midwifery and medicine and taught us how to communicate in a way that allows people to see birth in a different way. Whenever one of us learned something important about midwifery, she would share that with the others. I can remember certain births where I invented a technique, or other midwives may have used a technique that we'd never heard about, one that just occurred to us as necessary. Then, as we studied later in the library, we would find something that had been written more than a hundred years ago describing that technique despite the fact that it may not have been recognized as helpful in the modern day. I think midwifery was developed by people with common sense—people who were close to nature, who observed other species of mammals, and who saw that there were lessons there to be learned.

Some of my partners have been deep into the work of certification for midwives who received their training via apprenticeship, and we are solid in believing that that's possible. For a while there wasn't any sort of certification for the midwife who came in from outside the path of nursing and hospital education. We came out of a community context in which everybody educated themselves and educated one other in every field, and we midwives were just one sector. We had people who were suddenly learning how to be farmers and engineers, so that was something that our community was very familiar with. And you didn't feel inferior to anybody because you hadn't received university training. We knew farmers around here who could put an MIT engineering graduate to shame. A farmer who possessed, maybe, an eighth-grade education had the components of reality and experience under his belt. So we watched those things play out. Also in the community context, we visited and worked with many people in very poor countries, which gave us a bigger perspective. We realized that even though we were poor by American standards in terms of cash income, everybody in the country was way ahead of the people we saw in Guatemala, where many babies didn't live past their first year.

We also learned that people who are illiterate could be very wise and know things that people who are literate are very confused about. Guatemala is where I learned a technique that is now called the "Gaskin Maneuver," which is quite often a very easy solution to the shoulder dystocia delivery. I was fortunate enough to learn about it in 1976 from indigenous people, and since then we've never had an injury in the case of a shoulder dystocia. This complication means that the baby's shoulder is stuck behind the mother's pubic bone so that the birth process is impeded. The maneuver requires the laboring woman to be on all fours, which is interpreted by some as the knee-chest position. But it's not—it's "hands and knees," where the back is perhaps arched a bit, but the butt is not higher than the back. The maneuver opens the pelvis so that a baby who is stuck becomes dislodged just by the mother moving her body. In our experience it was just phenomenal how many babies we have seen born this way, where there was no injury to mother or baby. In contrast, it is commonplace for birth injuries to occur to mothers and babies when more invasive techniques for shoulder dystocia are used. So I've taken it as a challenge to teach that maneuver to the medical profession, and I've been working on it for twenty years. I've cooperated with two or three other physicians in the past and am looking to begin working with a professor of obstetrics as I expand his registry for people who have used the technique. It has been written up in two or three medical journals already and there will be more to come. There are still women having babies who are having treatments or maneuvers that are not so benign, all because of shoulder dystocia or fear of shoulder dystocia. This method is really pretty simple, and it has been around for a long time and developed by people who live in cultures where they are not so conditioned by the furniture.

I'm interested in midwifery education, medical education and health policy. I want to see 120,000 midwives practicing in the United States some day, and I want to see health care for everybody. I want to see an end to the malpractice crisis that does nothing but feed the wrong people without making medical care any safer. There has to be a system of compensation when there are errors, but hopefully we could create an atmosphere in which errors would be less frequent. We have to take the profit out of medicine. I want to see a day when we don't have medical advertising anymore. I'm working on these issues, and I'm also working on other issues like accountability, because these issues are so important. The fact is that both the infant mortality rate and the maternal mortality rate are rising in the United States. Both rates are much higher than they should be in a country that spends so much money on medical care. This is scandalous and should be a warning to the world as well as to us. I put in a lot of time now on the Safe Motherhood Quilt Project, which honors women who have died of pregnancy-related causes. This is a national effort to draw public attention to current maternal death rates and the gross underreporting of maternal deaths in the United States. The quilt is made up of individually designed squares; each one devoted to a woman who has died of pregnancy-related causes since 1982. We need to understand that it's difficult to accurately and completely count the number of maternal deaths that occur every year in any given country. But in the UK, the British have designed a system that is considered to be the gold standard in this area, and we ought to follow their lead and institute such a system here. We need to stop sweeping these deaths under the rug and learn by studying them how to prevent them.

I think that young folks who are thinking about going into midwifery should know that we're going to encounter some difficult years of transition until we get out of this for-profit system, and that the profession of midwifery is at risk. But I would also tell you to follow your dream. Don't be daunted by the challenges you see before you; seek out good mentors and don't give up. We can do this. You can't count on good luck, but you can certainly be grateful and recognize it when you have it.

Midwives are like a big family with many sisters

DIANE HOLZER

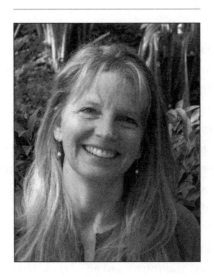

I was born into this world breech (butt first), and I have continued that trend by carving a life of doing things in my own particular way. I was born into a working class family in Detroit, and early on I learned lessons about inequality and racism. I spent my childhood years in the city where our family was one of only a few White families in an all-Black neighborhood. I was not allowed in the homes of my Black friends and they were not allowed in mine, so porches and the streets were our playgrounds. During the well-publicized riots in the 1960s, I remember playing with friends outside after curfew. We would dodge the National Guard tanks in the streets, hiding behind trees and laughing to somehow try to normalize the events that were occurring. During middle school my parents decided to move to the country, as was the fashion of the time, and so began my love affair with all things wild. I spent most of my time in trees and at the lake by our house. I often brought home injured wild animals to nurse back to health and became very good at it. I also spent a lot of time taking care of my younger brothers and the household, as both my parents worked. They commuted an hour into the city each day, and so I became very adept at cleaning, cooking and changing diapers. People said I had an innate ability to nurture and care for my siblings and others alike. But I wasn't ready to be tied down with family responsibilities, so at sixteen and still in high school, I left home to live on my own. I created a plan of study to meet graduation requirements and worked as a waitress to pay rent.

My avid interest in wilderness brought me to the University of Michigan where I studied wildlife biology and later to the University of Arizona where I studied ornithology, but I just couldn't keep myself in class. I began taking weekends off to go camping in the mountains outside of Tucson and simply did not return. Of course, it got in the way of my studies. At one point I gave up and went to live in the canyons of the southwest desert, by myself, for almost half a year. I brought a tarp from which I fashioned a makeshift shelter and a backpack filled with art supplies. Once again I found myself studying nature, but this time it was up close and personal. I became part of the routine of the wildlife around me and learned to walk in the rhythms of the area. It was a day's hike out of the mountains into the city for supplies, and I did this once a month, or friends who knew where I was camped would come up for the weekend to visit and bring supplies. Human contact was infrequent and I came to cherish it.

I had few friends with whom I kept in contact from high school. My best friend since sixth grade, Amy, with whom I'd shared an apartment in high school and hitchhiked across the United States and Canada working in apple orchards, sent word that she was pregnant and due to deliver in a couple of months. This news ended my stay in the mountains and found me traveling to Flagstaff, Arizona, to be with her while she made the transition into motherhood.

Flagstaff was another world, a community of people (hippies) who were devoted to the "back to land" concept while living in town. The heart of the community revolved around a local natural foods restaurant called Homeward Bound. Most people worked there, ate there, or just hung around outside of the restaurant. Amy lived in one of the communal households, which was quite full, and so I took up residence in the prolific garden in the back of the house. This was easy camping compared to the canyons outside of Tucson. Even though the house was in the city, the inhabitants had decided to be off the grid and without electricity, so kerosene lanterns provided lighting, and most nights were spent making music and cooking large communal dinners. There were several houses in the neighborhood, and it was just organically decided who was cooking, and there was one huge revolving set of dishware and utensils. They ground their own wheat and made bread a few times a week, which was always another cause for a get-together. For the most part they didn't use cars; instead they used bicycles to get around and bike carts to carry groceries, children, and laundry. So, of course, when they got pregnant they weren't going to go to the hospital.

The matriarch of the household was a beautiful strong woman named Elizabeth. She was studying to be a midwife with another woman in the community, Mary Ann, and together had begun to attend the births of the women in the community. Elizabeth was an herbalist, an avid hiker and handy with any tool. She was learning midwifery by self-study and apprenticeship. There were few books on natural birth back then, but Amy had read what she needed and felt confident in her body's ability to give birth at home. The birth was the first that I had ever witnessed, and Amy remembers looking at me at one point during her labor and telling me to breathe. It was a beautiful birth, and that was the seed for midwifery in my life.

In the course of helping Amy with new motherhood, I had gotten to know one of the occupants of the household, Bruce Ackerman, quite well. We seemed to share a common interest and sense of adventure. Bruce was an avid cyclist and the bike cart builder of the community, as well as the tofu maker. One summer day we embarked on a day ride about 30 miles outside of town, and as the day came to a close it suddenly turned into a freezing blizzard snowstorm. We took off our socks and used them as mittens and rode down the mountain in the snowstorm, and when we got home had to sit together under a blanket by the woodstove for hours to thaw. From that moment on, we were a couple.

Once Amy and the baby were recovered from childbirth and stabilized in new motherhood, I had hoped to be able to travel to South America. I had been called to attend a few more births while in the community, and birth at home became the norm. But I still didn't think about becoming a midwife. Meeting Bruce delayed the trip to South America for a while, but soon the urge to travel resurfaced and Bruce had to make the decision to travel with me or stay in Flagstaff and see if I would return. He opted to travel, and so began a life of being mostly inseparable for many years to come.

After spending time in remote Indian villages in Guatemala, teaching English in Lima, hiking the hills around Machu Pichu, and staying with many families all over South America, we found ourselves on the shores of Lake Titicaca—on the border of Bolivia and Peru—with altitude sickness for days. It was then that we decided to return home to the U.S.

Once again we found ourselves in a communal household in Ann Arbor, Michigan. But the inhabitants this time were students and graduates with lots of projects on their plates. Bruce got his first pair of shiny leather shoes (for work) and I got pregnant. As fate would have it, two of the inhabitants of the house were in midwifery study groups and one of the others was a cranial sacral therapist with a keen interest in women's health, midwifery and babies. Being pregnant and living with aspiring midwives once again brought home birth back into my life. I joined the local midwifery study group, and we arranged to have a special nine-month-long Informed Homebirth course taught to us by Harriette Hartigan and Anne Frye. We also took the Apprentice Academics course. I sucked up all the information I could during my pregnancy and even found myself taking a midwifery intensive course in El Paso, Texas with Shari Daniels, who ran the only midwifery school at the time with clinical experience built into the training. Seattle Midwifery School also provided similar services but could not assure preceptors for clinical skills. So with a huge eighth-month pregnant belly, I made a three-day bus ride to Texas to check out the Maternity Center. Shari took us to births, taught classes and was an intriguing, gutsy, and charismatic host and teacher.

I attended twelve births in the one-week training and witnessed several hemorrhages and other complications. I caught a baby and sutured a woman and left exhausted but happy for the experience. When I arrived in El Paso, the first thing that Shari had asked me was why I decided to change focus from animals to humans. This was a good question but there was no good answer. It was not a decision made consciously; rather it was a string of coincidences or calling that found me at a friend's birth, then another, then another. I was going to get the ultimate initiation as I settled in to give birth myself, and I would soon feel that ring of fire more deeply than I could even imagine.

The birth was intense: three days of labor and fourteen hours of transition. But finally that asynclitic (head tilted), posterior (face up) little girl decided to rotate, and was born into bright sunlight on Earth Day. I needed the two midwives, one apprentice, three aspiring midwife roommates, and Bruce to support me through it all. The fatigue caused bleeding that resulted in loss of two-thirds of my total blood volume. I couldn't sit up for a week and was severely anemic, but Bruce was there to help get the breast to the baby's mouth, and wheat grass juice quickly rebuilt my blood. It wasn't long before we wanted to be back in the mountains now that we had a little being to take care of. Our little one (and her parents) needed to be in the mountains to be healthy.

As fate would have it, just when it was time to head out West, we got word that Elizabeth—the midwife and friend from Flagstaff—was pregnant with her second and that she wanted us to come and help her with the birth. Elizabeth was living a nomadic lifestyle traveling the wilderness areas with her donkeys and family. They had set up a base camp near a freshwater spring, had little gardens, and set up a tipi where Liz could have the baby. She went into labor one morning as we were taking a trip to the spring, which was a steep hike down a canyon. We hurried up the canyon to make preparations and get the tipi ready. We had sent the instruments into town to be sterilized and didn't have them back yet, so we boiled water for a knife to cut the cord. Elizabeth is an amazing woman and a great birther, and her second little girl slipped out into the world with the prayers of the elements and the circle of her family and friends. It was a blessing to behold. In many ways the birth of Corona was the defining moment in my midwifery career. It was then that I was sure I would be a midwife. To share this sacred space with people I loved and trusted and experience my first "solo catch" in the wilderness, feeling so grounded and so trusting of birth, was a gift I will hold close to my heart always. It has guided me through all the hundreds of births that have come after this special, precious moment.

When our daughter Caymin began taking her first steps and could stand up and nurse while I was typing, I felt we were all ready to make the trip back to El Paso to study with the infamous Shari Daniels at her birth center. It was ironic to be moving to Texas from the Pacific Northwest because as an opinionated youth I would often announce that there were two places I would never want to live: Texas and California. I have now lived in both places for over a decade and am still learning the lesson of never saying never.

A whole book could and should be written on The Maternity Center in El Paso. It was like a constant TV series drama where pregnant women and their families with a distinct cultural reality intersected with young women from varied backgrounds who were on constant overwhelm; all are forced to depend on one another, learn from one another, and share very intimate events in their lives. The schedule was grueling. We had classes three days a week, and all the other days worked in the clinic and on call for births every second. We breathed, ate, worked and lived midwifery. There was nothing else except an occasional foray to the nearest gay bar where we would go for drag queen night and dance our hearts out. It was a great stress reliever. My class started with twenty-two people and ended with five. Only the overly committed could survive the program. In our heyday we had three clinics and were doing about 120 births a month. Though exhausted, we were learning all about birthin' babies.

I graduated with about 250 births under my belt, and was immediately hired by Shari to be one of the staff midwives who supervised and taught students. I had begun to feel comfortable with birth, but when I had to start teaching students I realized what I really did know and what I still needed to learn. Students are always asking great questions, and as a teacher it is good to know the answers; if you don't, be able to find them and get back to the students with the answers. I learned that I loved teaching and helping new students on their journeys to becoming midwives almost as much as being with the pregnant women on their journeys to becoming mothers.

And so the diet of midwifery continued. I stayed in El Paso, and as Shari closed her doors and moved, I went to work with Deborah Kaley when she began Maternidad La Luz, a birth center and midwifery school. Kaley had a vision to continue training midwives in El Paso but also to have a more sustainable work schedule for the students so that they weren't so burned out by the program. I still am part of the faculty of Maternidad La Luz, traveling twice a year to teach classes. I believe it is one of the best midwifery training programs in North America. Students receive a thorough didactic training and learn hands-on skills while learning the theory. It puts it all together in an integrated way much more easily than programs having to separate the theory from the clinical.

I spent almost a decade teaching midwives in El Paso. I met midwives from all over the world who found themselves drawn to that dusty border town. I met women from Brazil, Argentina, Mexico, Canada, Germany, and Belgium, and, most importantly, many of whom I still consider close friends. I feel I have an instant bond with someone who spent time there, even if it was after I left. The thing about attending lots of births is that you get to understand and really know the wide spectrum of "normal" that exists. A textbook will tell you that normal ranges from a certain parameter to another, but in reality the parameters are so much wider to the human experience. And while you get "normal" ingrained into your blood, you also get to experience the wide variety of complications or challenges that birth has to offer. I came away from my experience at the birth centers with a deep confidence in my ability to recognize and handle things that occur outside of normal. It was a major influence on who I am as a midwife. I got to learn in a circle of women who were also learning. Not only did we learn from the births that we attended, but in talking about births we got to learn from the births that our sisters attended. The information was a constant flowing waterfall that washed over us whether we were ready or not. Birth is an infinite teacher, always a mystery.

I had my second baby in El Paso, breaking my waters while at work at Maternidad La Luz one morning just at the end of my shift. I went home without saying anything to anyone and went into labor quickly. It had been a rare night of freezing weather and our pipes had burst, since in the desert the pipes tended to be run outside the building without insulation. So that meant no hot water. We took a walk to get ice cream, then Bruce and our daughter, Caymin, and I settled in to a day of hard work. I had always wanted to give birth with only my family around, and so Bruce and I decided that we would have the baby by ourselves without the assistance of a midwife. Given my history of hemorrhage, my friends were worried. But I was quite certain that I was not going to do that again and prepared my anti-hemorrhagic injections just in case. We knew we could always call someone if we needed some help. It was an incredibly empowering experience to labor with my husband and daughter (who was now five years old). I ended up having a second bag of waters and felt the need to break it to help progress at one point, and that was tricky, given how big my belly had gotten. But we managed well, and while Caymin sketched pictures of me in labor, or me throwing up in the salad bowl (that was very impressive to her) we grew ever tighter as a family unit. Cyril slid out into the world after seven hours of labor and no bleeding! We were elated. Caymin cut the cord and was the first one to hold him, and they have been very close all their lives.

With the birth of Cyril, I reduced my time at the birth center to one 24-hour shift a week, and that gave me time to attend the Southwest School of Botanical Medicine with Michael Moore. We spent lots of days camping and wild crafting herbs and making tinctures and salves and learning the medicinal value of the friendly plants of the Southwest desert. Caymin always accompanied me, and Michael was impressed that, on my own, I could schlep a baby while harvesting and teaching my little daughter. He was very generous with the noisy baby during lectures and allowed us to stay in the program even though we were a handful.

I met a fellow herbalist that had attended a midwifery Physician Assistant's (PA) program through Stanford University. In the Mexican culture midwives are much more than baby catchers, they are healers and bone setters and massage therapists. Often the midwives in El Paso would get asked to help with ailments that would come up in the family, such as cut knees with kids, high blood pressure with grandmas, and so on. Once again I found myself called to provide care for which I was not yet trained. I felt like I had a good base of knowledge in alternative medicine from studying and from growing up in a family that hardly ever went to doctors, but rather focused on good nutrition and healthy habits. But I really did not have much in the way of diagnostic or allopathic skills. Over the years I realized that I wanted to be like a Mexican midwife—a general healer— and expand my scope of practice to family care.

That desire and meeting the herbalist who had attended Stanford inspired me to apply for the Stanford Primary Care Associate Program. It was no longer a midwifery program but was a general practitioner program. So my family moved to California. I was not in California long before home birth clients found me, and so I started attending home births even while attending the PA program. It was tough but doable, thanks to a great midwife partner, Joan Green, with whom I had also attended home births in El Paso. She and I moved to California around the same time, and it was easy to just pick up our practice once we were there. While sitting in a coffee shop one day, we overheard a woman talking about how she couldn't find a midwife. We looked at each other and our midwifery practice was reborn in California.

Stanford was difficult for me. It is a highly competitive program with four hundred applicants for forty positions. My classmates were emergency room nurses and search-and-rescue paramedics. They were used to dealing with all kinds of medical problems and medications. I didn't even know what Benadryl was. I had mostly dealt with healthy women having babies, so I had much to learn. I befriended some very smart nurses who helped me get through the program. I had to find my own physician preceptor for my clinical skills, and through the midwifery grapevine I found Mike Witte, a pediatrician and family practice doctor with a history of attending home births and supporting midwifery. He worked in Point Reyes Station, a rural town of three hundred with surrounding ranches and farmland extending to the ocean. The population he served was a magic mix of Mexican farmworkers, ranchers and hippies. It kept life balanced and interesting. That is where I apprenticed in order to learn family medicine and where I still work today, fifteen years later. I feel that the program was an excellent complement to my midwifery and alternative medicine knowledge. I got the basics of diagnosis, examination and objective thinking. The hardest thing for me, however, was separating the subjective story that someone told me from the objective exam and my assessment. I learned to use a SOAP note (Subjective,

Objective, Assessment and Plan) that documents clinical assessment and examination data. In midwifery I learned to take the person as a whole and incorporate her thoughts and feelings along with my intuition and assessment in a holistic and circular manner that didn't separate one out from the other. The medical model of SOAP introduced a style of analytical thinking that challenged my brain to stick to the facts. At first it seemed so cold and disregarding of the "patient," but once I got used to the thought process, it deeply enriched my ability to support people through their healing process. You hear what the person thinks, you see what the body shows, and from that incorporate your own intuition and knowledge. Based on that, you can then create a workable plan for everyone involved. The experience changed me for sure; I have taken from the medical model pieces that serve my clients and me, and I use technology with much more ease. I have expanded my scope, and part of that is definitely borrowing from the medical approach. I love what I am now able to do. I have the honor of being with my pregnant clients and their families during the birth and when the postpartum care comes to a close, I can continue seeing them at the clinic for well-woman care, well-child care, ear infections and all the things that come up in family life. I am blessed to continue to be a part of their lives and watch the babies grow into adults. I can't imagine more satisfying work.

It was in 1986, while in El Paso, when I first got involved with the Midwives Alliance of North America (MANA). I attended a conference and was immediately hooked. One of the first newsletters that arrived in the mail said they were looking for a new president. I had been the editor of the "New Mexico Midwives Association Newsletter" for a few years and was involved in local politics, sitting on the El Paso Midwifery Commission, the Texas State Association Grievance Committee, and attending many meetings, so I figured I could help out the national organization by volunteering to be president. Well the first thing the smart women on the MANA board did was to make a rule that you had to be on the board for at least a year before you could run for president. So I waited for an opening for the West Coast regional representative to come along, and soon I began a twenty-year volunteer career on the MANA board. I never imagined that I would devote so much of my life to this. I loved catching babies and teaching, but politics were not my cup of tea.

It was while I was living in El Paso that the State of Texas decided that the midwives (of which there were well over 400) needed to be documented and accounted for. In order to continue assisting at births, the midwives had to register with the state by filling out forms and paying a small fee. As a consequence, the roster of midwives was decreased by about half. Most of the names that were dropped from the list were Spanish surnames, so we can only surmise that there were neighborhood midwives who only did a few births a year and who did not, for whatever reason, feel comfortable with the documentation process. I am sure that some of them had stopped attending births before the process and that some moved away. But it seemed like such a large drop in numbers meant that, for some, it was a barrier to practice and forced them underground. I personally knew of two such midwives who practiced in fear that one day they would be found. This seemed wrong to me, and I really wanted to be a part of a movement that could create an infrastructure for midwives, all midwives, including traditional midwives. I wanted to be part of an organization that would honor and respect our woman-centered beliefs, and support midwives to be able to collaborate with the medical system without fear of retribution. If we were going to have to live with laws that regulated us, then we had to be part of the process of making the laws, so that we felt comfortable following them. Midwives tell me all the time that they don't want to think about all that; they just want to practice and take care of women. But the stark reality is that birth is political, and we all need to take part in the process if we don't want to be swallowed up by the medical system.

Over the next decade (1990s), I was also a founding member of the Midwifery Education and Accreditation Council (MEAC), helping to develop the standards that are used for midwifery schools. We worked for ten years to submit our application to the Department of Education to become a federally recognized accreditation agency. In 2001, the U.S. Department of Education approved MEAC as a national accrediting agency of direct-entry midwifery educational institutions and programs that confer degrees and certificates. I sat on the MEAC Board of Directors for thirteen years (in tandem with being on the MANA Board). In 2002, when I became president of MANA, I needed to step down from MEAC. I also served six years on the Executive Council of the International Confederation of Midwives (ICM) as the regional representative for the Americas. It was no easy task to represent all of the midwives in the Americas. I still am the MANA liaison to the ICM and attend meetings each time the ICM Council meets, which is every three years.

One of the more interesting roles I had was to be on the steering committee of the Certification Task Force, which was a loose coalition of midwifery groups and individuals interested in developing a national certification process for midwives. While I was on the MANA board we created the North American Registry of Midwives (NARM) that became a separate entity. The next step was the creation of a certification process. The Certification Task Force worked by consensus, and after many meetings came to agreement on the basic structure for the process. It led to the first job analysis by NARM which, along with the MANA core competencies for midwifery practice, formed the basis of the credentialing process of the Certified Professional Midwife (CPM).

None of the volunteer work over the years has rivaled the length of time and commitment that MANA has taken. I feel like I had a very positive influence on the organization in many ways, some well-known and others not really known at all. I tried to be a leader who did not need aggrandizement or applause and worked on many projects in a silent way. Some of my accomplishments included: setting up a profitable structure for our annual conferences; being a champion of bringing traditional and international midwives to our conferences; working on the conferences that MANA sponsors annually in Mexico; helping to launch a credible and effective Division of Research that has a record number of midwife contributors and has become well-known in the scientific community for its dedication to researching normal birth; envisioning and helping to initiate a national public education campaign that targeted young women to let them know about the Cadillac care that midwives offer; and creating the initial design for a youth leadership project for aspiring and new midwives.

The changes that I have participated in and have witnessed over the last twenty years have been significant. The midwifery community now has a basic infrastructure where there was none before. We have a federally recognized accreditation body for our schools, we have schools that are accredited, and we have a nationally certified midwifery credential that is administered by a federally recognized agency. We have a growing population of certified midwives, and home birth is on the rise.

This change was made possible by a heroic dedication of many strong women who volunteered their time, sacrificed their families and sometimes their health to serve the midwifery profession. We have made midwifery a viable option for young women who want to become midwives. When I began attending births, there were less than ten accredited schools to choose from, no national certification to legally verify that I had any skills, and most of the states had no legislation that made it possible for me to practice legally. We worked hard to create these things and I am very proud of what we have done. There are many other people who have been just as dedicated as I have, and we all know each other intimately. We are like a big family with many sisters. Sometimes we bicker and even scream at each other, but in the end we always end up back in the circle holding hands.

Ultimately the most important thing is to move the profession forward, and each of us holds that goal next to our hearts, and each of us understands and respects and admires all of the personalities that it took to accomplish what we have. We deeply understand that it will take all of us and many more before we will be able to rest and say our job is done.

I feel that all of the stages of my life have influenced who I am as a midwife. My early years of learning from the women with whom I lived gave me the trust in birth that has never left me. Then to live on the Mexican border and serve hundreds of women who trusted birth themselves solidified my knowledge in the process of normal birth. I currently live in an area of highly educated women who have a hard time trusting in birth and getting out of their heads long enough to surrender to the process. I have attended over a thousand women in their birth journeys, and each is so unique yet so much the same. I have lived through a time when our national cesarean section rate was a third of what it is today. Technology has done great things for obstetrics and has also produced some detrimental effects. Reliance on technology, such as the fetal heart monitor, ultrasound and prenatal testing, has created more fear for women in their pregnancies and births. The testing always creates a time of waiting to make sure that all is normal. I used to spend most of my prenatal time talking to women about their diets, their lives, their hopes and dreams. Now I spend an inordinate amount of time discussing possible testing options, why they might want them or why they might not want them. The very fact of having so much testing in pregnancy creates fear and uncertainty because in order to explain why you may want to test, you have to inadvertently ask a woman to open her heart to the possibility of having a baby with a problem. Some tests are easier than others; some actually carry a risk to the baby, as in the case of amniocentesis. But each woman is unique in her need to feel safe in pregnancy and birth. In this world of informed consent, we need to talk to women about things we may not ourselves even believe just to keep up with all that there is to offer in maternity care. It is easy to see how women are losing their faith in their own bodies given the complexity of options in maternity care today.

We also live in a society that has gotten quite comfortable with controlling most aspects of our lives. We have gotten quite good at birth control and, if a woman and her partner are diligent, it is possible to delay childbearing as long as desired. This has resulted in many women having their first babies in their late thirties and early forties. In some ways this can be a great thing for a couple because they have achieved their academic goals and are well into their professional career. But in many cases they are just at the height of their professional careers and are not ready to suspend working to have a family. This problem, along with our economic realities, results in childrearing competing with a professional career, to say nothing of the decreased energy that a forty-year-old parent must experience compared with that of a twenty-year-old. Now, the ultimate control of birth is being brought to the spotlight, and that is the question of cesarean by choice. Some women are choosing to have surgical birth so as to make it fit into their schedules, so as to not interfere with any aspect of their sex life by having a baby pass through the birth canal.

Midwives have to bend with the trends of the times, such as older moms and increased prenatal testing, but our mission remains very much the same no matter what the current issue may be. I support women to have their babies in a way that will be empowering to them. I work in partnership with women to make the best choices for themselves and their families. Being a midwife is a lifelong learning process that enriches my life and gives back a hundredfold the enormous energy that I give out. I believe that midwives do need to be careful with this gift. We are important to the families that we serve, but we are not indispensable. We need to set boundaries in our service and be sure that we take time for our families and ourselves. For if we are not nurtured ourselves, we end up depleting our vital energy.

I encourage all young midwives to be sure to create a good support network. I think it makes good sense to create a group practice so that you can take a weekend off every once in a while, knowing that you have partners who can care for your clients while you take care of what you need for yourself. I encourage young midwives to realize that the birth is not about you, the midwife, but about the mother and her family and to avoid developing co-dependant relationships with your clients. We need to learn to build sustainability into our practices. Many of the older midwives have had to quit practicing because they were on call 24/7 for just too long. We need lots of midwives if we are to have a midwife for every mother. It is important to take care of ourselves and nurture each other. Our greatest resource is the connection we have with our midwifery sisters. Only they truly know what it is like and the support that is necessary to keep on keeping on. There is good reason why, through the years, lots of time has been spent on learning to get along with one another, learning to communicate. Take time to sit in circle with your sisters and express your heart, say the hard things, don't let things build up, and love one another. We need each other to keep midwifery moving forward.

Lastly I would like to encourage young midwives not to get complacent. Honor the work of the midwives who have come before you and pick up the torch and make it brighter. The infrastructure is in place, but there is still so much more we need. We need to attain legal status for midwives in all fifty states. We need federal recognition for insurance reimbursement. We need a health care system that covers all people and includes midwives as a corner stone of maternity care. We need mainstream recognition of the kind of care that midwives offer. We need home birth to really be a viable option for healthy women. We need a sustainable salary for midwives with insurance reimbursement for their services. We need many more studies on out-of-hospital birth and the midwifery model of care. And we need to support mothers to be able to stay home with their infants for the first year of their lives. There is so much work to do. We need a good exchange between the young midwives and the active older midwives to continue to advance the profession of midwifery in a woman-centered and empowering way. Find a partner today to teach, and learn and grow. Together we can move mountains.

You need two clamps and a pair of scissors

MARSHA JACKSON

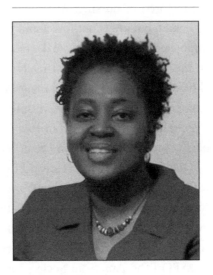

I grew up in Newark, New Jersey. My father was a self-employed mason contractor, and my mother was a stay-at-home mom until my older brother and I started school. My mom began nursing school in 1960 and eventually became a neonatal/labor and delivery nurse at a small community hospital. Sometimes when a baby sitter was not available, I was able to go to work with her. I probably did not go to work with her often, but those times really stand out in my memory. I enjoyed being around the mothers and babies, even though I was not supposed to be on the unit.

Along with caring for my family and pets, and spending time around mothers and babies, having family members that were business owners helped to lead me to midwifery and starting my own business. My dad had his own construction company. My maternal grandmother, who I always thought was a nurse, had a business that today would be considered an assisted living facility. Until I was an adult, I had actually thought she was a nurse. My grandmother had a short stature but was always very busy; she was a "take charge" kind of person and a wonderful caretaker of the elderly and of our family.

Prior to 1970, I planned on becoming a veterinarian. But when it was time to go to college, I decided I wanted to work with people more than with animals. I decided I wanted to be a nurse like my mom and my grandmother. I went to Howard University and majored in nursing. At that time, I knew I wanted to work with mothers and babies, but knew nothing about midwifery.

In 1974, when I completed my baccalaureate degree in nursing, I worked at Freedman's Hospital in the newborn nurseries. I really enjoyed working there. Freedman's was an old hospital that had an open maternity ward. It was a busy place, and there were many opportunities to talk with the moms. We learned a lot from each other. Freedman's Hospital closed in 1975, when I was out on my maternity leave after having my first baby. When I returned to work, Freedman's had moved into its new facility, now known as Howard University Hospital.

When pregnant with my first baby, my husband and I attended childbirth education classes at a local hospital. I was not enthused with the classes and knew that I could do a better job preparing families for childbirth. After I returned to work, I looked into becoming a certified childbirth educator and began the teacher-training program with ASPO (The American Society for Psychoprophylaxis in Obstetrics). I have always thought that was a ridiculous name for an organization. I was glad when the name was changed to ASPO/Lamaze.

During my childbirth education through ASPO, I began to learn about many different options for birth, and I also began to learn about midwives. There was an emerging home birth movement in the Washington, D.C. metropolitan area. Maternity Center Associates was a midwifery service that opened in Montgomery County, Maryland, and provided home birth services. I became a childbirth educator and began teaching childbirth classes in my home. I also established the childbirth education program at Howard University Hospital along with the Clinical Nurse Specialist (CNS) for Maternal Infant Care. I started getting to know the midwives in the area and began offering my services as a birth assistant for home births. I loved attending home births. Maternity Center always made a point to refer their Black clients to me for birth assistant services. We would usually figure out during the phone call that we were both Black. Clients would laugh, but appreciated when they figured out that they were steered to me because of our ethnic sisterhood.

In 1976, after working several years at Howard, I became the nurse-clinician for maternal infant care. As the nurse-clinician, I did staff development and worked with families that had babies in the Intensive Care Nurseries (ICN). I worked a lot with moms who were pumping and collecting breast milk for their premature babies. I will always remember the time I served as a wet nurse for a tiny one-pound baby whose mom was convinced that her baby would die and did not want to produce a milk supply. I was nursing my own young baby and pumped while at work. The preemie's mom Okayed my sharing breast milk with her baby. That baby thrived and was eventually discharged home. The mom did bring her back to the hospital to visit so we could marvel at how her tiny preemie had grown. She was about three years old the last time I saw her. It felt good to know I helped in this little baby's survival. Providing milk for her helped to save her life. It was like being a midwife to this little preemie, giving of myself to safeguard her and to help give her a good start.

My responsibilities as a nurse-clinician continued to expand primarily because the CNS position for maternal infant care was vacant. I requested a promotion to the CNS position since I received assignments that were given to the clinical nurse specialists working in other areas of the hospital. However, I was told that I did not have my master's degree and was, therefore, not eligible for the position. When I went on my maternity leave in 1980 for my third baby, I did not return to Howard University Hospital.

Judy Melson Mercer, Certified Nurse-Midwife (CNM), was the director of the midwifery program at Georgetown University. Judy was also a home birth midwife with Family Birth Associates, another midwife-owned practice that had opened in the D.C. area. I had thought about going into midwifery, but I did not want to go back to school without getting my master's degree. One night when I was attending a home birth in D.C. as a birth assistant with Judy, she was excited to let me know that the midwifery program at Georgetown was changing to a master's level. I was very excited, but our family was a two-income family. I did not have money budgeted to go back to school and we needed my salary. The midwifery program was full-time. Judy continued encouraging me to apply and reassured me that she would help me find some money. I probably would not have gone back to school at that point in my life if it had not been for Judy. I trusted her and began exploring options for loans for living expenses. In August 1980, about one week before classes started, Judy found a grant that covered my tuition expenses. What a blessing!

Before I even finished my midwifery program at Georgetown University in December of 1981, I received a call from a potential client requesting a home birth. I told her that I could not agree to do it because I still had to sit for my board exams. This potential client told me that she knew I would pass my boards, and she also knew that I would help her have her home birth. I felt a lot of pressure and it made me feel very uneasy. I did take my boards, passed them, and helped her have a home birth just like she had said. Through word of mouth, it became known throughout D.C. that I was helping families have babies at home. One family physician and one OB/GYN physician in the area referred clients to me for home births. Along with the client, I would attend one or two prenatal visits scheduled with the physician, and I would make one visit to the client's home before the birth. After attending the home birth, I would provide one postpartum home visit. As this worked well and without any advertising, I started a private home birth practice doing about one to four home births per month. Along with this home birth practice that essentially started on its own, I accepted a job with Cities-in-Schools in order to assure a steady income for our family.

Cities-in-Schools was a single-site adolescent pregnancy program that offered infant daycare, school for the teens, and health care services under one roof. This was a very challenging position because I was the first midwife hired. Kay Boyer, CNM, soon joined the staff to help set up the service. Kay was not planning to work as a midwife, but she had lots of connections throughout the city and across the country. This really helped Cities-in-Schools get its program off the ground. Kay's husband, Ernest Boyer, was also a nationally known educator and U.S. Education Commissioner under Jimmy Carter. He provided expertise in setting up the educational part of the program along with other local educators. This was an exciting position for me as a new midwife. I felt I knew the basics, but I had to represent a new service. What I did or did not do would affect this new program and all midwives in the community. I felt a lot of pressure to assure that things were done correctly. Cities-in-Schools hired a great medical staff, which included a nutritionist, a nurse, another staff midwife, several social workers, and an office clerk. This team worked well together, and the team quickly got the program up and running.

I have always been a fairly quiet person, and so I try to avoid conflicts. As a midwife, however, I quickly found out that was not possible. I have the distinction of being the first CNM to have hospital privileges at Georgetown University

Hospital. That was a very difficult position for me. The staff was not sure how to interact with these midwives from Cities-in-Schools. Our service was set up so that we consulted directly with the attending physician, not the residents. The attending physician had an OB Fellow working with him. I remember the moment I had to hatch from my shell and become more outspoken.

I had admitted a young teen mother to Labor and Delivery (L&D) in active labor. Her labor was progressing very quickly. We had an external monitor on her to record a baseline strip of the fetal heart rate and we monitored contractions to document fetal well-being. The mom moved around a lot and it was difficult to get a good recording. We could hear a few variable decelerations, but there was good recovery back to the baseline. The OB Fellow had mentioned to me that I might put on an internal electrode. I told him I was getting her admitted and that she was moving very quickly in labor. The OB Fellow came back in the labor room very angry, shook his finger at me and with a loud voice said, "Didn't I tell you to put a fetal scalp electrode on the patient? Do it now!"

I could not believe how he spoke to me in front of the client. He was unprofessional and disrespectful not only to me, but to my client. I excused us out of the room and told him, "Don't you ever speak to me like that. I am not a child. My mother and father never spoke to me like that. So don't you ever try that again. Right now we need to focus on the patient." Later, the nurses later told me that they were amazed. They said they had never heard anyone talk to him like that before. I had to be very assertive and forceful. This was out of character for me, but it was very important that I establish ground rules. He was not used to working with midwives, and I was not secure in my role as a midwife. My client delivered and had a healthy baby without putting on a fetal scalp electrode. I also made it clear with the Fellow after the birth that he had taken the situation to another level. Since he did, I told him that if he ever attempted to speak to me again in that kind of tone, he would not have to deal with me, but he would have to deal with my husband…and my husband is a really big guy. After that spring evening in 1982, I had no more problems, and, in fact, the Fellow always made a point to speak to me. The situation forced me to be more assertive and to speak up for myself. I also became a better negotiator.

Another event in my early years truly affected our family. It was our decision to have our fourth child at home. I did not become a midwife until after our third child was born. I wanted a home birth with our third child, but my husband thought it was a crazy idea. In 1983 when we were pregnant with our fourth, I was a midwife providing home birth services for families. I believe that my clients helped my husband decide to try a home birth. When I was not home, my clients would speak with my husband on the phone and share their home birth experiences. After our wonderful home birth, my husband became an outspoken supporter for home birth.

I believe being a home birth midwife has made me a better midwife. In the hospital it is easy to call for help. A neonatologist and an obstetrician are always close by. In the home setting, I have to use more discretion and determine if that "sometimes gray area" should be considered normal or abnormal. It can be very lonely in the home setting. As a new grad, I transferred some clients from home to hospital who I would not transfer today. That comes with experience and confidence. Midwifery does keep you humble. When you feel that you are confident with your skills and assessments, something usually happens to make you realize that there is always something else you need to learn.

My family has always been very supportive of my midwifery practice. It was sometimes hard for our family, particularly when the children were small. My children would worry that I might not be home in the morning if they heard the phone ring during the night. The nighttime phone calls were also disruptive to my husband's sleep. Since we did not have family living close by, we had to depend on our friends to help with childcare when my husband's job required him to travel. We were the first among our friends to have children. In some ways that was good because it made our friends more available. I remember standing at the door waiting for a friend to come watch the kids so I could dash out to a birth.

When I pause to think about what events played a major role in influencing my midwifery practice, it causes me to reflect on a seemingly low point in my midwifery journey. In retrospect, a lawsuit that I was involved with through Cities-in-Schools (CIS) helped me become a better midwife.

This case stemmed from a client I worked with at CIS between 1984 and 1985. I was the Chief Nurse-Midwife and had frequent contact with the family because I followed up on appointments they missed. Thus, the family knew my name well. This family filed a suit because the teenaged mom delivered a baby with cerebral palsy, and the family needed money to provide the care this child needed. CIS was initially not named in the suit, but was included when it was discovered that the physician scheduled to do the birth did not have professional liability insurance. We were short staffed, and the midwives were only providing prenatal care. The physician was called when the mom went into labor, and he delayed responding to the labor call. When he arrived at the hospital many hours later, the mom had been taken in for an emergency cesarean birth. The baby was diagnosed with cerebral palsy. I was brought into the suit with CIS because the attorneys were looking for the deep pockets. I had the deep pockets because I had a $1million/$3million professional liability policy. As soon as the attorneys found out about my insurance, I was also named in the suit. Many of the attorneys who reviewed the case apologized to me for our poor health care system. I had had very limited prenatal visits with the mother and, in fact, had not seen her since 34 weeks gestation. I had done nothing wrong, but I had the deep pockets.

This was a very difficult time for me early in my journey, but it did help me to get acquainted with the medical-legal system, helped me to develop skills to critically evaluate midwifery practice, and caused me to find ways to deal with stress. The outcome of this case was that my insurance paid $100,000, Cities-in-School's insurance paid $15,000, the hospital's insurance paid $1,000,000, and the physician without insurance paid only $5,000 and continued to practice as an OB/GYN. Through this experience, I have become an expert witness and began to review cases for attorneys. Reviewing cases helps to keep my practice safe.

Early on in my midwifery journey, I became active in the American College of Nurse-Midwives (ACNM). I was curious to know how the organization functioned. There were few midwives of color when I became a part of ACNM. What I quickly learned was that we looked out for each other. I did not get to go to the annual meeting every year when my children were small, but whenever I went, I was active with the Ad Hoc Committee on Minority Affairs, currently known as the Midwives of Color Committee.

I have always been a spiritual person, and prayer is a very important part of my life and in my midwifery practice. As I have matured, I always pray for guidance in all my actions. This has become important in my practice. I am not one who prays with all my clients, but I pray for all of them. If clients invite me to pray with them, I do, and if clients include prayer in their birth plan, I am pleased to pray with them. As a midwife, I have to be confident, trust my gut feelings, be a good listener, and be ready to deal with stressful situations. After dealing with those stressful situations, it is also important to have a safe place and way to air those feelings. Prayer helps there too.

After I had been practicing as a midwife for about six years, Alice Bailes, CNM and I joined forces to establish BirthCare & Women's Health, Ltd. We started BirthCare as a home birth practice. Alice and I were childbirth educators in the D.C. area and also midwifery classmates at Georgetown in 1980. We started BirthCare on Alice's back porch after the 1987 ACNM annual meeting in Orlando, Florida. I was looking for a partner to expand my home birth practice, while Alice was looking for someone to hire for a practice she was starting.

It was fate that we got together in Orlando. When I arrived at the hotel, Alice was one of the first persons I saw. We sat together, and immediately she pulled out an ad she had composed. I looked at it, and she asked me if I was interested. I read it, thought about it a little. I told her I would not be interested in working for her, but I would consider being equal partners. She thought about it and said, "That sounds good. I would consider that." From that point on, we did not pay attention to any of the speakers. We were busy planning BirthCare. This would be a difficult challenge for our family. If Alice and I went into practice together, I would have to take a cut in salary. As a nurse, I could easily make more money and work more regular hours than I could as a CNM in private practice.

I realized that starting my own practice was taking a risk. I felt it was important for me to be clear that this was what the Lord wanted for me and my family. I felt that I was a more experienced midwife and that I could leave Cities-in-Schools to start my own practice. I had to have faith that our family would be able to survive if Alice and I pursued getting BirthCare off the ground. I was torn because if you attend graduate school, you expect to make more money. Our family had gone further into debt for me to become a midwife. Starting BirthCare was a big risk. On paper, it just did not seem like the right financial move for our family, but I realized this was God's plan.

Over the years, BirthCare has truly been a blessing for me and for many families in the D.C. metro area. I still cannot say that it has been a financial blessing for my family. I could have made more money working some other place. However, BirthCare has been a blessing in other ways for my family. Although being a midwife requires some long hours, having my own business has offered me some flexibility. As an owner, I have a little more say in scheduling and business finances.

I really work too much. It has not been easy to do all the things that need to be done to keep BirthCare functioning. I have always said that with BirthCare I have learned so many things that I never wanted to or had any desire to know about. But, you do what you have to do. To make the business run, we had to learn about political issues and had to be proactive in addressing those issues. In D.C., around 1990, there was a very interesting case that developed about vicarious liability for physicians who worked with midwives. The National Reciprocal Insurance Company (NCRIC), a company that provided professional liability insurance for physicians, began charging a surcharge to physicians who worked with midwives. This move by NCRIC had the potential to make it impossible for physicians and midwives to work together. When we approached the local D.C.

Chapter of ACNM to get some help to change NCRIC's position, the chapter initially did not support the effort. It affected our practice more since we were in private practice. After we continued to stir up momentum, local midwives became involved. There was a well-attended, two-day public hearing in D.C. to address this issue. One of our clients, an attorney, assisted us in mobilizing our clients and other midwives. Our attorney for BirthCare, the late John Grad, was the lead attorney. The D.C. Superintendent of Insurance rejected the surcharge rate increase, making it illegal for physicians to be charged a surcharge for vicarious liability. We continue to be active in political issues because if it affects midwives, it affects our practice.

Since our practice was primarily a home birth practice, we also had to keep our radar up regarding home birth issues. I became more active with the Home Birth Committee when the ACNM seemed to ignore home birth. Home birth was not mentioned in written documents or other public relations materials from ACNM. Since home birth is BirthCare's area of expertise, we needed our professional organization to support us. We became very outspoken about home birth and stayed in touch with ACNM to express our concerns. I was soon appointed the chairperson of the Home Birth Committee and served in that capacity for six years (1991–1997). During that time, the Home Birth Committee became a standing committee of the ACNM, we found professional liability insurance for home birth, and revised the manual for home birth into a "Handbook for Home Birth Practice." We also spearheaded both a retrospective and prospective study of home birth practice in the United States with certified nurse-midwives. In addition, we compiled a home study program for midwives attending home births published in the *Journal of Nurse-Midwifery*.

At the 1998 ACNM annual meeting in San Francisco, I became a Fellow of the ACNM. It is truly an honor to be recognized by my professional organization as one who has made significant contributions to the practice midwifery. It is nice to pause for a moment to smell the roses. As a fellow, I get to put more initials behind my name—FACNM!

As a midwife, you help hundreds of families have babies. It is such a special time when you can help your own family members and your own children have babies of their own. The first family member I attended was my niece Jennifer (really my cousin, but I am like an aunt to her) who birthed at our birth center in 2002. Jennifer birthed really easily, and it was very special having her five-year-old daughter, Lauryn, hold the flashlight for me and her mom. Lauryn still speaks fondly about that moment.

I was at the hospital birth of my first granddaughter in 2003. It was a wonderful experience. I did not tell the staff that I was a midwife, but I was very assertive in assuring that my son and his partner had the birth that they wanted. It was not until after the birth that three nurses came in the room, and recognizing me, said, "Hey, you were my midwife!" Everything changed from that point on, and the nurse that had given me a hard time during the labor said, "I thought you looked familiar, you used to work at D.C. General Hospital." I replied to her, "Now you understand why I did not let you push us around and put us out of the room." She smiled and was helpful the remainder of our time on the labor and delivery unit.

My oldest daughter and her husband planned home births with me in attendance for both of their children. I had another midwife attend the birth with me for support. With their first birth in 2005, they labored at home for several days and transferred to the hospital after an extended time with ruptured membranes and a labor that reached a plateau at five centimeters. She birthed fine in the hospital with her first baby. Their second birth took place in 2007 and was the perfect home birth. My bedroom tends to be like a family room. My daughter and her husband planned their birth to be at our home. It was very special that my grandson was born into the loving hands of his dad assisted by my hands. It was such an amazing experience for me and our family. I look forward to sharing in the births of other family members and of my grandchildren that are yet to come.

Also in 2005 I received a great honor. Linda Janet Holmes, the guest curator of the Smithsonian exhibit "Reclaiming Midwives: Pillars of Community Support" called me one evening with an invitation to participate in the exhibit as a modern day midwife. Linda is the author of *Listen to Me Good: The Life Story of an Alabama Midwife* and has done extensive research of midwives in the United States. Linda and I talked like we were old friends. She asked me to get together things that I had collected over the years, including an authentic birth bag and other supplies that I had taken to home births. I pulled things together, and a display case was set up that included an old birth bag that I had used with all the supplies I took to a home birth, awards that I received, some photos, and a brief write-up about me.

The exhibit ran from November 2005 through August 2006 and traced the story and practices of African American midwives from the seventeenth century to present. The exhibit celebrated the impact and work of "granny" midwives, included an emotional display of still photographs by Robert Galbraith from the 1959 midwife training film, "All My Babies," and followed the work of midwives into the twentieth century and current day midwives. As part of the exhibit, there were many community outreach activities in which I participated. These activities included individual presentations, tours of the exhibit, and panel discussions.

During the opening ceremony, I had the pleasure to meet and take photos with Claudine Curry Smith, one of the last granny midwives in Virginia. She co-authored the book, *My Bag Was Always Packed: The Life and Times of a Virginia Midwife*. She died in March 2006, before the exhibit ended. It is wonderful to remember how happy she was at the opening of the exhibit and how much she remembered about midwifery. Ms. Claudine's family was surprised that she was so lucid that day. I am sure it was because midwifery was such an important part of her life. During the community events, I also got to meet many women interested in midwifery and got to see many of my past clients who came to see the exhibit. I also received communication from the museum about past clients who happened upon the exhibit and were surprised to find "their midwife" on display. It was truly an awesome experience and a high point in my midwifery life.

I learned so much about my sister midwife ancestors. I have always felt closely bonded to granny midwives particularly when I entered midwifery school. It was after I became a midwife that I learned that my paternal grandmother, Uzella, was a midwife in Charlotte, North Carolina. My grandfather shared that information with me after he found out I was a midwife. I was really excited to learn that, and it made me feel like there was an inner reason for me to feel so connected to midwives. It was in my blood!

As a midwife today, I have encountered many difficult and stressful situations, but I have been spared some of the adversity that my granny sister midwives encountered. They are the ones who paved and smoothed the rocky way that I still travel today on my personal journey. I am so thankful for the granny midwives.

Over the past twenty-eight years, I have helped over two thousand women and families birth. Through my work with ACNM, I have become a trustee with the ACNM Foundation. This is a new experience for me, and I am learning a lot about fundraising, which is necessary for midwifery to continue making an impact in women's health care.

Midwifery is an amazing profession to have. I feel so blessed that I provide a service that I love for women and families. Through the years I have met so many amazing people and have become a part of so many families. It is always exciting to hear back from families I have helped birth. Now I am moving to the next level—helping the babies that I have helped birth have their own children. When I started midwifery, that possibility never entered my thoughts.

I did think that the longer I was in practice the easier it would get, but I have not found that to be true. I have learned a lot about running a business. Over the past few years, we have had some turnover of midwives at BirthCare. It is somewhat distressing that it is very difficult to find midwives willing to work the hours necessary to provide the services. BirthCare has been a successful business for more than twenty years because we are very frugal and operate on a cash basis. We try to avoid going in debt. This makes it impossible to promise our employees large salaries. Profit-sharing with our employees does increase our employees' gross salaries. Because our expenses vary so much from year to year, it is difficult to project our budget for the coming year. The realities of operating our own business remain challenging.

Through the years I have learned so much about midwifery and about myself. It is an awe-inspiring and wonderful journey with lots of ups and downs. As an experienced midwife, I have gained wisdom and share it with the many students, staff, and families that I work with daily.

The following pearls have helped me through my journey:

Birth is simple. Basically, you need two clamps and a pair of scissors. During the exhibit at the Smithsonian, this point was very evident. A birth cabin was a part of the exhibit, and surprisingly the birth supplies that were set up included two clamps and a scissor, which is what I carry today in my birth bag.

Set out on faith and realize your dreams. Alice and I started BirthCare by bringing together our midwifery skills, our birth bags, a shared belief system, and some common sense. We did not take out a loan to start BirthCare. The only equity we used to start the business was sweat equity. Neither of us had much in financial reserves nor was interested in putting any personal finances at risk. We did occasionally miss a few paychecks to make the business work.

Turn a negative into a positive. Listen to criticism but don't let it break your spirit. When I was in high school, my teacher told me that I would never make it in college because I was a poor reader. I could have believed him and decided not to pursue my education. Though I did not read as fast as many of the other students, I could read and understand. That negative statement from my teacher motivated me and made me set out to prove him wrong. Being somewhat shy growing up, I could have internalized that statement and believed it. But, my family instilled pride in me and always told me I could do whatever I set out to do. I had many role models in my path to encourage me to pursue my dreams. Staying focused helps you to overcome.

Be smart with your hands and your senses. Students should work hard to master hand skills, such as Leopold maneuvers, assessing the cervix, and supporting the baby when the mother gives birth in different positions. Don't be afraid to smell things and listen to your inner voice. Develop the ability to decipher the message, be it through your hands or other senses.

Learning to sew as a child is an important skill to develop. I never knew that the time my mom took to teach me to sew on the machine and by hand was preparing me for a midwifery skill that I needed. I always enjoyed sewing and became a pretty good seamstress. I made many of my own clothes, including suits, coats, and my wedding dress. I took much care to hem neatly and line the clothes that I made so that they would look neat, inside and out. Today, if someone needs a repair after birth, I do a really good job. I can see how the tissue fits back together if there is a jagged tear. The other midwives sometimes call me if they have a difficult repair to do and need help.

God's grace allows you to do what you do. Marsha does not do this alone. God favors me and has given me this gift of midwifery to share with others. His grace gives me the courage, strength, and ability to be a midwife. I am thankful that God hears my prayers and the prayers of others to help keep me going.

As a midwife, it is very important to have balance in your life. It is very easy for midwifery to consume your entire being. Having a supportive husband helps to keep me focused and gives me a reality check periodically. I am very active in my church and enjoy being a part of the music ministry. I am also part of the diaconate of my church serving as a leader there. My spiritual foundation helps to keep me grounded.

My midwifery journey has been so rewarding. Over and over again I get to experience mountaintop experiences with families. We share memories, and my extended family gets larger and larger. What a blessing it has been to be guided into such a wonderful profession. I owe homage to my granny sister midwives and I bask in such a rich legacy. It is an honor and a privilege to be a part of such a well-respected profession and a challenge to be part of such a misunderstood facet of the health care industry.

What an experience the journey has been and continues to be. I will know it is time to give it up when I stop feeling the "birth high." It is harder to get up at night and spring back after a birth since I am getting older. But I still look forward to births and miss births if it has been several days between them. I am still passionate about midwifery and work hard to keep our service available for women and families. I will stay prayerful and ready for all the miracles that I get to share.

Every woman wants a healthy baby

JENNIE JOSEPH

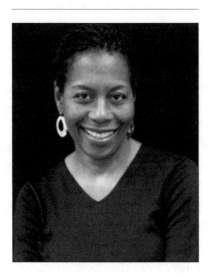

I was born in Cambridge, England, in 1959. I was the first child of my parents Eric and Sylvia Joseph, who had recently emigrated from Barbados to settle in England. I was born in a rural area. My father was in the Royal Air Force and traveled extensively with them. We moved from base to base quite frequently. So I grew up as a military child. I grew up in areas where back in those days there were no people of color around us. We were always the only Black family in the area, in the town, in the city, in the region, probably in that half of the country, an unusual situation for that time. I remember quite distinctly feeling so different, always being the only Black person in the hallway, on the bus, in the crowd, or in the school for most of my life. We also lived in Germany for a while, and my brother was born there. My parents still live in England. I have been in the United States since 1989.

I am clear that my life was moved for me, without any input from me at all—my destiny was midwifery. I don't recall choosing, thinking or wondering. It was just as if it was automatic. I do remember becoming interested in babies. That was when my brother was born. I was nine years old at the time. I had it very clear in my mind that I was going to mother and be in charge of that child. It was a very interesting feeling at nine; I don't really know where it came from except that I just felt tremendous ownership of him, and even though he is a forty-year-old man now, I still have that same sense today! Perhaps that began my interest in babies, but for sure, I knew at sixteen I wanted to be a midwife.

I was called to be a midwife. It is as clear as day. I knew I wanted to do it. I barely knew what it was. I knew very little about how to get it done, but any time a career officer or teacher would suggest to me that I should choose secretarial work or teaching, or even nursing, my immediate thought was, *No, I am going to be a midwife.* I knew that very clearly, very strongly. In England, school finishes at age sixteen; you graduate at sixteen and are expected to be ready to go into the working world or into further studies in college or university. So at sixteen I was stuck, because there wasn't any kind of midwifery program that I could enter until age twenty. So I had to kill some time, but I didn't waver. I knew what I wanted to do. I did some training in nursery, daycare, childcare, and then I went to college and studied for two years to be what is called a "nursery nurse" which is essentially someone who works with children and cares for them through their development up to age five. I did that for a couple of years. I was just treading water, waiting to be able to get into midwifery. I also did some nanny work. I worked in children's nursery schools and hospital nurseries. I did whatever I could do to be around babies and hounded the midwifery program at Edgware General Hospital so much so that they let me in at nineteen. And so I *finally* began my midwifery career.

During my career as a midwife I have practiced in hospitals, community settings, birth centers and home births. I have never done any other kind of work until I came to the United States, where I added entrepreneurship to my arsenal of midwifery skills. I had to become an entrepreneur. I had to become a business-woman because midwifery, just like medicine in America, is about business. I love and still yearn for the days when midwifery was purely vocational, when it was done from the heart and for the joy and the love of it. And although I do still operate that way, I have struggled so much financially as a result. Unfortunately I have never been able to mesh the idea of being financially well off for doing my passion, my calling, my service, something I love so much that I would do it anyway. I started a non-profit corporation in 1998—Commonsense Childbirth, Inc.—in order to reach women from all walks of life and to be able to find grants and donations to continue my work. As a product of the British National Health Service I have had a hard time with the fact that health care is not necessarily a right in the United States. Much of the care that I have provided over the years has never been compensated, and those grants and donations—well that's another story! Subsequently, I have yet to become financially stable or comfortable. Having decided that this is something that *is* achievable, not to mention *sensible* if I wish to continue living in the United States, I am now working toward the goal of making midwifery work for me financially, as well as for the women and families whom I serve.

My early midwifery practice began in busy London hospitals, where I was considered an unusual type of midwife because I was a direct-entrant (non-nurse) way back when there were not any direct-entrants as a matter of course. In those days, the direct-entry program was a pilot program. I was one of the first few women in the country that was allowed the opportunity of entering into midwifery without having a nursing diploma. So I was really and truly unusual. When I graduated from the midwifery program I involved myself in the "business as usual" of being a hospital-based midwife for many years, but I also worked as a domiciliary midwife, or what we call community midwifery, where I would visit mothers at home, conducting postpartum checks after their discharge from the hospital. I also ran prenatal clinics in the community, usually at a family practice office or community health center. I also attended the very occasional home births that happened in our area. In those days I was simply part of a system; I did not have much thought about any other way of being a midwife outside of that system. I was paid by the hospital on a salary as opposed to a per-birth or per-visit fee for service. I was aware of the fact that the system of care was very much the same for each woman, yet I wanted, even then, to individualize care for them. I read *Spiritual Midwifery* when I worked in England, and I could not even begin to relate to what I read; nonetheless I was intrigued. I didn't translate any of it into my practice at the time, but I remember thinking, *hmmm . . . that is interesting.* I had no idea that I would end up in the United States nor have the pleasure of meeting Ina May Gaskin and many other women mentioned in the book.

My American midwifery, on the other hand, was very much influenced by the direct-entry midwives who I met when I arrived in Florida. I imagined that we were one and the same because they were not nurses either. I naïvely assumed that that was all there was to it. What I discovered and what influenced me greatly when I came to the United States was that the direct-entry midwives were quite adept at delivering babies with very little resources. For example, they did not have boxes and boxes of supplies and medication, back-up situations, and physicians waiting for their call. It was all very strange in my mind. I remember very distinctly when I first went to see a birth center and was shown around the quaint little house; I was horrified! I was thinking, *Well where is my stuff? What would I do without all of the stuff?* I was shown a little cart with a few baby blankets, a bulb syringe and some tincture bottles, and I was totally surprised that you could deliver a baby without *stuff*! And yet as I began to work inside of that system and learned from one of the most amazing midwives that I have ever met, Char Lyn Daughtry, I learned that you needed very little because you really weren't doing much of anything. The mother was doing the work. So those influences became really powerful for me because I watched and soaked in every facet of delivering a baby without interfering with anything. It shaped the way I developed into an "out of hospital" midwife. The family involvement also touched me to such a degree, I realized I had spent the previous ten years missing out on the joy and the empowerment and the growth of the family through birth.

Culturally speaking, I had never separated or really thought about the impact of culture on birth. Working in hospitals for the most part, birth was just a routine. There wasn't any influence from anything other than the standard model that says we need to get this woman on this table; we need to get the baby out of her so we can get this next person on the table; we need to get the next baby out so we can get the next woman on the table, and so on. When I was able to work in an out-of-hospital setting in the United States and see how individual the births could be and how each family had their own way of handling and guiding their birth, my heart sang—it was such a privilege to be able to see that. The cultural mores, the family traditions, the standing for independence that I saw in the women whom I served doing home birth in Florida opened my eyes to a whole different way of being and living and a whole different way of practicing. And even though those influences came later in my midwifery career, they shaped and molded me into the midwife that I am today, more than twenty-six years later.

I learned to be a good midwife from my original teacher in England. She was a dear lady, and at the time I thought she was quite ancient. I was nineteen, so she was probably all of forty! She told me one thing that I have never forgotten—that I wouldn't make it in midwifery because I didn't have enough patience. Imagine! My approach was, "Well I will show you." And I am still doing that today because she was right. I really don't have much patience, but I love this work so much that I have managed to put that particular character flaw aside when it comes to being with women and being with birth. She also taught me to keep my hands in my pockets, which is quite a challenge inside of a hospital environment. I thought I was doing exceptionally well with that until I came to the United States and *really* saw what it meant to keep my hands in my pockets. I learned the skills from watching women birth their babies. They taught me more than I ever learned in a hospital or from a textbook. I am a very good teacher myself; I can *teach* midwives, I can *train* midwives, but I learned how to *be* a midwife from the women.

I remember a birth I did in Florida when I first arrived—with a woman who had more faith in me than I had in myself. She was determined that she was going to have a home birth. She was also determined I was going to be her midwife. And I had never experienced that kind of thing before. I was used to being paid to do my job at a hospital where we all understand the nature of the transaction; you show up in labor and a midwife delivers your baby. This, however, was quite a different approach. She asked me specifically, she solicited my services; she encouraged and cajoled me into taking on this work *with* her. She viewed me and spoke to me as an equal partner in this work. And that was a dynamic that I had never really experienced. When she labored I watched her. She sat on the floor cross-legged and she rocked and she moaned; and she moaned and she rocked; and she rotated her body in a circular movement, and she chanted, and she rocked, and she moaned some more. Her contraction would build and she would rock and move and moan louder, and her sounds would wane as the contraction went away. I just sat in awe of this woman doing this work and managing her birth. No questions, no "Can you? Will you? Can I? Should I?" Nothing. She just managed her birth. And as she got closer to having her baby, she got her self situated in the position she wanted to be in and she pushed her baby out, and even though I was there to help guide her, she knew what she was doing and just got on with it. I never had seen anything like that before and realized then that women *knew* how to have their babies. At the same time I realized it wasn't about me. What a revelation!

I have seen women do any number of things in labor; things that they had no clue they were going to do, things that I would never have imagined that they were going to do, yet their bodies would guide them and they would find their way. I have seen women fighting and railing against their contractions. I have seen them open and accepting their contractions. I have seen them frantic and scared. I have seen them overjoyed. I have seen everything—a complete gamut of emotions. I have seen the power and the ability of women as this exceptional event takes place. I have been privileged to be part of that and to witness that and to be with that. That has been my addiction ever since I first saw it.

I delivered my own son twenty-two years ago in an English hospital with a midwife. Midwives, I should say, were part of a system not unlike midwives in American hospitals, and the shift changes and the busyness at the time confused me such that I don't know who actually delivered my child. I was already a midwife myself at the time. I was working from the paradigm of already knowing everything there was to know about midwifery because I had been a midwife for five years. So as I got close to delivering my baby, I was quite sure I knew what to do. I had been teaching classes to women so they would know what to do, so I knew what to do, too. And my birth took me totally by surprise. Now in retrospect, I am also surprised at how little I took on in terms of being involved and being a part of my own birth. I birthed my child within a system that said it was okay to hand over the experience, albeit to another midwife, but hand it over, regardless. So when my water broke before my labor started, I thought that I was just going to fall right into labor, but I didn't. My water broke on a Tuesday night and I delivered my son on Thursday morning. I had the most drawn out, excruciating, posterior primigravid labor that you could imagine. I decided halfway through that I was going to die. I decided that everybody was wicked and mean. I decided that nobody had ever experienced anything like this before! But what happened for me when I delivered my son was the realization of how very powerful I was. I remember thinking that without that birth I would have never become the midwife that I am now. The experience allowed me to realize that I had no clue what I was talking about when I was teaching women about how to have a baby. I was able to teach from a different perspective after that. I was able to sympathize and empathize. Without experiencing that birth I would have had no base from which to teach, from which to support, from which to share. I was able to recognize that no matter how bad it is, you survive it; you come out the other end. It gave me courage when working with long labors to help women to know that it would finish, that the baby truly would be born. It gave me a place from which I could really relate to other women. It influenced me enough so that even though I continued for another five years working in the hospital, I was able to develop the individualization of care that has now become such an integral part of how I do my work here in the U.S., at this time and in this place.

It is difficult for me to say how being a midwife changed my life because—for my entire adult life—I have not been anything else but a midwife. If I look at the impact of midwifery on my life, then midwifery has indeed taken its toll in many ways. But it has also given me such reason to be, to have joy, to keep going—such empowerment and ability to know why I get up everyday. The real toll it has taken has been on my family. Midwifery took precedence over everything in my life; midwifery took precedence over me, myself. I lost myself in midwifery. I became Jennie-the-Midwife, and neglected Jennie-the-Person. I neglected my husband and my son in pursuing my passion. If anything, midwifery changed my life in the possibility that if I wasn't a midwife, there might have been more balance in my life. So going forward is a challenge. But that is also my goal: to still be this midwife-person serving women and to do what I love to do, but with balance and to find ME to birth ME because it's my turn now.

Being a midwife involves taking risks. As a Florida midwife, I took on many risks. I took on that I would be a maverick working outside of a system that says normal is physician care, normal is hospital care, normal is surgery, and normal is pathology. And in saying no to that, I took on women who were willing to go outside the system. Yet I took on, sometimes, risky women in order to help support what they wanted and allow them the opportunity to do what they needed to do. But putting me in that situation was foolish, and luckily I have had no repercussions. As for fear, I have never been scared in the process of being a midwife, whether delivering, advocating, pioneering or campaigning. Perhaps that is why I love it so.

The most important lesson I have learned has been to let things unfold, to allow the birth to take its course, to allow the women to have their way. Being a support and being there were so much more important than any medical, technical wizardry that I could use. I have learned that women are strong. I have learned that women are hardy, that women have power. I have learned—and I know inherently—that every woman wants a healthy baby, no matter who she is. Every woman wants a healthy baby, no matter what she is doing, no matter what she is saying, no matter what she looks like. *Every woman wants a healthy baby and every woman deserves one.* And that is what I know.

In the United States the power of the hospitals, medical establishments, insurance companies and physicians, along with the impact of racism, classism and sexism have greatly influenced midwifery and the position we find ourselves in today. Women have bought in to the idea that they cannot deliver their babies their way. They have been duped into believing that they have no say, so much so that the majority do not even see that there is anything actually wrong with the current maternity care system in the USA. The midwifery movement has, therefore, been a fringe "alternative health care movement", an unusual aberration, something that has been looked upon as quite unnecessary and just not suitable for the majority of the population. People that choose midwives are seen to be bucking society, going against the grain, putting their children at risk, doing it because they don't have any money, or insurance, or just plain being foolish. I don't believe that is the case. But I see how the society has been able to make that stand. It is all about education, after all. It is also about having the midwifery movement be uniform, be united, be strong and be safe so we can continue to present ourselves powerfully to our constituents, the women and families of America. One of the things that I am very clear about is that midwifery needs to be all-inclusive, that inside of the profession we don't find ourselves with the same issues to deal with: politics, racism, classism and so on. So we have a challenge, because in our education of the public we need to be able to show uniformity and cohesiveness about what we do and why we do it, and how the benefits can be enjoyed by *every* person in every facet of society in the United States. From the day I arrived on these shores and realized what was happening in America, I have fought for women of color and families of color to be able to have the chance for normal, healthy birthing and have outcomes that, at the very least, match the general population in the country. As I have learned and understood the history of Black midwives in the United States, my heart has been broken and has not yet been healed. Because as the Black midwives were eradicated from providing the community services that they provided from slavery times onward, the situation has become dire for Black mothers and infants in the United States. And sad to say, many people in the African American community do not even know that this has happened and that it is still happening now. They do not understand the detrimental impact that losing their community midwives has had on their communities' health. I fight that battle daily, continually, because it has to be fought.

As long as we have a situation where two to four times as many Black babies as White babies are born prematurely or too small, or are dying before they reach the age of one, then I have to fight. As long as Black mothers—regardless of their age, economic status or educational levels—are nearly four times as likely to die in childbirth nationwide as their White counterparts, then I have to fight. As long as we have these health disparities, then I have to fight. And as long as people do not know about these deplorable statistics, then I have to fight.

When I started working in the field of infant mortality, specifically Black infant health, I had no idea how very deep the problem was, how the roots of the situation have been so firmly positioned that it has become okay for that kind of statistic to stand. People say "Oh dear, I didn't know" as if that is enough, and actually do not have any agenda or interest in it changing. Well it has to change. Even if the situation worsens, as it tends to where African American infant mortality is concerned, nothing tangible happens in terms of really addressing it. So having taken on that cause, and having fought long and hard, I can now say that I have a system and a situation, at least inside of my own practice, that has been proven to make a difference in effectively reducing those disparities. In my midwifery practice I run an outreach clinic for indigent women alongside of the birthing center, and over many years we have had very few low birth weight babies. On the average our babies weigh seven and a half pounds. The average gestation is thirty-nine weeks, and even women who do not choose to deliver with us in the birthing center but prefer a hospital birth, do well. A 2007 Study was conducted on one hundred of the women in my clinic who were at risk for poor birth outcomes. I am so very proud to say that the study proved what we already knew: No low birth weight or premature babies were born to African American or Latina women enrolled in the study. In contrast, the U.S. rate of low birth weight for infants of all races at that time was about 7%, and approximately 14% for African American infants. In addition, the national prematurity rate hovers around 12% for all races, and is up to nearly 18% for African American infants. So we know that what we do is making a substantial difference. I have developed a system of maternity care called The JJ Way™, which has been studied and evaluated as a best practice maternal and child health care model. This model can be translated into clinic settings, family practice settings, HMOs, any practice where practitioners are willing to change just a few ideas about how they provide prenatal care for women. These few tenets and using a midwifery-based model of maternity care have made the difference, literally, between life and death for risky pregnancies.

I consider it one of my most significant accomplishments. The JJ Way™ incorporates four main tenets, which I believe are essential for healthy outcomes across the board. The first is ACCESS. Without this we can achieve nothing. If a client cannot find her way into our care, then she cannot avail herself of what we have to offer. I implemented an 'Easy Access' approach to my practice: regardless of ability to pay, you will be seen for an initial prenatal visit. The second tenet, therefore, is CONNECTION. Once I have you present, my goal is to establish and support a connection, a bond, between you and your unborn baby, your provider(s) and whichever helping agencies are necessary to ensure the healthiest possible outcome for your pregnancy. The third tenet is KNOWLEDGE—teaching a woman and her supporters about pregnancy birth and beyond, helping her in practical, meaningful ways, and reaching her at her level leads to the fourth tenet, EMPOWERMENT. With true listening and encouragement throughout their pregnancy, women develop their own sense of power and control and make the best choices for themselves, their families and ultimately their communities.

I have also accomplished a method of delivering babies that I feel very strongly has had a positive impact on how things have turned out for my clients. I have developed ways and maneuvers, certain systems that have helped me, where had I not done things that way the outcomes may have been different. I feel that I have accomplished the acquisition of skills and techniques that came through experience. I want to have my program made available to everybody and anybody. I want to have people using and working in my system—the JJ Way™ system. I want to teach the midwives how I do my little techniques and procedures. I want to share my knowledge and my experience. I feel like America has not embraced midwifery totally, fully, and completely. Yet we are making headway.

I am definitely passing the torch to younger midwives because, as I have become older, I have realized that I cannot do what I want to do all the time, every time. I have also realized once again that it is not about me. It is about empowering others. I so much enjoy working with and teaching younger midwives. I realize the pride that comes with seeing those midwives grow and become accomplished and independent. The *Sage Femme* wisdom I would pass on to younger midwives is to totally be yourself, develop your own way, incorporate what you have learned, but just *be yourself.*

The image that best describes me is a passionate and fervent activist. I am an instigator, workaholic and totally driven. I can no more NOT do what I do than fly. I HAVE to do what I am doing. I have to be involved with working in this field—working with the women and families, changing and improving, and redirecting the path of midwifery in the United States. The image I seek for myself is peaceful, settled, balanced and accomplished, and yet I also know that I haven't got there yet. So it is difficult for me to describe myself. I recognize that the change, the development of me as a person, as a woman, continues to mirror the development of midwifery in the United States. So, perhaps I am in transition now, wise enough to finally realize that yes, *I* am about to be born, willing to let go and breathe myself out gently and softly . . . do you see the head?

The American public has been hoodwinked

MAKEDA KAMARA

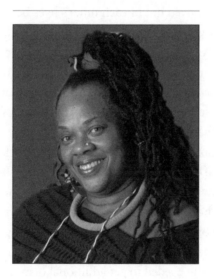

I grew up in a tightly-knit Afro Antillano community in Panama in Santa Cruz, a small, segregated section of Gamboa in the Panama Canal Zone. I am the youngest of five children born to Gladstone and Ometa Millett, a third generation migrant worker family that has followed the imperialist job market since being brought to the shores of the New World. Gamboa was often referred to as "a town behind God's back" due to its perceived remoteness from the city. One still has to cross a one-lane bridge to get there. Gamboa, located at the mouth of the Chagres River, was dammed to form Gatun Lake and is an integral part of the Panama Canal Zone. When younger, I wasn't aware that I lived in a rainforest, a place that has the largest biodiversity of butterflies in the world. Right now Gamboa is a big hub of eco-tourism in Panama. But back then it was just home. We are known as *Afrocaribeños* or *Afroantillanos*, the second wave of Africans brought to Panama. The Colonial Africans were brought over during the fourteenth century. As a matter of fact, one of the first slave revolts in the New World took place in Panama in 1512. Panama, because it runs east-west and joins north-south, was a big hub of getting slaves from one place to the next. The second wave of Africans came from the Caribbean to build the Panama Canal around the turn of the nineteenth century. That's where my family came from. My great-grandparents were brought over to build the canal. They were the diggers and builders of the Eighth Wonder of the World. Ours was a very close-knit community of around five hundred people; we lived out of each other's lives because we knew that we only had each other. It was there that I learned that individual freedom is bound by group responsibility. You simply can't do what you want to do irrespective of others and your community. I learned the importance of family, kinship and extended family. It was a very poignant time and a special time in history. We were—and I was—raised by the village. Who you were was not based on what you had but by your character.

My mother, like most of the women in my community, knew about herbs and healing. She had lots of expert knowledge regarding birth, breastfeeding, healing herbs and what we now call attachment parenting. Seeing women breastfeed and hearing a baby being born during the night were the norms. I just thought that was the way of the world. I recall being badly burned by an explosion of our kerosene stove. It was bush tea, cocoa butter, home remedies and TLC that cured me. Mom knew when she needed to get additional help and when it was within her reign. Bush tea of some sort was the medicine *du jour*. It also helped that we ate only what was in season. It amazed me when I came to the U.S. that all sorts of fruits and veggies were available all the time and able to be stored for long periods without spoiling.

Midwifery was definitely a calling; and it has definitely been a journey. As a kid I wanted to be a teacher. I remember my mother bringing a blackboard home once from her work as a domestic up the "White people's hill." I was in my glory. My friends and neighbors became my students and I the teacher. Midwifery definitely was not on the radar screen. Although in retrospect, teaching and sharing with women and families is what we do. I miss my hometown very much. It no longer exists as a place, but it exists in our hearts and souls. My life there gave me the foundation for a life of service and community. Through my mother and her *comadres* (co-mothers) I learned that when you struck a woman, you struck a rock, I learned to love and trust women, and most importantly I learned to live lightly on the planet. We weren't rich materially, but we were rich spiritually; I never thought of myself as poor. I had everything I needed: a very loving mom, wonderful siblings who blazed a remarkable path for me to follow, and a village that nurtured and educated me and helped shaped my character. Yeah, that little town behind Goddess' back in the rain forest at the Chagres River was a little piece of heaven on earth.

I migrated to Brooklyn, New York, in October of 1966. It was quite scary. We had all imagined that the U.S. was like paradise—the land of milk and honey. Reality is a trip. Brooklyn was definitely a concrete jungle, cold and unfriendly. Worst yet, teenage girls didn't play after coming home from school—there was no community, no sports and my mother wasn't there. The Black world was changing: the anti-colonial movement in the Caribbean and Africa was taking hold, and the Civil Rights Movement in the U.S. influenced us all. I proudly remember winning a prize in the eighth grade for a paper celebrating the independence of Trinidad and Tobago. We all had been proud of Ghana's independence. As fate had it, I ended up at Brandeis University in 1968 after Martin Luther King was assassinated on April 4, and many of the White universities opened their previously closed doors to qualified Black students. That window of opportunity opened, and I happened to be in the right place at the right time. I became involved in the Black Power Movement and ended up going to Africa after graduating from college. It was there in Africa, in Tanzania, that I got the calling to become a midwife/healer, changing the world one baby at a time from an extraordinary friendship and experience.

I stayed with exiled former Black Panther members living in Dar es Salaam, Tanzania. One of the sisters was pregnant and had an unassisted home birth with such ease. A seed had been planted and a strong mental note imprinted in my soul. I then moved to Weru Weru village outside Moshi, the second largest town in young Tanzania. Moshi is the home of Mt. Kilimanjaro. How blessed to shower every morning and see its majestic peaks. Weru Weru is about seven or eight miles outside the town. Then it was a distance to maneuver. Without access to get to the market and the one and only food store, my access to meat, dairy, soft drinks, and so on was nil. Noticeable changes in my health began manifesting. I met this beautiful sister from the village and we became good friends. We couldn't speak each other's language but communicated through gesticulations and spiritually. I had found a community and a woman friend. I would go with her in the evenings and gather around the village bonfire listening to stories I couldn't understand but could feel the nuance of, and listen to drums and participate in dancing. Through her I was able to witness my first birth; it was history after that. I just knew that that was meant for me. A seed had been planted. In Tanzania I learned a lot. My experience there added to my sense of community and purpose. Mwalimu Julius Nyerere, the president at the time and father of African Socialism—"each one teach one"—had transformed his country from a trusteeship with high illiteracy rate to a country with wide literacy through an education campaign. He devised an educational system that was African-centered. His motto was that education was not for high-powered jobs but for service in building young Tanzania and Africa. I moved to Uganda after finishing my contract in Tanzania and there I continued teaching. Uganda, known then as the pearl of Africa, is located over 5000 feet above sea level on the equator. It is the source of the river Nile and has to be one of the most beautiful places on earth. I also had an opportunity to work in Africa Basic Foods (ABF). ABF was a company started by Dr. Williams, an African American doctor who had lived and worked with Kwame Nkrumah—one of the fathers of Pan Africanism and the first president of Ghana. The goal of the company was to combat *kwashiorkor* (severe malnutrition) with soy-based foods to complement local diets. This further nurtured my interest in midwifery, maternal and child health and nutrition. I became a vegetarian and avidly studied the relationship between diet, exercise, spirituality and well-being. I had gone to the Motherland wanting to be a historian and returned with a calling from the Most High. My identity had been crystallized and my passion stoked; midwifery, healing arts, public health was my path.

Prior to my trip to Africa, I had been accepted to Harvard Graduate School of Education but deferred entrance until my return. After graduation, I taught high school at Roxbury Community College before moving to Ann Arbor, Michigan, in 1976 to pursue my degree in public health. There were several concurrent events occurring at this time, whose leaders had been affected by the Black Power struggles: The Women's Liberation Movement, the natural foods movement, vegetarianism, alternative birth movement, anti-apartheid movement, Rastafarian movement and the rise of vibrant up-and-coming post colonial African and Caribbean nations. All those movements affected my vision shaping my midwifery walk.

I got involved with Ann Arbor Safe Alternatives to Childbirth, setting up women's feminist health centers, and the Afrocentric Women's Health movement in Detroit, Michigan. However, my mainstay was the continued evolution of our freedom struggle here in the West. A focused Afrocentric cultural and political movement was rapidly evolving and the cultural community in Detroit was a vibrant one. Many of the movements in the White progressive sector did not intersect or coalesce with the Black movement at this point in time. In fact, many of them were parallel movements. A lot of changes were happening in White America with the changes in the draft laws around military service; college education was no longer valid deferment. Hence, White middle and upper class youth were being drafted. The Black Power Movement gave life to the Women's Liberation Movement (many of the women involved had honed their organizing skills in the Civil Rights Movement.) While there were people of African descent involved in midwifery, our reasons and aims were informed by different experiences. Ours was forged as a struggle against genocide, unequal health care, unconscionable acts against Blacks and other people of color for "medical" science and freedom. In Detroit, the Pan African Congress Division of Health had Uzazi Chama (an Afrocentric approach to childbirth education). Many were choosing home birth and breastfeeding along with a repudiation of the racism and poor maternity care. Our aim was to stem the genocide in our communities and strengthen our families with natural living and childbirth practices—getting back to our roots. Many of us no longer felt safe using the existing medical institutions available to us. My first births were born from the trust of the women that I could "do it." As Umsalama, my big sister, once aptly stated, "We were dumb and lucky." I just read a how-to book for my first births.

My partner at the time was vehemently opposed to my getting involved in midwifery. "Why get involved in something illegal?" he said. "Why not become a doctor?" I couldn't get him to understand the differences. While I understood his and his family's concerns, I was on a mission.

In 1983 the Childcare Providers of Afrikan Descent (CPAD) held their yearly conference a few days before the Black Women's Health Project's first national conference in Atlanta, Georgia. It was a life altering experience; sisters on a journey. Umsalama (Sondra Abdullah of CPAD) had arranged a workshop for us with The Farm Midwives in Tennessee. Any doubts that I had about my calling were eliminated during those aforementioned experiences. The problem then was the how: *Which path? How do I find a preceptor? How can I leave to go to the few midwifery schools around at that time? How…?*

Despite the existence of home birth, it was difficult for African American women to find midwifery apprenticeships. There was much subtle racism in White progressives. However, with the urgency of our mission and on the backs of the Grand Midwives and our ancestors, I knew that I had to persevere, regardless of the obstacles. I decided to continue self-study and apprenticeships but also to pursue nurse-midwifery to increase the accessibility of midwives to our sisters in our communities. That affirmation now in the universe, I went to The Farm workshop. I can remember my initial hesitancy the first time I went to The Farm. But the work and spirit of The Farm folk was genuine. I fell in love with Ina May, her family, The Farm and its people who were working on creating a new tribe with a different set of material and social relations. My ancestors, Mother, our struggle, the Continent, my early life experiences, first births, love of humanity and Goddess spirit within me: all have and continue to guide my life.

In learning to be a good midwife, my first realization was the simplicity and unique normality of birth and how complicated we have made it by trying to improve it. Despite our love of technology, what humanity has created only functions at 30% efficiency when compared to the body's functions. Birth is a fine-tuned process evolved over thousands of years. I came from a town where there was no fear around birth. It was just a part of life as was breastfeeding. Women nursing freely in the open were the norm and the expected. Handling of babies was restricted not only to the birth mother but the community as well. Even at eight-years old I was taking care of the neighbor's babies. I remember this baby girl's birth that took place one night in my building. I couldn't wait to come home from school to go pick her up and bring her outside. That kind of responsibility and trust from the adults reinforced the normalcy of childbirth and childrearing.

How ironic that we dreamed of coming to the "world" (U.S.) without realizing how much more of a natural rhythm of life we had. Physiologic female phases were not medicalized or made to be seen as a curse. Yes, I had dysmenorrhea but my menstruation was not a curse just a part a woman's life as is birth, breastfeeding, nurturing, and so on. As my knowledge of nutrition and lifestyle choices in relationship to menstruation widened, I further embraced my menses as a center of power of my woman's expert knowledge. All the centers of our power as women have been medicalized and perceived as an accident waiting to happen. How can we tap our gifts if we cannot tap our sources of power and strength? Imagine a world in which women embrace the sacredness of the phases of their lives, and babies were born peacefully with their souls intact? In such a world, our children would be born without violence and would be intolerant to the injustices in the world to which many of us, today, are desensitized. The safeguarding and protection of women and babies are essential to justice and peace on earth. The resources of the earth are plentiful; no one needs to suffer if all things are equal and our connectedness in this chain is the norm.

There's a wonderful book I read in the 1970s by Jean Liedoff, called *The Continuum Concept*. She's a medical anthropologist who studied birth among an indigenous group in South America. Here in the U.S. we are always living in so much fear of what may happen. But one of the things Liedoff learned when observing birth and childcare was what she called "the continuum concept." In the Stone Age jungle culture to which she returned four times, she observed that children were allowed to flourish, based on their own interconnectedness with family members, activities of daily life, and the environment. Thus they didn't feel the need to constantly fear that something would harm the children. They strongly believed that babies and children were part of life's continuum and thus can sense imminent danger.

In 1993, I finally finished my nurse-midwifery studies after an on-and-off, thirteen-year journey, which included my children's births and nurturing, self-study, home birth practice and apprenticing with midwives here in the U.S. and in Africa. It was a great experience. The initial period of midwifery rebirth in the '70s was electric. There was a lot more autonomy. The Midwives Alliance of North America (MANA) and the Childcare Providers of Afrikan Descent (CPAD) were born and growing. There was a dramatic change in childbirth and breastfeeding practices in the U.S. It was still only a very small percentage of the population who birthed at home. Sitting at the table and affecting a wider sphere of influence on birth was part of the vision of MANA. How to do it without loss of autonomy was a slippery slope. How do you institute standards of care, seek reimbursement, define educational paths to midwifery, and a woman's right to choose? For us in Africa-America, how do we coalesce while increasing the critical mass of African American midwives and sitting at the table as equal partners in the movement? Even more simply, how can we create an environment of trust so that we can work for the common good of all women? My mantra whilst on MANA's Board of Directors was to open our struggle to the citizenry through grassroots organizing. I insisted that it was important to struggle on many levels at the same time. My experience as an African descendant in the U.S. meant that I constantly had to be on guard *vis á vis* the system. The power structure has an uncanny ability to adopt, become adept at and redefine concepts to suits its purposes. That's how it maintains power and control. This is essentially what happened to successes and changes from the struggles of the '70s. Childbirth classes, birth assistants and many of our hard-fought victories of the past are redefined and offered in hospitals the country over. They no longer resemble what they were. Surgical deliveries are now becoming the norm, VBACs (vaginal birth after cesarean) are not allowed, and physiologic births are a rarity. The lack of unity of vision and turf issues among CPMs, CNMs, and CMs has weakened our collective power. Birth centers are closing, CNM hospital-based practices are closing and manner of practicing has been altered. There is restriction on our trade. The majority of African American midwives cannot find jobs despite representing only 2% of the total pool of CNMs. I was one of the founding mothers of the Cambridge Birth Center in Cambridge, Massachusetts. At the time (1990s), we provided approximately 70% of the births at the hospital. The birth center still exists, but its transfer rate to the hospital is high; family practice doctors and obstetricians now do most of the births in the hospital, and surgical deliveries have increased from about 14% to over 30%. In another major urban city hospital in Boston, midwives are forced to have a "collaborative" practice with physicians or lose their practice. A woman can have prenatal care with a midwife in the community health centers but can't be assured of a midwifery delivery in the hospital. The midwives must supervise residents in the delivery. At first it was a choice, but now it is "or else." The sad part is the lack of choice for the unsuspecting women. The "powers that be" wrested control and definition of the movement because of our lack of collective unity as midwives, our inability to build grassroots citizen supports, and lack of autonomy in our profession. Once CNMs were allowed to practice in hospitals, we did not fight for complete autonomy to expand our base of support or to ally with our other sister midwives. The litigious nature of our society is a great concern to me as is the increasing prenatal screening in the case of "what ifs" that breeds fear in childbirth. Even in home births, families want reassurance. Another concern is our lack of business sense as midwives. I personally am not as good at the business part of our profession as I should have been at this stage. I am learning as I get older, but it might be too late. I wish I'd been more savvy in my youth. *Ces't la vie.*

Midwifery has also allowed me to see that as long as I'm on this Earth, breathing air and drinking water, and marveling in all the different wonders and miracles of the universe, I have a responsibility to leave this world a much more beautiful place than how I found it. That it is my human responsibility. First, one has to have a vision that makes a difference and is spiritually grounded. That vision must be disciplined and trained in service and sacrifice to the Most High. That vision modifies and transforms one's personal and group behavior. As a midwife, even though I feel like everyone should be able to have a physiologic birth without intervention, I think what's important is that I've learned that even if a birth doesn't go the way that I think that it ought to have gone, that a woman's choice ought to be respected and it's all part of the process. You just have to go with the flow. I've learned to be more humble realizing that it's not about me. My job is to accept my responsibility as a steward of the unique normality of birth as a primary mammalian experience. I think it has made me a much better human being, given me a capacity to be free.

I had a lot of resistance from my inner circle in my midwifery walk. Folk wanted me to become a doctor. Why be a midwife when you can be a doctor? I wanted to be a midwife. They are two distinct professions. They come from different vantage points. And even today I sometimes think, wow I should have just gone on and become a doctor, I wouldn't have to be going through a lot of the B.S. that midwives have to go through having to always validate their existence. But if I'd gone that route, I know that my education and my world-view would have been different. To be *with woman* through the life cycle is my calling. Even today, I see birth as only a small part of the scope of a midwife's practice. Returning an equal balance between the matriarchy and patriarchy is part of the midwife's role also. Not only women's lives, but men and children's lives and the Earth's life are being held captive by this existing imbalance. Being a midwife means all of these things together because midwives of the past were not only there for women during childbirth, they were social workers, public health workers, educators, health care providers, they defied unjust laws and rulings. In Africa and during the epoch of the Grand Midwives in the U.S., midwives had esteemed roles in their communities because of the various capacities in which they served. I wouldn't change that because, even today I feel in my own way, I serve in these different capacities in my own community. I wouldn't trade that for anything in the world. It is risky, midwives are judged harsher than OB/GYN providers, we are under much more scrutiny, and we are still not an autonomous profession here in the United States. We are still, constantly, not only fighting for existence but also fighting to salvage the unique normality of birth. With all this technology that we have people tend to forget that we've only been driving cars for just over a hundred years. But we as humanity have been around for millions of years so birth is a process that has been fine-tuned. It works most of the time whether someone's there or not. Yet, as a society, we value and have more trust in things—our iPods, our cell phones—than something that has sustained human-ity since the beginning of time. It doesn't make sense!

The struggle against patriarchy has impacted the modern midwifery movement; midwifery is basically women's work. And over the years we've had capitalism, feudalism and all these isms and schisms that are based on the patriarchy. In some ancient African cultures, the patriarchy and the matriarchy coexisted harmoniously. Among the Akan, Nubian, Meroe and many of the matrilineal cultures in Africa, a midwife's role was an honored one. As a result of slavery, colonization and imperialism we know very little of the mother culture of Africa from whence we all came.

I have a friend, the former ambassador of Grenada to the United Nations who is now a professor at Brandeis University, Dessima Williams, PhD. She wrote an article in the Boston Globe a few years ago about worldwide economics. She wrote that there was over 363 trillion dollars made in the world economy from unpaid labor, 70% of which was women's work. So it's really a question of power, control and definition. Sexism affects women's work. Women are sometimes the biggest offenders. We have bought the ticket. Just like how we as Africans and African descendants have internalized racism in a negative way and turned it against ourselves in the form of self-hate, women have internalized sexism. Worldwide midwives have various definitions of who we are: TBAs (Traditional Birth Assistants), CNMs, CPMs, etc. We have all these degrees of separation. This to me is just a reflection of the kind of dissonance that's created by the baggage of powerless groups.

The most important life lessons that I have learned over the years while practicing midwifery is the willingness to know that I am part of something bigger than just myself. When you are part of a birth and the woman gets connected to her Goddess energy and all is still; everyone present becomes transfixed and is forever changed by the power unleashed by the birth. Whatever your spiritual or religious belief; whatever your name for the universal consciousness that governs us (Jehovah, God, Goddess, Yahweh, Allah, Buddha, etc.), birth as designed by evolution is a transcending experience. One leaves there not believing but knowing there is a Goddess—something bigger than us.

For me, as a Black midwife, even within the context of women owning their births, I have to look at the fact that here in the United States, Black babies still continue to die three to one compared to White babies. Our babies have less of a chance of surviving because they are born prematurely, have low birth weight and our mothers regardless of class, education or income are at risk. As an African descendant midwife my role is to flip this switch by struggling to eliminate the social and racial determinants of health. I thought that there was going to be a real change in America after the civil rights, Black liberation and antiwar movements of the '70s. I just knew we were moving toward structural change but the paper tiger has rebounded. Yet I take faith in Gandhi's words. In history there have always been tyrants and despots, but they always fall. One simply has to commit to non-cooperation with unjust laws and be willing to accept the consequences of one's action. Many of the social changes that have occurred in the U.S. such as, public education, voting rights, women's rights, all came from Black sociopolitical movements. White women have benefited more from affirmative action than Black people have, but public perception is different.

One of the things I hope to see someday is a midwife for every mother. I hope to see a much more responsible society that takes care of its mothers, youth, elders, that respects and honors the reproductive rights of women, and their families. A baby that is attached to its family will be attached to its community, nation and world. There is an organization called the World Association for Breastfeeding, which looks at breastfeeding as a reproductive right and breast milk as a natural resource. It is a way of redefining value because if breast milk is viewed as a natural resource, and women produce that resource, then women should be paid for women's work. Norway, after studying breast milk as a natural resource, went on a countrywide education campaign to all segments of society and computed its worth as part of the gross national product. They also instituted some structural guarantees and incentives for women and their families. Women attending the International Confederation of Midwives triennial conference in Norway in 1983 were amazed that the discussion on national TV about the Prime Minister (who was a woman and pregnant at the time) was not about how she will govern, but rather, how she was going to fulfill her breastfeeding responsibilities. What better way to insure your nation's prosperity and future than to invest in mother, babies and families?

We have MacDonaldized birth. The American public has been had, they've been hoodwinked. We cannot have babies and have women believe that in six weeks they can resume the life they had before. I've had the opportunity to be a participant in over a thousand births during a twenty-five-year span. Each has been different with its own twist on normality. Presently as Director of the Imani Family Life Center, my aim is to use birth and women's health to bring families and communities closer. We offer various services that address the needs of families, including direct care. I hope to use my organization as a grassroots vehicle to increase awareness of the social, political and economic determinants that form and shape our lives, seeking solutions to disparities in health care, birth and breastfeeding. Our mission is to use the awareness garnered through the organization to create small living democracies in our community, which will create a ripple effect throughout the larger culture. To quote Exodus 1:20, "God made the midwives prosper and the people increased in number and in strength." I believe that we are the ones we've been waiting for.

When it comes to younger midwives, my advice is patience, humility but most of all love. During the early years of midwifery you were chosen by older midwives who sensed the "calling" in you or you were "called" to it. If I had any nugget of wisdom it is that it has to come from the heart. This is not an easy path. Trust the process without being cavalier; know your circle of safety. It is important that you remember that it is not about you. You can't take credit for the good births or the bad births. You are only the hands of the Most High, I daresay, and stand on the spiritual nature of this noble profession. Asoka Roy, a CNM from India and the midwife to the Gandhi family whom I had the honor to stay with during a Midwifery Today Conference, shared some pearls with me. It was her humility and love of GODDESS that shone in her that most impressed me. Midwifery is something that you have to love to do. And it has to be tied with one's social, political and spiritual consciousness, humility, and respect for women and for the family. Birth belongs to families and the community. Birth is a manifestation of the culture. How you are born and how you cross over is cultural and reflective of society's values. As a midwife, you are welcomed by a family to share in a very transforming, spiritual moment. So you really have to be very humble and understand why you're there. Regardless of your beliefs, it is not your birth. You are the invited guest in an untenable situation. You are there to honor that family's choice doing work over which you have no professional autonomy. You are caught between a rock and a hard place. So you've got to be willing to fight, to struggle. You know there's a lot of joy, and a lot of pleasure, but you also have to be prepared to struggle.

I never see myself as a wise woman. I just think that the longer you are on the planet you have a history that feeds your wisdom. However, I know a lot of older unwise folk so it's not a given that all who have eyes will see. I have had an opportunity to be invited into the lives of some remarkable people. I always say that I am just as good as the woman and families I serve. I am always very grateful that my ladies have taken me in, they and their families have trusted me, and I've become their friend. I have this one family in particular that I've been a midwife to for at least twenty years. They are a family of seven, and I was the midwife for the last four children and I can remember going to that family and seeing those children grow up. I think the youngest is maybe fifteen now, and the amount of love that I have gotten from that family, I can't even say it in words. I can recall during my lows going to their home knowing I'd be met with lots of love. I just feel very grateful for the women that I've served and how they have made me become a better human being. I am grateful that they have shared with me, they've allowed me to grow, they have loved me and they have allowed me to love them, and our lives have become intertwined and forever changed. Recently I attended a dance conference in New York and saw this woman. I said, "Your face looks so familiar." She said to me, "you delivered my baby." And I said, "I did?" And she said, "Yeah, nine years ago." She said, "We were in dance class together and I was pregnant and you came over and you rubbed my belly and said 'you're having your baby with a midwife, right?' And I looked at you and said, 'no I'm seeing a doctor.' And you said to me 'honey, you need a midwife' and the next day, I called my doctor and came to see you, and in a month we had the baby together." I looked perplexed. She said, "Oh you probably don't remember me because I didn't have locks at the time and moved to DC." I said, "I may not have remembered your name or your face but I remembered your spirit because the minute I saw you I knew there was a connection." Boston is a really small place and when I go to the store and I see my women and families I'm just happy. You cannot convince them that you are not their doctor; they say, "Oh there's my doctor." In the play, *Mississippi Delta*, the lead woman was called a "doctor midwife." I guess my ladies see me like that. In the tradition of the old Grand Midwives: Maude Collins, Onnie Logan, Gladys Milton, Phyllis Carter and all these great midwives that came before me on whose shoulders I stand; my Mother—Chichi Millett, grandmother (Sarah Elizabeth), my aunt (Rosana Alvaranza) and the powerful women in Santa Cruz, Gamboa whose determination and courage helped shape my spirit; I say *asante sana* for all the love. The Grand Midwives who delivered all those babies under unfathomable circumstances are the real wise women. I'm just humbled to even be mentioned in that company, because they are the *Kentakes* (Queen Mothers) whose tradition of struggle, humility, service and sacrifice continues to inform my midwifery path...*La luta continua*. We will win. It is the victory of good over evil.

She is the center

ABBY J. KINNE

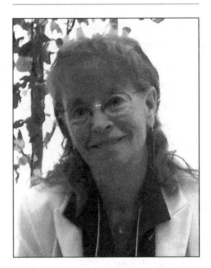

I grew up in Glenside, a small suburb of Philadelphia, Pennsylvania. My father was a brilliant chemical engineer from Philadelphia, who knew more about more things than anyone I have ever known. I adored and admired him. My mother was a very Victorian "lady" from the Deep South, born in New Orleans. My parents met at the University of Heidelberg in Baden-Württemberg, Germany, where my mother was studying to be a translator and organist. She spent several years in pre-World War II Germany learning German by living with a local family. I have one brother, two years older than I, but as a child, he was seriously ill with asthma, so in many ways I was treated more like a firstborn and often left to my own devices.

Although we only saw my maternal grandmother once a year, she had a tremendous influence on my life. Unlike my mother, she had a no nonsense approach to life and a keen interest in medicine. Her dream for her two daughters was that they would become a dentist and a pediatrician. Although neither one followed her lead for long, I felt her presence and approval as I began my midwifery career.

By the time I was eleven or twelve, I thought I wanted to be a doctor when I grew up. My dad helped me build a huge tree house in our backyard. I used to dream of turning that tree house into a medical clinic where I would begin my practice as a physician.

I never thought about becoming a midwife. I don't think I even knew what a midwife was. My husband, Fred, and I were young struggling students at Syracuse University when I became pregnant with our firstborn. Living just off-campus, we were very much involved in the social revolution of the '60s. The lesson of this first pregnancy, as it is for many women, is what we did NOT want our childbirth experiences to be. With no money or medical insurance, I received prenatal care at the hospital clinic, never seeing the same physician twice or establishing a relationship with my caregivers. However, we were excited about the prospect of becoming new parents and took childbirth education classes designed by Grantly Dick-Read. We thought we were ready!

My first labor was unusually fast for a first baby—a total of only seven hours—and I was only in the hospital for three hours prior to birth. Fred was not permitted to be with me in labor; in fact, he was not permitted even to be on the same floor with me! I labored alone in a large ward, separated from other screaming women by only thin curtains. As I struggled alone to cope with my intensifying labor, I could hear the nurses yelling at other laboring women who were crying out in pain. I determined at that moment I would not cry out myself.

I felt humiliated when they shaved my pubic hair and gave me an enema—routine practices at the time. I remember vividly sitting on the toilet after that enema, my contractions so strong it was difficult to remain on the toilet. Shortly thereafter, I returned to my labor bed and felt something warm and wet come out between my legs. I was alarmed. I thought the baby may have just slipped out onto the bed, but I was afraid to look. I pushed the call button for the nurse who told me my water had just broken and that the baby was rapidly descending.

They rushed me to the delivery room. I am sure they were surprised that this primip (first time mother) had progressed so rapidly. They had me sit on the delivery table so they could administer a saddle block—a spinal anesthesia similar to an epidural. I could feel my baby's head on my perineum! I was sitting on his head! I wondered why I needed a saddle block if he was almost born but was too timid to question the doctor who I had only just met.

Thrilled to have my newborn son in my arms at last, I began breastfeeding. Looking back, it is surprising I chose to breastfeed. I did not know a single soul who had breastfed her baby. All too soon, they took my son to the nursery for observation.

Two years later, when we learned we were expecting our second child, we were determined to have a better experience. By now, Fred was the manager of the bookstore at the Syracuse University Medical School. This afforded him the opportunity to be exposed to a wide range of information about childbirth which he shared with me. One of the most significant things he shared with me was information about the La Leche League (LLL), a support group for breastfeeding mothers.

I began attending LLL meetings and, like a sponge, I absorbed all they had to offer. I even began exploring the possibility of becoming a La Leche League leader myself. I learned of the women who had founded LLL ten years earlier in Franklin Park, Illinois. I was excited to learn that many of them had given birth at home with Dr. Gregory White, author of *Emergency Childbirth*. Being pregnant at the time, I was inspired by the stories of their births. I even tried to talk my private obstetrician into helping us at home, but he would have no part of it.

The local hospital had just opened the first rooming-in unit in the city. My second labor and birth were a huge improvement. I only labored for three and a half hours, arriving at the hospital just before giving birth, and I refused a shave, enema and saddle block this time. Again, they took my daughter to the nursery after the birth, but since I had signed up for rooming-in, I consoled myself that she would soon be back in my arms and we would never be separated again! However, the nurse came back shortly and told me they were sorry but our daughter had been placed in the wrong nursery, so I would be unable to have rooming-in. "But," the nurse said, "you are young and will have many more babies, and you can have rooming-in the next time." Of course, my reaction was that my baby would only be born once and was separated from her mom for most of the next three days!

In the years that followed I *did* become an LLL leader. I loved the work and helping other women successfully breastfeed their babies. I became active in the organization, honing my leadership skills as I moved up through the ranks, eventually becoming chapter president and holding several statewide positions.

During the '60s this country saw an emerging birth revolution. Couples, responding to their frustration with how unnatural birth had become, were demanding less medical intervention and more family involvement. Hospitals began permitting fathers to accompany their partners in the labor and delivery room. Most hospitals were now offering rooming-in to encourage maternal-infant bonding, and many were encouraging mothers to breastfeed their babies. However, somehow their progress was just not fast enough for us. We always seemed to be several steps ahead of them, wanting more than they were ready to offer us as parents.

When we contemplated having a third child, home birth was a serious consideration. We had developed strong beliefs about the importance of bonding. We believed our older children should be able to witness and participate in the birth to reinforce what we had taught them about the normalcy of breastfeeding and birth. During most of my pregnancy we scoured the surrounding area for a home birth midwife, to no avail. By now I had developed a good relationship with my obstetrician. When we learned he actually lived in our neighborhood, which was only five minutes from the hospital, I begged him to help us. Again, he did not feel comfortable with the idea of home birth. However, he did agree to no episiotomy and early release from the hospital.

This third baby *should* have been born at home, though. My labor was only forty-five minutes long—start to finish! I remember not feeling very hungry when we sat down to eat dinner that evening. Fred cleaned up after dinner while I lounged on the couch and timed my "Braxton Hicks" contractions. Soon I realized they were pretty consistent, so we thought maybe we should consider going to the hospital. It was my due date, after all.

I decided to go upstairs to the bathroom before we left. I had to stop twice on the stairs to kneel down for strong contractions. Hmm…these contractions were hard and close. When I got up to the bathroom, I passed a large blood clot, about the size of the palm of my hand. I thought, "Bloody show." Fred raced outside to get the car.

The contractions were so close I again had to lie down on the floor at our front door. My mom, who was staying with us so someone would be there to watch the children when I went to the hospital, tried to help by attempting to put my shoes on as I tried to relax and breathe through that contraction. I remember just feeling annoyed that she was distracting me by trying to shove my shoes on my feet. As I went out the door she thrust a towel in my hands to sit on in the car in case my water broke.

It was only a five-minute drive to the hospital but it seemed too far. And yes, my water broke on the way. We raced up to labor and delivery, and they took me directly to the delivery room as the baby's head was already crowning. As I rushed in one door, my obstetrician rushed in the other door. The first thing he did was an episiotomy! My daughter was only halfway out when I said, "Hey, why did you do that?" He looked downtrodden and replied, "Oops, sorry. I forgot."

On the positive side, he did follow through on his promise about early release. He whispered to me that both my daughter and I were fine and that I could sign out "Against Medical Advice" in the morning. Because of that we would not be admitted. So my daughter and I stayed together in the recovery room all night and left early in the morning.

Just nine months later, I learned I was pregnant with our fourth child, without having had a period. It seemed that the more I learned about birth control, the stupider I became about employing it, or maybe I just became more cautious about what I put in my body! With our rapidly growing family, we decided to leave our campus home and move to a sprawling, eleven-room farmhouse on an eighty-acre farm in the beautiful rolling hills an hour south of Syracuse and a hospital.

However, during my monthly appointments with my obstetrician, he expressed concern about my ability to make it to the hospital in time, given my history of fast labors. In fact, he pointed out that each labor had been half the length of the previous labor. If I followed this course, my labor with this baby might be only twenty minutes long! When he suggested that we prepare for the possibility that this baby may be born without the benefit of medical intervention, it did not take much to convince us to plan on giving birth to this baby at home. He told us that as experienced parents, he felt it would be safer for us to plan on a home birth rather than give birth in the car at 70 miles per hour on the freeway. Fortunately, he never suggested that we induce labor to insure that we would be in a hospital when my labor began, as might happen today. He remained patient when I went past my due date by one week, two weeks, three weeks, and was approaching a month late.

By now Fred and I had done years of research about how to have a home birth without a physician. Unlike today, books about home birth were almost non-existent. We began reading *Williams Obstetrics* and maternity nursing texts that Fred found at his Medical School Bookstore. I wrote to couples who had given birth at home, including some of the founding mothers of La Leche League, to glean what I could from their experiences. From our reading and conversations, we developed a list of supplies. Fred went to every prenatal appointment with me so our doctor could teach us what to do if something went wrong. He had come to know us quite well over the course of my pregnancies. He seemed to respect our commitment to home birth and our dedication to self-education. Or perhaps he was just relieved that we would not be asking him to attend our birth.

Our closest friends, Dick and Sandy, agreed to help us when I went into labor. Sandy would provide food and childcare for our children and Dick would film the birth for us. As my due date came and went, we had several false alarms when Dick and Sandy raced to our farm, but hours later the contractions always stopped. When labor began for the fourth time on a sunny, crisp fall afternoon we called our team again. But when I was still laboring at bedtime, I sent everyone to bed, not wanting to feel guilty when I had cried "wolf" yet again.

It was a long, lonely night. The contractions were so strong I found it hard to convince myself that this was another false alarm, but why was this taking so long? Was I afraid to give birth at home without a midwife or doctor? I didn't think so. As the household awakened in the morning, I was clearly in active labor. Fred attempted to check the dilation of my cervix but could not tell what he was feeling. As the morning wore on, he began to worry, although he never let me know this, and I was too preoccupied with my labor to give it much thought.

Soon after lunch almost twenty-four hours after it began—I finally felt like pushing. As I pushed, though, one of the outer lips of my vulva began to swell ominously. As the baby's head began to appear, Fred worried that the dark and wrinkled bulge he saw on my perineum was the placenta, not the baby. Was this why I had labored so long? Remember, he had never seen a baby born from the foot end of the table. But moments later, our daughter slowly emerged, pink and healthy. Our older children were thrilled to see their new sister being born, just as we had imagined.

But as the placenta emerged, instead of feeling better I felt worse. My vulva continued to swell, and it became clear I was developing a huge hematoma—a bruise. When we called our obstetrician, he suggested applying ice. When it was still growing thirty minutes later and I began to feel weak and dizzy, he suggested we come to the hospital to have the eight-centimeter hematoma drained and cauterize the bleeder. The good news? Having been born at home, my baby daughter was considered "contaminated" and so we shared a private room. We had our rooming-in at last.

And why did this labor last so long, in spite of all the predictions of a precipitous labor? When I viewed the home movie of our birth a few weeks later, I discovered she was born "sunny side up" or posterior, with her face up instead of down as most babies are born. And she showed no signs of being a month overdue, either. Had labor been induced on my official due date, she would have been born a month early.

In less than a year, a promotion for Fred necessitated a move from our beautiful farm in upstate New York to Ohio. Fortunately, we were able to find a home with enough space for our family and a field for my yearling colt. In no time at all I had hooked up with the local La Leche League groups and became involved on a statewide level again. One of the local leaders was married to a general practice physician who became our family doctor, a good thing since within a year we found we were expecting our fifth child. In spite of the complication with our home birth, we were spoiled now. We would definitely be planning another home birth. Our family doctor assured us that the hematoma that developed with our fourth baby would not likely occur again. However, he was unwilling to attend our home birth, so the search for a midwife began again.

Although we were unable to find a midwife to attend our birth, we did find a childbirth educator who taught "emergency childbirth" as part of her curriculum. How fortuitous this connection became. Not only did she teach our class, she agreed to attend our birth, and became our baby's Godmother. As a result, our families became permanently entwined. We also invited a filmmaker to record the birth for us.

Labor began on a rainy fall day, shortly after lunch. My mom had taken the two older children out to lunch to "get them out of my hair," unaware that I was in labor. My two-year old napped, but my three-year old must have sensed something was up, as she never left my side. Progress was rapid, but I managed to reach Fred, who assembled our birth team in plenty of time. Our oldest son, Rick, assisted the filmmaker. Our daughter, René, sat by my side, wiping my brow with cool cloths, along with our daughter, Stephanie, three, who gently stroked my legs with tons of baby powder. Our daughter, Heather, two, wandered around wondering what was going on. Just four hours after it all began we had a beautiful baby boy. It was a perfect birth and we had a beautiful film to prove it.

Word spread like wildfire throughout La Leche League and the surrounding community that we had had a home birth and had filmed it. Within weeks, we were getting phone calls from other couples who were interested in home birth, wishing to see our film. We planned a film showing at our home for a group of these couples. Soon, this group morphed into a home birth support group.

We met every weekend, offering each other support, sharing information we had unearthed and sharing our film again for new couples joining the group. Fred and I wrote a booklet entitled *Handbook for Home Birth* which contained all the information we had gathered over the years: how to make the decision about staying at home; recommended supplies; obtaining backup medical care; what to expect in normal birth; and recognizing complications and what to do if they occur. Many of the couples in our group invited me to attend their home births because I had been so supportive of them during their pregnancies. I was thrilled at the opportunity. What a blessing!

We were even asked to speak and share our film at La Leche League conferences. As word spread, the phone calls changed from requests to attend our group and view our film to "Will you be our midwife?" I said, "Me? A midwife? I am not a midwife!" To this, they responded, "But you have attended more home births than anyone in town. Will you please be our midwife?" And so began my midwifery journey.

My growing library of texts in obstetrics, maternity nursing and midwifery were my constant companions. I hooked up with a labor and delivery nurse I had met at one of the home births I attended. We found we had a lot of knowledge to share with one another. For example, she taught me how to take blood pressure and do internal exams; I taught her about labor, baby care and breastfeeding. And every birth I attended served as a source of growing clinical experience.

1976 was a difficult year for our family and a turning point for me personally. I was diagnosed with vaginal cancer as a result of my mother having been unknowingly given diethylstilbestrol (DES) in her prenatal vitamins when she was pregnant with me. DES had been discovered as an effective treatment for miscarriage. In their infinite wisdom, drug companies decided to test-market prenatal vitamins containing DES on the assumption that if the drug prevented miscarriage in women at risk, why not prevent all miscarriages by adding it to prenatal vitamins?

I was told that I had a 30% chance of survival for a year even if I had a total hysterectomy. I had the surgery but refused radiation and chemotherapy. I also became a driven woman. With five small children, I felt I did not have time to die. I was determined to accomplish as much as I could in whatever time remained for me. I was also angry that once again my life had been dramatically changed by the supposed wisdom of the medical profession in their attempts to manipulate a totally natural process.

Late in 1976, just a few months following my surgery, a core group of individuals from our home birth support group decided to plan a conference for couples interested in home birth. We found a location on Ohio State University's campus and invited Dr. Mayer Eisenstein, president of the American College of Home Obstetrics at the time, as our keynote speaker. We hoped to attract a hundred attendees so we could pay Dr. Eisenstein's travel expenses. In fact, over 500 people attended our conference! Fortunately, we had the foresight to create and distribute a survey to all conference attendees about what their interests were in home birth. As a result of the survey, we decided to create a 501(c)(3) not-for-profit organization—Center for Humane Options In Childbirth Experiences—CHOICE, founded in January 1977.

As an organization, we created an educational prenatal care program for clients, provided childbirth education classes, a free lending library, a parent support group, an apprenticeship program for aspiring midwives, referrals to practitioners, and public speakers for community education. We held monthly workshops about midwifery, often taught by supportive local physicians, to broaden our base of knowledge. We held weekly peer review sessions so we could learn from our experiences at births. We even rented office space to house our library and conduct our programs.

The next decade of my life was dedicated to raising my family, honing my skills as a midwife, expanding the services of CHOICE and reaching out beyond our own community. The demand for midwives in Ohio grew by leaps and bounds, but the midwives available to serve these couples were few and far between. We traveled to all corners of this state to attend home births and even went to West Virginia on occasion.

This was tough on my family. Hardest of all was being on-call at all times. Fred used to say that my being a midwife was worse than me having a lover! We could be in the midst of making love, and if the phone rang, our lovemaking was interrupted. This, I am sure, left him feeling like he was never number one in my life. For a short time, as an organization, we tried to develop "on-call" times, allowing each of us to have guaranteed time with our families. However, we soon found that when it was our turn to be off call, we would say, "If Mary goes into labor, call me anyway," so we finally gave it up.

For the children, it meant sometimes missing important events in their lives—birthday parties, school programs, sports events, and even Thanksgiving dinner or Christmas morning. On the positive side, I think our children grew up to be truly altruistic human beings and have a healthy view of childbirth.

On one occasion, our oldest son, Rick demonstrated to us just how deeply affected he had been by having a midwife for a mother. He was sixteen at the time, and we had been living in a barn with an open floor plan. I taught childbirth education classes there each week. There were no walls in the barn, and the children had to retreat to their rooms in the loft to quietly read or play so I could teach class. On this occasion I had been at a birth that day, but the baby had been born, so I called home to ask Rick to tell my students that I would be late. I suggested that he show them a birth video while waiting for me to arrive. When I arrived home, I discovered Rick teaching my class, using my outline! He told me he had heard me teach it so many times from his bed in the loft that he knew it all by heart. He even asked one of the women if he could palpate her baby. Now, how many teenage boys would have done that?

Being a midwife also posed some dangers for me, and by extension, my family. In January 1978, I got a call from a first-time mom in labor. She lived over two hours away. While talking to her on the phone, I noticed a weather alert on the 11 P.M. News—a blizzard was on the way. I drove to the home of my partner so we could travel together. I parked my car, and we started out in the midst of a heavy rainstorm in her old Ford Pinto. As we headed south on the limited access highway, the temperature dropped dramatically and heavy rain turned to snow. About an hour south I noticed that my partner was no longer able to keep up with traffic. She said, "I have the accelerator all the way to the floor," but as we approached a town along the highway the car was barely moving at a crawl. We pulled over to the side of the road. Fortunately, a couple of fellow drivers stopped to help us.

While these Good Samaritans had their heads under the hood of the car, I ran into the town to find a pay phone (this was before cell phones) to call the mom in early labor. To my dismay, her husband said she was working hard, and I could hear her making pushing noises in the background. I advised him of the situation and told him that he should decide if they wanted to go to the hospital, given that we may not make it in time for the birth.

I then ran back up the road to the car. The helpful fellow travelers told us they were not sure what was wrong with the car and that they were unable to fix it that night. I told one of them we were midwives on our way to a birth and asked him if he would be willing to take us to the birth, over an hour and a half further south, on his way home. Much to our amazement, he agreed. Progress was slow due to the rapidly worsening road conditions. When we were finally only a short distance from the couple's home—out in the middle of nowhere—we saw a sign by the side of the road that said "High Water." We looked at each other, laughed inappropriately, and said, "High water? What does that mean?" Within seconds, "BAM" the car hit the water and the engine immediately died! There we sat in the middle of a lake with the deep water lapping loudly on the doors of the car like a boat at sea in a storm! Eventually, our driver got the car going again, and we got to the laboring mother's home. As we raced to the mom's bedside, she was just about to give birth. The birth went beautifully while our driver warmed himself by the woodstove in the living room.

It turned out that it was the worst winter storm in Ohio history—"The Blizzard of 1978." Enormous snowdrifts covered cars and houses, blocked highways and railways, and closed all airports for two days. More than 5,000 members of the Ohio National Guard were called to duty with heavy equipment clearing roads, assisting electric utility crews, rescuing stranded persons, and transporting doctors and nurses to hospitals. Forty-five National Guard helicopters flew over 2,700 missions across Ohio rescuing thousands of stranded persons, many in dire medical emergencies.

When we finished the birth chores and went back into the living room, our driver was gone. Vanished. We wondered, "Was he simply an angel sent to deliver us safely to the birth in time?" I am sure every midwife has a story like this.

In 1977 I developed the Apprenticeship Training Program for CHOICE, authoring *The Birth Attendant Handbook*, which was finally published in 1983. In 1987, I developed the Monitrice Training Program and authored *The Monitrice Training Program* in 1988. Over the years I have trained approximately sixty apprentices and forty-five Monitrices, most of whom are still practicing. I have served CHOICE as Executive Director, Midwife, Midwifery Coordinator, Monitrice, Monitrice Instructor, Childbirth Educator, and public speaker.

As more midwives began to practice around the state, I co-founded the Ohio Midwives Alliance (OMA) in 1984. I served as President of the Ohio Midwives Alliance until 2008 and continue to serve as Editor of "BirthWrite," OMA's quarterly newsletter. I was Conference Director of the OMA Midwifery Conference in 1985 and served as Chairperson for OMA's Legislative/Legalization Committee, initiating political contacts and presentations at the state level, and writing proposed legislation and proposed rules and regulations.

In the early 1990s we were offered the opportunity to address the state legislature because we had attended the home birth of a grandson of former Ohio Governor Richard Celeste. Though I had never had much interest in politics, in 1991 I compiled *Midwifery: An Informational and Educational Packet*, which was presented to Governor Celeste's Advisory Committee on Midwifery Care in Ohio. This group included senators, representatives, and state board representatives. Interestingly, the greatest opposition on the Advisory Committee came from the state Nursing Board.

In 1985 Fred accepted his first assignment as a newly ordained pastor, and we moved to the small community of Raymond, northwest of Columbus, Ohio. A volunteer emergency squad served this community. When they heard that the wife of the new pastor in town was a midwife, they approached me about joining their Emergency Squad. The Emergency Medical Technicians (EMTs) on the squad, mostly men, had no interest in "birthin' them babies," and were therefore relieved to have a midwife available to help them. They even offered to pay for my education. I became a licensed Advanced Emergency Medical Technician (Advanced EMT) in 1986 and served that organization as Newsletter Editor, Treasurer (1987-1989), and Vice-President (1993-1994).

In the years I was on the Emergency Squad, a baby was never born in the squad, but I had an opportunity to teach the other EMTs an annual class about Obstetrical Emergencies, giving them an opportunity to practice "catching" a baby using a bucket and a model baby. They loved it. I continue to provide educational workshops on Obstetrical Emergencies to EMTs to this day.

As I began to reach beyond my own community, I joined the Midwives Alliance of North America (MANA). I served MANA from 1986-1988 as Statistics and Research Committee Chair, working on the development of a computer version of the MANA statistics form. I then became their Membership Chairperson from 1993 to 1995 and served on the Executive Council of the MANA Board of Directors as Treasurer from 1995-2001 and as First Vice President from 2001-2008.

During my years on the Midwives Alliance Board of Directors, I was given the opportunity to represent MANA at the International Confederation of Midwives (ICM). ICM only meets every three years, so I attended their meetings in 1999 (Manila, Philippines), 2002 (Vienna, Austria) and 2005 (Brisbane, Australia). These years were both fascinating and personally challenging for someone whose world was so limited. I felt a strong need in preserving the recognition of apprentice-trained midwives globally. I became the Chair of the ICM Education Standing Committee, working to broaden the International Definition of a Midwife by the World Health Organization (WHO) to include apprentice-trained midwives, not just university-trained midwives.

With the same purpose in mind, I contributed to the development of the North American Registry of Midwives (NARM) National Registry Exam. In 1991, I successfully completed the NARM Registry Examination. During 1994 and 1995, I served on the NARM Certification Task Force as Skills Validation Chair, developing national certification for midwives. In 1994, I became the first NARM Certified Professional Midwife (CPM) in North America.

As my husband and I approach retirement, I have chosen to limit my involvement in the midwifery movement to serving my clients and continuing to teach the apprentices who will soon carry the torch forward. I believe that in my lifelong career as a midwife, I have acquired a set of skills unique to midwives that are essential to pass on to my apprentices.

Although I have always been committed to expanding my knowledge and skills as a midwife, providing the most educated and experienced care possible, I believe that midwifery has something unique to offer the women we serve. From my perspective as a mother first, I have tried to impart to my apprentices the importance of establishing an intimate relationship with the mothers they serve. This includes the smallest things: from how you touch a woman and the gentle way you hold her wrist while taking her pulse to the intimate way you stroke her body to help her relax in labor. I have learned that when you are with a client, she must feel as if she is the only person in your life. She is the center, as she should be.

I have also tried to teach my apprentices to recognize and trust their intuition. We all have this ability, but especially in a science-based field we tend to trust science rather that listen to our hearts and trust the message it brings to us. This can sometimes be a difficult skill to attain—and some apprentices never do acquire it—but if you trust it and listen carefully, it will never fail you.

As I move into the waning years of my life, I move there with confidence that these special women, who are stepping up to the plate to fill my shoes, will be able to do so with energy and grace. I may not live to see midwives become the caregivers of choice in this country, but I have no doubt that women will eventually demand the personalized and intimate care I sought for myself when I began this journey.

Our mothers got chewed up in the institutional process

KIP KOZLOWSKI

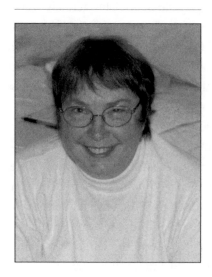

My great-great-grandfather was Hiram Harrison Lowry, the educator and missionary who founded Peking University. My great-grandfather was a physician missionary in China. My grandmother was a nurse, my grandfather an educator who ended up the superintendent of schools in Oberlin, Ohio. My dad was a salesman, and a good one. I come from a long line of missionaries, educators, doctors, nurses and salesmen. How could I *not* be a midwife?

My childhood family was fairly dysfunctional—frequent divorces, alcoholism, and abuse—all the usual. Through it all I had the blessings of strong, loving grandmothers and grandfathers, a mom, a stepmother and a dad who did their best, and a sister who shared it all.

My career path was set at age four when my dad asked me to bring him some aspirin for a headache. Solemnly providing that service made up my mind to become a nurse, and I still remember the moment clearly. My saving grace came at age six— another moment of epiphany—when all the letters suddenly became words and *I could read*. Books are my companions, teachers, guides, friends and escapes.

We moved yearly—sometimes twice a year—so I was always the odd girl out. People frequently ask me how I got the name Kip from my given name Barbara. When the time came to leave for nursing school, I sat in my great-grandmother's rocking chair and made up a nickname for myself, so that it would sound like I had been popular in high school. The ploy actually worked, and I *loved* nursing school and all the extracurricular activities that came with it.

Those were the old days, when becoming a nurse meant "walking to school five miles, barefoot, uphill both ways." We had the first summer off—after that it was straight through the three years. I took college courses that first year, along with basic nursing courses (making perfect occupied and unoccupied beds, changing bandages and dressings, medications, massage, bed baths, and so on). The next twenty-one months worked more like an apprenticeship. We spent two or three months in each area—Medical-Surgical, Obstetrics (OB), Pediatrics, Operating Room, Emergency Room, Psychiatric Unit, and Ward and Team. We worked as student nurses on the floors five days (or evenings, or nights) a week and had classes at the hospital in the relevant specialty. Ward and Team came senior year, and it meant we were in charge of a ward at night for that three months. It was a tad stressful, but we sure learned!

When I finished nursing school in 1966, I was offered a job in one of my hometowns—Oberlin, Ohio. Allen Memorial Hospital was then a small 62-bed facility. I was hired as the Evening Supervisor of Obstetrics—pretty heady stuff for a new grad. I oriented under a dragon of a head nurse and a saint of a night OB supervisor, who taught me about the possibility of tender loving care for laboring women. I had two labor rooms, one delivery room, twelve postpartum beds in two wards, two semi-private rooms, and a thirteen-crib nursery. I supervised myself, mostly, with the occasional help of an aide, and when things were really hopping, a Licensed Practical Nurse (LPN). I did labor support, called the doctor in from his home or office at exactly the right moment, dripped ether if the anesthesiologist didn't make it, cleaned the instruments, did the postpartum care (including evening care with its backrubs for every mom), mixed up all the baby formula, prepared the bottles, fed any preemies or babies whose moms weren't up for it, did meds, changed the dressings of the rare cesarean mom, charted and did rounds. It was excellent training in multi-tasking!

My husband and I married one year after my graduation, and in 1967 we moved to New York City. He was a Navy Corpsman stationed at St. Albans on Long Island. I got a job at Columbia Presbyterian in Manhattan in the brand-new Neonatal Intensive Care Unit (NICU). It was the second in the country and the first to train nurses in this new specialty. It was challenging and fascinating, and I loved those teeny-tiny babies.

After only six months in New York, my husband was transferred to a ship out of San Diego. We lived in Navy housing, and I worked at the County Hospital of the University of California at San Diego in Labor and Delivery. It was the days of three-to-four postpartum days in hospital, and lots of drugs for labor. I was a radical (or so I thought) and was teaching Lamaze. I believed all the rest of the medical model though. I remember (oh Lord, please forgive me) berating a mother who wanted to go home after only one day, telling her how dangerous birth and its immediate aftermath was.

After a few months, Dr. Louis Gluck came to town and opened a Neonatal Intensive Care Unit in our hospital. I was immediately transferred into NICU. Not too long after that, I became pregnant, and my husband left with his ship for Vietnam. Of course, with all this experience (Labor and Delivery, NICU, teaching childbirth classes), I knew it all and so was very confident and prepared for birth. My husband made it back to the states in my eighth month, in time for our daughter's birth. And guess what? I *didn't* know it all! The reality of birth was an enormous shock. My first contraction doubled me over, and they came hard every three minutes after that. (We all know that only happens in soap operas.) My contractions *hurt*, a *lot*, even though I was *breathing*! My entire labor was 4 hours and 14 minutes. (The rule is: "*First labors take 20 hours.*") I went home in 24 hours because I couldn't rest in the hospital. Breastfeeding was hard—my nipples really hurt—"*tenderness*" my ass. (The rule is: "*Breast feeding is natural and will only hurt if you are doing it wrong.*") I was beginning to rethink this whole business.

We moved to Portland, Oregon right after Kate was born. Joe was discharged from the Navy and started college on the GI Bill. Being a corpsman had reawakened and solidified his dream of becoming a doctor. I stayed home with our baby until she was one year old and then started working part-time nights at the Oregon Medical School Hospital in the Neonatal Intensive Care Unit. Joe went to school full-time and worked part-time evenings as a lab tech at Good Samaritan

Hospital so we could trade off childcare. I went back to teaching birth classes—a bit humbled, but still very dogmatic. As part of my ongoing birth education, I attended an International Childbirth Education Association (ICEA) Conference in San Diego in 1972. One of the workshops offered was on home birth, and I righteously went to it to explain to those poor misguided women just how dangerous birth was—blah, blah, blah. Well, apparently the saying that "When the student is ready, the teacher appears" is true, because I walked out of that workshop a different person. It was a huge and disconcerting "Ah ha moment" for me. *Of course*, birth works. *Of course*, women do best when in the security of their own homes. *Of course*, midwives. *What was I thinking?*

As you might imagine, this changed things a bit for me. I stopped teaching birth classes and became a La Leche League leader. We moved to Chicago so that Joe could go to medical school. I became pregnant with our second child and started attending Home Oriented Maternity Experience (HOME) meetings in women's homes. I planned a home birth with the Chicago Maternity Center much to the disapproval of most of my husband's teachers and classmates—but fortunately not his. The official dismay was escalated when a local hour-long news program (a forerunner of "60 Minutes") called "Two-on-Two" did a piece on home birth and asked if we would be the filmed home birth couple. We were told by the school that we could do it, but only if they didn't mention that Joe was a medical student! The birth and the filming went off beautifully, and the film crew was so impressed with the difference between what they were seeing in the hospital and our birth that they sent us flowers and cards.

Life after our home birth became a bit schizophrenic for me. Here's where being a Gemini helps. I went back to work when Lizzie was thirteen-months old, to start an NICU at the hospital where Joe was a student. The rest of my time, I was politicking for change, for home birth, for natural birth. More and more I felt a desire to *prevent* babies ending up in an NICU rather than *treating* them there. When I became pregnant with our third child, I was grateful to quit work at seven months and start living what I believed twenty-four hours a day.

When Joe finished his internship we moved to Lansing, Michigan, where Joe started his family practice. In 1978 we had our fourth child and third home birth. I was teaching independent childbirth classes aimed at helping women get a more natural birth in the hospital, as well as working as a birth photographer, a doula, and an assistant with the local home birth midwives. At the same time, I teamed up with two marvelous and like-minded women Libby Bogdan-Lovis and Susan Ekstrom. Libby was an anthropologist who was one of my childbirth class students and has become a dear friend, and Susan was a brilliant academic. With anthropologist and author Brigitte Jordan as a consultant, we formed a group called the Consumer Task Force on the Childbearing Year. Together we stirred up as much agitation as we could manage. We taught childbirth classes, put on local and regional conferences on birth issues, did monthly meetings at a large local church and brown bag lunches at Michigan State University, talked to classes of any sort, attended every medical and policy meeting we could get into and generally made pests of ourselves. Because of our efforts, a local hospital opened an Alternative Birthing Suite that truly offered alternatives. Unfortunately, only two doctors used it regularly, my husband being one of them.

By 1984, I felt I needed to do more. Being an activist, birth educator and doula was becoming more and more frustrating, as I saw even "educated" women getting run over by the system and having limited options if they chose to birth in the hospital. Trying to teach childbirth classes that aimed to help women find their way to a natural, drug-free, mother-managed birth in the hospital *and* act as a doula to further facilitate that outcome became intolerable. It just wasn't happening. Over and over, we saw our lovingly taught, lovingly supported mothers get chewed up in the institutional process. I left for midwifery training at the School of Allied Health Professions at the University of Medicine and Dentistry in Newark, New Jersey. It was one of the dwindling number of schools nationally that offered a Certificate of Midwifery for which a Diploma of Nursing was an acceptable precursor. Nurse-midwifery schools were rapidly dropping that option in favor of requiring a bachelor's of nursing degree, and I was afraid if I waited I would be out of luck. Our youngest daughter was only six and our oldest was eleven. My husband became a single parent for a year. I made it home for occasional weekends, but that was it.

It was a crummy year. The model of midwifery I learned was not what I thought it would be, and the responsibility I felt was terrifying. I thought my head was on pretty tight when I entered the program. I was almost forty, had four kids and loads of relevant experience, but I still came away at the end with a medicalized approach and a boatload of fear. However, I did have my certificate as a Certified Nurse-Midwife (CNM) and a new understanding of the whole problem of how maternity care is done in our culture.

When I came home with my shiny new midwifery certificate, I was ready to change my little world with new tools. The first thing I did was call the local community college. I explained that I was a CNM and offered to help teach obstetric nursing to associate degree nursing students. I was asked, "Do you have a master's degree?" "No," I said. I was asked, "Do you have a bachelor of nursing degree (BSN), and are you working on a master's degree?" "No," I admitted. "Sorry," they said, "then we can't let you teach." I have to say that *really* pissed me off. This was a big heads up that letters after your name can—and often will—count more than your skills, abilities and knowledge.

Getting privileges at our local hospital was an interesting process. Somehow all the doctors and unit heads that knew me (and Joe), and knew where I had been and what I was doing, were dumbfounded when I showed up on the hospital doorstep and knocked for admittance. They didn't realize I was going to want to *practice*. New protocols had to be written. Actually, this turned out to be to my advantage. Since they didn't have a clue what kind of animal I was, they let me have quite a bit of input. For instance, I explained that I was trained and licensed to do newborn care, so they wrote in newborn privileges! This is not a common part of most hospital practices. I was backed up against a wall by a hostile family practitioner after a committee meeting to discuss granting my privileges. He told me I would get them over his dead body. My husband agreed to be my primary backup, and a friendly obstetrician agreed to be backup for Joe on this venture, and I was in.

My first hospital birth, and first birth as a graduate midwife, happened days before my privileges were formalized. I was thrilled and scared to death. She birthed beautifully. She had a second-degree tear that needed suturing. My hand was shaking so hard I could hardly place the stitches, and it took forever. When it was done, mom and baby were happy and I was ecstatic. I flew out of the room, high on birth juice, and came up hard against the horrified faces of the labor and delivery nurses and the Unit Head. "What have you done?" they gasped. I had done a birth *without privileges*! Although they were outraged, nothing ever came of it. I practiced there for nine months. At the end of that time, my little practice was just beginning to take off, but many of the nursery nurses didn't even know I was on staff. I began to learn the importance of marketing.

Apparently this life I chose for myself this time around inherently includes lots of change. In the first ten years of my midwifery, I had that little hospital practice. I also worked at a teen well-woman clinic where I learned how to call a teen's home and sound like I was chewing gum so as to sound like another teen, and how many young girls are sexually active without their parents' awareness. I even learned to do male exams.

Then my husband had a very creative mid-life crisis that involved moving out west to be a ski instructor and work in a small mountain clinic. There I did home births up in the mountains with an eccentric and wonderful *male* midwife who also substitute-taught school, sold fish, worked construction and did mountain rescue. I met a marvelous variety of women, learned more about the range of *normal* in normal birth and the importance of good food for pregnancy.

The midlife crisis wore itself out and we moved back to Michigan. I joined three of my friends who were direct-entry midwives in their home birth practice. Each woman, each birth, each midwife provided more education. My friend, Mitzi Montague-Bauer, and I started a doula service. This proved to be useful to me in many ways. Without the intolerable weight of responsibility for the outcome that my midwifery education had placed on me, I was able to relax and see more. Mitzi is a very pure and spiritual woman with infinite patience. Me, not so much. But I had some skills that she didn't. Interestingly, each woman got the doula she needed. I learned that regardless of plans the right people will be present at a birth.

My mother died, and I stopped doing midwifery and used her legacy to open a women's bookstore. I sold a few books, but mostly I learned more about women. The bookstore became a place where women came to talk, and I found a bottomless well of pain. I taught classes called First Menstruation, with my thirteen-year-old daughter, for mothers and daughters, and found the thrill of encouraging the discovery of women's innate power. I learned I am a hopeless businesswoman.

After three years people started asking me to attend their births again. I invited a friend who trained as a nurse in Germany to work with me. Midwifery was part of her nursing education, and she is a wonderful massage therapist. We decided to explore adding massage as an integral part of prenatal care, so our clients got a full body massage at almost every visit. I'm not sure we ended up with any useful data, but our clients sure loved it! Many lessons came out of this experience. The importance of a good head for business was made clear yet again. A good mix of TLC and observation is clearly the best for improving outcomes, and a good backup system is an important piece of optimal care. This last piece was the weak link in our situation. Lansing was not open to out-of-hospital birth options.

One of our clients came to us for a home birth because her first birth had included a shoulder dystocia that had been very scary, but that had ended up well. They thought the dystocia was a result of unnecessary intervention in labor and something they wanted to avoid. With this next baby the mother once again had a moderate shoulder dystocia. It was my first. The baby was born limp and quiet. While my partner wrestled with the oxygen, the parents started screaming and yelling in tongues, and I gave the baby mouth-to-mouth. The baby promptly came around and pinked up beautifully, but her muscle tone was less than I would have liked. Even though she was doing fine, and my partner felt she was fine, I was completely rattled. We took the baby to the hospital, where they admitted her to the NICU. She stayed there for six days, even though she was fine when we arrived and tested healthy on every test. I was devastated. I spent those six days panicking and crying, sure I had done a terrible thing, wondering how I *dared* have the audacity to put myself in the position to be the difference between life and death. Why would *anyone* want to be here? Of course, I realize that much worse, sadder, harder things happen to mothers, to babies, to midwives, but for me it was incredibly frightening and painful—and more than enough trauma.

Months later, when a client who was two weeks past her due date suddenly dropped several centimeters of fundal height and palpated as having very little fluid, I found that getting good consultation and referral services was difficult. I got an ultrasound without problem, but when her AFI (Amniotic Fluid Index) showed almost no fluid, I called several physicians, trying in vain to get her admitted for care. Finally, one doctor agreed to see her, but he wanted her to come in the next morning. I was adamant about getting her in before she started labor so she could be observed carefully. We managed to arrange for admittance that night. They put her on the monitor for evaluation, and she had her first contractions, resulting in a severe and slow-to-recover fetal heart deceleration. The next contraction showed the same. The decision was made to do a cesarean section, a decision with which I heartily concurred. The baby boy was born quickly and healthy—with a cord that was so friable that it pulled apart when the doctor went to cut it! That did it for me.

I contacted our few clients and helped them find other midwives. I thought long and hard about this whole stupid idea of trying to change the world. I am not particularly brave or selfless. I decided to try another strategy to "Use My Midwifery to Do Good." I called Clarice Winkler, another Michigan midwife I knew only slightly but knew had lots of home birth experience, a great reputation and who now had a hospital practice in a town about forty-five minutes away. As fate would have it (synchronicity again), she had reached a point in her solo practice where she needed a partner, having received the go-ahead from the hospital just the day before to hire another midwife.

Clarice and I worked together for three years in that hospital practice. We had an amazing amount of latitude for a standard hospital. We worked in an office with our backup doctors but had our own "wing" that we decorated with daylight light bulbs and baby pictures. We got one room designated as the

"Midwife's Room" on the Labor and Delivery floor. We put in a homey bedside light and posters. We managed to keep that door closed most of the time and get on with some plain old midwifery, even within the constraints of the institution. The nurses tended to either love us or hate us. Fortunately they self-selected who would work with us most of the time. The doctors gave us a lot of space, too. We decided they really didn't want to know what we were doing. For the most part, they just showed up when we called them. It was a win-win situation. We got "legitimate"—they got our practice statistics to add to theirs—making theirs the best in the hospital. And, of course, our clients got really good care. Oddly enough, I found being in the hospital made it easier for me to practice non-intervention and be less afraid. Again, I think it was a sense that all that responsibility didn't rest just on me. With a feeling of a safety net under me, I was able to be a cautious and careful safety net for our clients, without going overboard.

One hard lesson came when a client with very heartfelt and strong desires for her birth came to us. Her first birth had been awful for her. Her care providers had not been with her during her birth, and no one listened to her. She got medication that she did not want, and then her baby came very quickly. There was much rushing around and carrying on, and she tore badly. She did not want to repeat that, and I worked hard to be sure it didn't. I stayed with her all night in the hospital, smiling reassurance in the dark, walking with her and coaching through every contraction when labor became intense and scary for her, catching her baby gently over an intact perineum. I was very pleased with myself. When I came into see her the next morning, she was furious with me! She told me that I had put her through hell by not giving her medication when she needed it and expecting her to be a hero, all in all forcing her to undergo a very "male" model of birth. I was crushed. I learned that "you just never know."

Three years was enough for me, though. One month we had twenty babies due, which was busy for us. Several of them were induced for one reason or another, and I found myself thinking how nice it was to have that control over the timing. This did not strike me as a good thing. The environment was changing, too. We had added a third midwife, and the hospital was beginning to pressure us to "produce" more. It is hard to explain to bean counters that changing what we were doing—our individualized, time-consuming, continuous care—would change our results and their "product," namely, quality midwifery care. It was getting harder and harder for me to keep my mouth shut, and when my contract was up, I moved on with both relief and regret. Fortunately for the women who wanted options, Clarice stayed on with other midwives for six more years. I admire that stamina, patience and will—certainly good things in a midwife—but I didn't have it. Of course, the fact that I could rely on my husband to support me gave me choices not every midwife enjoys.

Threads running through all my years were birth photography, jewelry and products for midwives. I had several very small businesses that I took to midwifery conferences. Probably my most notable and successful was Midwives Market. I made midwifery-friendly bumper stickers, cross-stitch kits and pattern books, buttons, magnets, and carried hard-to-get books and videos. I enjoyed this tremendously, and though my business skills had not improved, the pressures were very low. Unfortunately, this business backfired when, after my "retirement" from active midwifery, I spent three days at my booth at a Midwives Alliance (MANA) conference next to Jennifer Gallardo from Andaluz Birth Center. She was introducing her wonderful waterbirth video, "Born in Water," and for all those days I heard and watched that video, over, and over, and over. It made me crazy—crazy enough to decide that I simply *had* to come home and try one more time to open a birth center in Lansing. Be careful what you wish for!

Some old friends and new acquaintances joined me in the planning. Since we had been working on this on and off for twenty years, some of the groundwork had been laid. We decided to attend a National Association of Childbearing Centers' (NACC) "How to Start a Birth Center" workshop. When we introduced ourselves on the first day and told them where we were from, Kitty Ernst, President of NACC, snorted and said, "Good luck. You'd do better to go back and work on legislation in your state." We are all naturally stubborn, and probably nothing she could have said would have made us more determined to succeed.

We came home and began work in earnest. This time everything came together. I found the perfect building and talked three other experienced and wonderful midwives into joining me. Clarice was ready for something new. Geradine Simkins and Nancy Curley were "retiring" in Traverse City. I managed to create such a convincing picture that all of them agreed to come, the bank gave me a loan, and the potential landlord held the building for me until I got through all the township foolishness. We had an experienced and extraordinary birth educator and doula to teach our classes and to start and facilitate our Mother's Support Gatherings. We found a woman with business skills (I learned that lesson!) to manage the day-to-day office and pay the bills. We completely renovated the building and opened officially December 29, 2002. Our first baby was born on January 20, 2003.

What I had planned was a birth center that would be completely independent and as good a place for the midwives as for the mothers. I set up the salaries so that they were fairly competitive with smaller hospitals. Following Jennifer Gallardo's lead, we set up a schedule that was wonderful—one week a month a midwife was on first call, one week second call, one week in the office, and the fourth week *off*. There would always be two midwives at each birth. Client visits lasted one hour. Birth preparation—based on normal, drug-free, mother-managed, undisturbed births, was part of the package, as were a prenatal and a postpartum massage. A well-respected obstetric (OB) group at the city's largest hospital agreed, much to my amazement, to be our backup physicians. I knew that our set-up assured the best possible arrangement for mothers and babies. I knew that once the word got out we would be swamped by all those mothers who were so unhappy with their previous birth experiences. I just hoped we could keep up.

Enter reality. We elected then, and have kept, the policy of not taking insurance. The clients pay us up front over the course of the pregnancy, and we issue them a superbill of charges after the baby is born. They then pursue reimbursement on their own from their insurance carriers. This has proven to be a problem for many clients. In Michigan, Medicaid will not pay for any out-of-hospital births. Insurance companies for the most part have been very reluctant to reimburse birth center charges in full. Blue Cross and Blue Shield has been particularly difficult. It is hard for people in general—and us in particular—to understand why the insurance companies wouldn't be glad to pay our $3800 fee instead of the average $8,000 to $12,000 hospital fee—but, of course, that is naïve thinking. In any case, my planning was way, way off base. After one year, Nancy and Gera moved back home after having helped get us organized and off to a great start. Soon after, our birth educator Susan Kuchnicki left after setting up our many wonderful mothers' groups. We simply could not afford their salaries. Three of us stayed—two at severely reduced salaries. I got my *first* paycheck in 2009, six years after we opened! When we told our young mothers in June 2004 that we feared we would have to close the birth center due to lack of funds, they immediately went into action. "Not an option," they told us. They said we needed to be there for their future babies—and for their children's babies! They had garage sales and marches and other fundraisers. I took out some more loans. Bless my husband's support. Our OB group moved into private practice from being a university-affiliated group and decided not to back us any more. We were forced to make arrangements for hospital transfers through the OB residents program when we needed to transport. This has worked out well, much to our surprise. Somehow we always managed to squeak by, week after week, month after month, and finally year after year. We have been open now for over six years, and have attended over 400 births. We have added a third part-time midwife, Shelie Ross. Mitzi joined us as our office co-coordinator, and we hired a more experienced money manager, all of whom also work for peanuts. We midwives teach our own birth classes. We are still squeaking by, but we are still here and growing.

So I ask myself, *What am I trying to accomplish here?* I feel sad and frustrated that so many women don't "get it." They don't even see why experiencing their births is a worthwhile goal. Culturally, of course, it makes sense for so many reasons. From the day we are born, and any day after that, we are taught that our bodies are poorly functioning, capricious, damp, smelly, embarrassing, weak, and unreliable. Women have bought into these cultural messages and internalized them.

"We like a quick fix."

"We don't care for symptoms."

"Being numb beats pain—always—unless you are working out."

"Sex and motherhood are mutually exclusive."

"Control is possible."

"If you do everything right, the outcome will be as you desire."

"Pregnancy and birth are medical conditions beyond the understanding of mere women."

"Women today are too fragile to undergo the horrifying rigors of childbirth."

"Wanting a 'good experience' is selfish."

"Babies don't remember."

"Babies are fine with the way we do things."

"Everybody does it this way."

"I had (did) this or that and I'm fine."

"I have a birth plan, so it will all go as I want."

"My doctor is really nice."

"Well, I'll do it the 'regular way' for my first baby and then I'll see."

The list of ways in which women don't "get it" or are indoctrinated not to "get it" goes on and on and on.

Years of standing by, of listening to thousands of birth songs, birth cries, complaints, years of seeing joy, blood, sweat and tears has taught me differently. A mother and her baby are wise together. We can teach them steps to many dances, and that is useful, but we cannot know the music they will get when the time comes, and they must be ready to dance to that. All we can do then is love, admire, reassure and quietly watch as best we can to keep them as safe as we can. For each woman, the decisions that are made about her pregnancy, her birth, her body, her baby, will be played out on her body—she *must* be enabled to make those decisions for herself. Women have the best chance of making the "right" choices for themselves. Women can give birth. Babies can get born. Some women just know this, and when they are exposed to the possibility, they light up.

I'm infinitely tired of politics. I have chosen to make my own little world and invite like-minded women to join me. We just try to do it right as we understand it, to provide a space where women can be treated as well as loved pets, for heaven's sake! I feel blessed (most of the time) that things and people came together to let this dream survive. I realize that we are a very small David, with a very large Goliath lurking around, but I am content to just do this little piece. I know that the young women whose lives are changed through their own experiences here will carry the torch.

A clear separation between a woman's body and the law

CASEY MAKELA

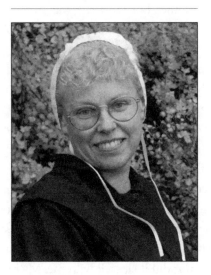

grew up in New England near the shores of the great Atlantic Ocean, in snug coastal towns in Maine and Connecticut where a person's sense of self was Yankee to the core. The firstborn grandchild of Irish immigrants who went through Ellis Island, I was brought up on the rich lore of determined family members who were proud of the struggles they had endured to become Americans. They instilled a deep respect for the American ideals of hard work and perseverance in their children and grandchildren. Mine was a deeply spiritual family. Women were celebrated in my family, and it was always a special feeling as a child to be reminded that I was the firstborn daughter of a firstborn daughter of a firstborn daughter of a firstborn daughter. There was almost magic in the uniqueness it implied, and it was that much more so when my own first-born was also a daughter!

My childhood was largely divided between the library, the ocean and learning music. I loved to read and learn and explore. Books (medical and obstetric especially) provided me with knowledge that was otherwise unavailable—if not outright unapproved of—in the conservative private schools I attended as a youth. The ocean, with its churning majesty and tidal pools teaming with life, provided endless opportunities for exploration. Playing music set my imagination free through hours of melodic self-expression which usually led to soul-soothing daydreams.

My maternal grandmother, born in 1913, was an obstetrical nurse for thirty years. We were very close, and her compassionate example of what it meant to really care for people left a lasting impression on me. As I got older and began to form my own ideals and search for my life goals, I found myself curious about how childbirth might be different in our "modern" times for women, than from what she had known herself as a young woman and how it could be improved. I was intrigued by the concept of midwife-attended home birth that I had read about, and I was sure she would feel the same—natural birth sounded so normal. But although my grandmother was forward thinking for a woman of her time, I was shocked by the comment she made during a conversation we had on this matter when I was in my teens. She said that birth should, of course, be medically managed just exactly as all hers had been. Being under anesthesia was how babies *should* be born. Midwifery was archaic; doctors knew best. This was not a point of view that I expected, nor did it sit well with me. My heart told me that there had to be a better way. Fortunately, the natural birth movement was well on its way and the information was inspiring!

I went to school for nursing, but my heart yearned to work in obstetrics. I found it extremely difficult during clinical rotation in a large busy metropolitan hospital to see birth treated the way it was back in the 1970s. By special permission, largely due to my honor roll status, I was allowed to work and spend all of my extra time on the Obstetrics Ward. I had expected the experience to confirm my desire to work there someday—but it turned out very differently. Up to that point I had suspected that the stories I had read describing the mismanagement of birth in hospitals were probably exaggerated. Yet, much to my dismay, I found out first-hand they were actually true. I witnessed labors being started or stalled to better suit doctors' personal schedules (including being on a golf course or at a country club), women being strapped to labor beds and not allowed to walk around during labor, fathers not allowed in delivery rooms but cloistered in waiting rooms like inconvenient afterthoughts, infants suspended by their ankles and spanked on the bottom, then separated from their mothers and whisked off to the nursery ward to be bottle fed, among other things. Those stories were not just sensational exaggerations after all. Knowing that birthing women deserved a better experience and not wanting to be a part of an unchangeable establishment, I abandoned obstetrics, completely disillusioned, and reconsidered my life and educational goals.

For a few years I worked part-time in geriatrics and with hospice, where I felt I could actually do some good. But, once my own children were born, I finally left nursing altogether to devote myself to my family and the work of midwifery, which was quickly evolving in my life. It was a choice that offered no job security or retirement, but I never looked back or regretted it. I wanted to be part of a solution for safe, natural, non-medical birth, even if it meant being all by myself with no professional status.

During that time I taught childbirth education classes and attended home births of friends and friends of friends. At first it all seemed so hush-hush and outright scandalous to go against what our doctors and families thought was "safe and responsible." But being young and determined to reclaim birth as our right, it made real sense to me and my community of home birth sisters, supporters and friends to just do what came naturally rather than go to the hospital. Our bodies, our births! I also had the chance to apprentice with nurse-midwives for a time, and I learned a great deal about gentle, responsible management in home birth settings. Theirs was a busy practice that provided a unique opportunity for which I will always be grateful.

Choices in childbirth were always clear for me personally. I did not want to just read about the joys and advantages of home birth, I wanted to have first-hand experience. I felt strongly that to represent home birth and birthing freedom, one ought to have personal experience of it to be better able to effectively speak and teach about it. Birthing my children at home gave me a sense of self that defies explanation. This was especially true of the unassisted birth of my son John in 1986, which I wrote about for the magazine *Midwifery Today*. Unassisted birth—intentionally giving birth without the assistance of a professional birth attendant—was a very controversial choice to make back then. It was somewhat socially difficult to bear at the time, however, the benefits of the outcome of that birth far outweighed the criticism and scrutiny. While all my births taught me the pure power of being a woman, my unassisted birth revealed the ultimate of feminine mysteries and meaning of self-accomplishment. That birth was mine alone.

As time went on, I longed for there to be a school where students could study midwifery from a traditional, community-centered perspective, but such a program did not yet exist. Midwifery was typically taught as a medical extension of nursing in Certified Nurse-Midwifery (CNM) programs which represented childbirth management as a medical procedure. There were simply no schools of authentic, birth-friendly traditional midwifery. While there were a few good books available that provided information and even instruction about the management of natural childbirth, more was really needed. An accessible, structured academic program that could round out an apprenticeship really seemed like a great idea. It was clear that more midwives were needed, but education was needed too.

I was particularly sensitive to the need for education because the lack of specialty education was one of the many challenges I faced in becoming a midwife in the way that I envisioned for myself. But a positive attitude was always more serviceable than perpetual discouragement. Goethe once wrote: "Until one is committed, there is hesitancy, the chance to draw back . . . . Concerning all acts of initiative (and creation) there is one elementary truth the ignorance of which kills countless ideas and splendid plans: that the moment one definitely commits oneself, then providence moves too. All sorts of things occur to help one that would otherwise never have occurred . . . . Whatever you can dream you can do. Begin it; boldness has genius, power and magic in it." This was a powerful and inspirational statement for me that often provided an encouraging reminder to persevere.

Once my family settled on our farm in Michigan in 1984, I initially avoided setting up a home birth practice. There were no midwives in northeastern Michigan that I was aware of, so I would have had to work alone, and I was not comfortable with that. But despite my reluctance, the need for midwives was so great in this area that it was unavoidable that I would become a resource. Actually, women at that time had great difficulty finding a doctor to care for them during pregnancy. There was only one obstetric (OB) clinic one hour north of my home, and they were not accepting new patients. None of the general practitioners were accepting pregnant woman for care either—it was really an awful time for women's health care here. I assisted many, many families and provided much needed resources, and so my practice was extremely busy. I traveled to births as far away as twelve hours round-trip, working alone. It was exhausting.

Things got better when I finally met Karen, another home birth midwife who lived about two hours away. We established a beautiful, lasting friendship which swiftly developed into a partnership. We birth-worked together for over twenty years and covered huge distances, including Michigan's Upper Peninsula and even Canada until the Border Patrol finally put an end to that! My dear friend had the same commitment to midwifery that I did, and when I decided to establish Michigan School of Traditional Midwifery (MSTM) in 1988, she broke with the pack and stood by me to support the project through thick and thin. She eventually became the school's assistant educational director working with hundreds of students. Together we lived the principle of historian Laurel Thatcher Ulrich: "Well-behaved women seldom make history." Karen Kamyszek, (Certified Traditional Midwife) CTM, passed away in June of 2007, but not before seeing the dream of a school devoted to traditional midwifery founded and state licensed. My personal story would not be complete without including this memorial to Karen, my beloved spiritual sister and loyal friend.

Midwifery was not my only occupation throughout most of my adult life. I have been a professional musician for thirty years and for over ten years was a touring artist with my husband and the Michigan Touring Arts. Our award-winning children's musical program was called *Casey & Mac—Songs & Stories for Little People*. We performed in hundreds of theaters and schools. We recorded an album under that name and were among several artists who were selected to work on a special recording project to benefit the prevention of child abuse. The album, *If We Dare to Care*, featured a collection of Michigan's favorite children's recording artists and was narrated by Isiah Thomas. My husband and I were honored with an award from the National Association for the Prevention of Child Abuse in the 1990s for our work with children as well as many other awards for our work for homeless shelters and family-centered special interest and relief groups.

My husband Bill, (otherwise known as "Mac") and I raised seven children together, and because of our performing schedule, our children traveled and even performed with us. Although our children's lives were educationally rich and diverse, ultimately our schedule and personal points of view created problems with school officials. They could not reconcile themselves to the fact that I considered myself to be our children's primary educator and public school the place that simply filled in the gaps. Needless to say, in the interest of peaceful conflict management and the pursuit of educational liberty, we decided to home school our three youngest children. It was a decision we never regretted. Through the experience we learned that family liberty certainly extends beyond the birth-place, or at least that it should. Home-based education is part of the natural evolution of birth freedom and attachment parenting. At first I was unsure of my ability to be an effective home schooling parent. But thanks to the loving encouragement from a local family who had home schooled their daughters I was able to get beyond my jitters the first time the public school bus pulled in front of our house, stopped, and then drove away with three unoccupied seats because our children were not onboard. To this day I hug my good friend Debbie in gratitude for her faithful support of my launch into those uncharted waters. Today, I can reflect that it was an important, well-made choice for those three. I didn't "ruin" them after all. One daughter attends Wake Forest University School of Law (accepted at age twenty-two), the other runs her own successful body casting studio and doula practice, while our son started his own excavating company and attends college part-time for business management. Their stories of achievement are very inspiring to me. I am on several speakers' bureaus, which give me an opportunity to share my experiences in home schooling and always, of course, include commentary about midwifery.

One might wonder what the performing arts could possibly have to do with midwifery and birthing freedom. Public platforms in any venue can provide valuable chances to speak out about one's personal special interests, and I took every opportunity to speak out about the fact that freedom in birth leads to stronger, more confident families!

I am also a writer and an author. Over the years, I have written articles on homesteading, home schooling, cooking, simple living and livestock management for a diverse range of periodicals, as well as articles about herbology and other birth-based subjects for mothering and midwifery magazines. In 1994, I wrote *Milk-Based Soaps* as part of a fund-raising campaign for the Michigan School of Traditional Midwifery. The school needed revenue, so I just diversified a little to meet that need. The result was notable and well worth the effort.

Unfortunately, midwifery is not an occupation that always provides a steady monetary income, especially practiced from a Christian, spiritual viewpoint such as mine. In my practice, a family lacking funds is still just as deserving of services as anyone else—mine is a vocation practiced as a calling, or some might say a ministry, which is community-supported by various means and in varying degrees. Compensation has not always been monetary, and some of my dearest treasures are more lastingly meaningful than money ever could have been. For instance, my spinning wheel was compensation for a birth years ago. The lessons that came with it resulted in warm hats for my family, relatives and Christian missions ever since. Another example is one of my guitars—a beautiful little instrument. Because it was old and rather road-weary from being passed around and treated as generally worthless, it was relegated to cold closet storage, and the family felt sheepish offering it to me as payment. But it has sat on my lap now for over two decades accompanying the songs I have sung to thousands of children and families. It always seemed as though that guitar was the only right choice to be with me, serving families in my musical profession. By *letting go and letting God*, I can say that I have been richly blessed!

I never allowed myself to be frustrated because midwifery couldn't exclusively support me, and I never wanted to betray midwifery into the hands of legislators in a quest to gain financial security. Instead, I explored creative diversification to compensate financially and, in doing so, always incorporated a means of heightening public awareness in the interest of natural, non-violent birth. For instance, both my natural soap companies—Killmaster Soapworks and The Quaker Soap Company—have product lines (such as the Universal Mother soaps), which donate proceeds to mother/child-friendly initiatives around the world. This accomplishes two things: first, it serves as a public awareness platform that can direct general attention to my special interest in natural birth, mothering and breastfeeding. Secondly, it generates actual revenue for those types of organizations. Just the soap companies alone produce thousands of pounds of soap annually that have my slogan included on the label—"Peace on earth begins at birth." That's a lot of bars of soap with a message for people who may otherwise not ever have known about the issue. I even wrote an article for a midwifery magazine entitled "Mother's Milk Soap," which was reprinted in the 1990s in other magazines unrelated to birth as a point of curiosity through which attention was again directed to natural birth and breastfeeding. This is a public relations success! Writing, music, soap-making: all of my businesses are operated with a component for creating public awareness of midwifery and the joy of natural birth.

Beyond those many peripheral endeavors, midwifery is at the center of my very being. It is a dimension of mothering that is intrinsic to me, and in that maternal sense it defines my life and directs my focus. It has allowed me to not only see and share firsthand the power of purpose in the women I serve, but it has also illuminated my relationships with my daughters. Most of my girls have attended births with me from the time they were quite young. Their innocent perspective was very beautiful and often soothing. At one birth, my daughter Hannah, then age twelve, invited the nervous dad to color with her in a coloring book she had brought along to pass the time. This was the family's first child, and it was a long and difficult labor. Whenever the father needed a break, he would go downstairs and actually color with Hannah for a few minutes. I was amazed by that. They finally welcomed their hard-won firstborn son and named him Andrew. The next day at the postpartum visit, Hannah brought a decorated folder with her. She handed that folder to the proud father. The folder cover was colorfully entitled with careful lettering ("Waiting for Andy") and contained all of the pages they had colored together. It was her gift and one I was not even aware she had created. As he looked through the many pages, joyful tears quietly emerged. He hugged her hard and thanked her for such a treasure.

At births I worked with my daughters in a knowing way that needed no language or words to communicate thoughts or needs. It was a unique experience that only existed with them, especially Marion. My Marion always seemed to be one step ahead of a need at any given time. Her presence was silent as a shadow, her ministrations thoughtful and timely, and her depth of understanding profoundly transcending surface reality. She welcomed life with joy and accepted death with peaceful understanding. She sometimes even knew with uncanny clarity what adults could not yet see. She learned from firsthand experience not to fear birth but to trust in the process as being normal and to be accepting of all outcomes—even when "truth" is misrepresented with cruel and unjust bias. Marion studies law now and hopes someday to become an attorney to advocate for women's rights.

My devotion to midwifery extends beyond birth itself. Serving women exclusively in the birthplace was never enough for me. My heart yearns for women's freedom in birth so intensely that I wanted to do more than just attend women in birth; I wanted to create resources for authentic, traditional midwifery that would be long lasting and serviceable. With help from likeminded midwives who shared the same dream, I founded a traditional midwifery school to help ensure that community-created traditional midwifery would never be left by the wayside as an antiquated memory. Then I created a collective resource base where the ideals of midwifery existing outside of legal definition would be supported and preserved; where the occupation was represented as one of moral standing rather than professional designation; where midwifery would be preserved in the ideal of a vocational art, not a medical science. This led to the establishment of both the Michigan School of Traditional Midwifery in 1988 and then the American College of Traditional Midwives (ACTM) in the 1990s.

My motivation is clear. Medicalized birth in America denies women the truth about the general normalcy of the birth process. Our medical system does not regard birth as a safe or even natural body function. They'd go broke if they did. Compounding this is the complete lack of reproductive education in schools, though we can vaccinate girls in sixth grade now to help protect them against an STD! Finally we have the media, which, for the sake of ratings and the promotion of sensationalism and theatrical heroism, usually portrays birth as some terrifying life-or-death process from which the woman, who was apparently completely uninformed to be able to deal with the event in the first place, must be rescued in critical time. That birth is such an easy target for misrepresentation and that fear is profitable both in movie ratings and ticket sales means that the minds of women are easily sabotaged into fearful self-regard. This warped image of childbirth generates not only media profits but also generates increased revenue for the greatest profiteers of all time—institutionalized medicine. Our U.S. medical system, where women face a soaring cesarean section rate of way over 30%, and as high as 50-60% in certain institutions, stands first in line to reap the financial rewards from those women who are fearful of birth. It also benefits from those who, under law enforcement, are forced into medicalized care, often against their better judgment, because freedom of choice has been legislatively denied them. Our northeastern Michigan hospital that has been "heralded for excellence" has a "no compromise" 100% c-section policy for all women desiring to have a VBAC (vaginal birth after cesarean), no exceptions, and there are no medical alternatives otherwise available within a four-to-six hour drive. It is a medical monopoly at its finest, on just my local level alone.

It is unacceptable to me that free choice in childbirth is not a basic, standard, legally defensible human right. It is unconscionable to me that there are some states that even have laws mandating that women can only birth in a legally-defined environment with legally-defined medical personnel in attendance. Doing otherwise invites aggressive legal prosecution for both the families—who face charges like child endangerment—and the midwives who attend them. How can this be tolerated in this "land of the free"? Why can't birthing women be part of that great mass of American citizens who can expect their privacy to be respected, and themselves to be able to live the ideals of liberty and the pursuit of happiness? How on Earth can birth be categorically reduced to a medical malady, subject to standards of legislated protocols? It defies all logic and staggers the mind!

Trying to legalize midwifery under a professional designation, creating licensing procedures state-to-state and/or legally defining midwifery as a medical title are certainly ambitious undertakings, but they are not solutions to the problem. None of these things serve birthing women's rights. The issue should never have been the legalization of midwifery; it should have been the legalization of a woman's right to choices in childbirth. Where she births and with whom should transcend legislative authority. That's the battle that desperately needs to be won. There must be a clear separation between a woman's body and the law. Restore women's rights to own birth and leave midwifery out of the political arena.

Even if I am left as the last voice crying out on this issue, I will not be silenced. My daughters and granddaughters are depending on a reasonable defense of their birth choices, and I will be there for them and every woman who chooses to define birth for herself. I won't stop speaking out on this because birth freedom is worth defending to my very last breath. I wrote about my dream for midwifery in an article for *Midwifery Today* in 2006, entitled: "Traditional Midwifery, a Traditional Vocation." There is also a Birthing Freedom Petition on the ACTM website which has generated signatures of support from around the world. If it accomplishes nothing other than public awareness of the problem, then at least it's something.

When they choose to, women should be supported to take responsibility for their births and educated to believe that they are absolutely capable of birthing, with or without assistance, in most cases. This is also why I feel it is so important to not lay claim to any birth as a midwife. Midwives should ideally refuse to be congratulated for a "job well done," but instead gently restore that praise back to where it rightfully belongs—to each and every woman who was perfectly capable of birthing her own child with or without you. This leaves a mother feeling capable, competent and vibrant with her own inner strength, not a grateful dependent on her deliverer. She is the bearer of life and, as such, the only one deserving of any credit. In this, the real truth about birth is admitted and honored. I don't need to submit a tally of birth outcomes to justify my occupation as a midwife because I do not care to align myself with or try to appease a medical model or agency of approval. My work is with women and families. My obligation is to empower them to do what is their moral right to do in choosing natural home birth. My calling is to educate and enable women to know that they are fully capable of bringing forth life free of the implication that "qualified" assistance is needed to "save" her in case of "what-if." I am a midwife, not a fear monger. I won't betray my calling by making women victims of fear. They have the media and medical institutions for that.

As an educator, I believe that midwifery students should be taught that creating confidence is about instilling faith in ability, not faith in pre-established protocols dictated by some governmental mandate largely set up by liability insurance designers who have a profit-motivated agenda to protect.

I am so proud of our students. Many of our Michigan School of Traditional Midwifery graduates have gone on to make noteworthy contributions to birth work. I have worked with hundreds of midwifery students from around the world, and it is my earnest desire to welcome each and every one as the important contributors they are and have the potential to be. I have never approved of the degrading nicknames or titles such as "newbie" that have been bantered about over the years. Those women, newly interested in midwifery, need to be nurtured and encouraged to pursue their goals and be likewise respected for the effort they are making to do so. My heart is greatly warmed by the depths to which students immerse themselves in the study of midwifery. The heart and soul commitment and earnest desire that I see demonstrated through their hard work and dedication assures me that there will be capable women in the future who will represent midwifery for the sake of birthing women's rights rather than for a professional mainstream agenda. This gives me hope that someday women's basic human rights will be fully restored to them, and that they will have the freedom to make choices for their own births with true personal liberty, defining for themselves where they birth and with whom.

Midwifery has been a journey of faith for me that has paralleled my spiritual faith journey in many ways. I have evolved and matured in both. As a Conservative Christian Quaker, peace, non-violence and the defense of birthing freedom are principles I will spend the rest of my life defending. I'll always seek out new ways to impart the great truth of birth as a natural, normal body function. For instance, once my children were grown, I still wanted to contribute to children's education in some way. I began writing children's stories about life on a farm and, in doing so, incorporated the subject of birth in most of them. With my family's help we began publishing those stories, fully illustrated with photography of exceptional quality, for free online as "Quaker Anne's Children's Stories." Providing safe, wholesome online learning resources for children was one part of the project's motivation. But the other motive was to have the opportunity to portray birth from a natural perspective as it normally happens on a farm. Children can see a chicken hatching from an egg, or a horse, goat, sheep or dog being born, bees in their hive—all with simple unembellished narration depicting the normalcy of birth.

The years have certainly passed quickly for me as a midwife and a mother. I feel it especially now as a grandmother and when I attend birthing families having their tenth or eleventh babies—and I have been there for all of them. Or when someone approaches me in public and reintroduces their adult child, saying, "Do you remember Jimmy?" That always makes me smile! These are individuals whose birth I attended so long ago that he or she is now also a parent. I often encounter these adult children and hope that birth has been a good and honest experience in their lives, wondering as well if it will be so for their children. I have become especially humbled by the passage of time because I sometimes now attend birthing women who are the daughters of mothers I once attended in birth. Although I have attended hundreds of births, I find that I don't measure time in numbers of births anymore. Instead, I am beginning to measure time by the generations I have served and assisted as a midwife. It seems a strange reality.

Looking back over the years and replaying the history of midwifery in my life, I can't help but hear the lyrical echo from the famous song "Truckin" by the Grateful Dead: "What a long strange trip it's been." In some ways, that really sums it up in a nutshell. But through it all, midwifery has been my life's work and very meaningful to me regardless of the sacrifices. I don't regret a moment of it. I have worked with birth in every dimension possible and have witnessed and experienced miracles and grace, pain and sorrow, peace and contentment. No matter what, I have clung to my trust in God's design. I have faith in birthing women and wish that the white dove of peace may descend upon every one of them as they make their birth journeys, each in peace and without fear.

A shoelace in my glove compartment

LINDA MCHALE

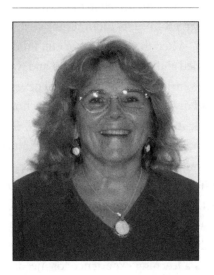

I grew up on the edge of the woods in New Jersey. My sister and I spent hours in the woods catching frogs, toads, lizards, snakes and the occasional baby bird. We would bring the creatures home and try to convince our mother to let us keep them. Luckily for them, our mother would make us release them after a few days. Once my dad ran over a rabbit's nest with the lawn mower and accidentally killed the mother. The tiny babies became our charges. My mother got toy doll bottles and made them formula. We all took turns feeding them and tucking them back into the warm blankets that were heated with a hot water bottle. Being gentle was paramount. These little bunnies lived and were eventually released back into the wild.

I learned respect for living things that has never left me. In fact I feel a kind of communication with them that was established when I was young and has served to educate me throughout my life, especially when it comes to birth. Animals seemed to be attracted to me and would literally follow me home, but allergies kept me from having a dog or cat of my own. I wanted to be a veterinarian, but as I got older I realized that my allergies would not let me attain this goal.

By the time I was in high school, my family finally did get a dog, but I did not feel that attached. When she got pregnant, my interest was peaked as I gently petted her belly and talked to her. During those years, smoking cigarettes was a hip thing to do, but it was not allowed in school. I was caught smoking in the girls' room and got suspended for three days. This was the time our dog decided to give birth! This was the first of many times I found myself in the birthplace by "accident." I watched as each little beagle emerged from its mom. Enthralled, I offered soft words and gentle stroking to mom. When the babies came out, I did not take them from her or dry them. I just watched and offered her support and water. After that, whenever any of my friends' pets were giving birth, I went whenever I could.

In 1975 when I had my first child, there were no choices for birthing women. I had read Grantly Dick-Read's books and *Thank You, Dr. Lamaze*. I went to the local obstetric (OB) group and told them I wanted a natural birth. During an OB visit, the doctor did a vaginal exam and found out I was five centimeters dilated. "How about if we induce you this weekend?" he said. The fact that I wasn't due for almost a month didn't seem to be a problem to him. I declined his offer and told him I wanted to go into labor on my own. As it turns out, my daughter Jasmine, was born ten days early at 6 lb, 2 oz.

Jasmine's birth was a learning experience for me, as is everyone's birth. The labor started with my water breaking and no contractions. Hours later, the OB called back and told me to come to the hospital. They started Pitocin to initiate contractions and three hours later Jasmine was born. I was amazed to see her. She was more beautiful than anything I had seen before. I could have looked at her all day. To say it was love at first sight is not strong enough. They stitched up my episiotomy, and I just held her, content. The bad part happened when they took her from me to go to the nursery. I hadn't thought that far ahead. It took me hours to get her back. I was crying and my heart was breaking. I vowed to never have another baby in the hospital.

Six months later, my neighbor Diana's water broke on my couch. I thought it was another sign that midwifery was coming my way, and both Diana and I laughed heartily. We had planned for me to watch her son when she went to the hospital to have this child. Early morning her husband called and told me he was bringing him over. I sat nursing my baby Jasmine and talking to the big brother to be. Five minutes later the dad, George, came knocking at the door yelling "Help me, she's having it!" I popped Jasmine off my breast and called to my husband to take care of the kids. I ran next door in my bathrobe to see Diana clutching the doorjamb, totally dressed and making pushing noises. "Lay her down and take off her pants," I told George. He helped Diana to the bed and I washed my hands. After we got Diana's pants off we could see the baby coming! What a thrill. I connected with Diana, and our conversation seemed more like monkeys grunting back and forth to each other than anything else. We both had our hands on the baby's head, guiding the baby out and then up onto Diana's belly and chest. There was a glow of light all around us, and we three adults stopped and stared at this newest of human beings. It felt holy. It felt right. We were not afraid or rushed. After awhile, I remembered that a placenta would come next, so I went into the kitchen and got this huge bowl big enough for spaghetti for ten people! I had never seen a human placenta before. I had already given birth and not even seen my own placenta.

We decided to call the ambulance because neither of us knew how to tell if everything was all right. My mom called the local newspaper, and they sent someone out who took my picture with the baby and wrote an article entitled, "Neighbor Helps Out," that was in the Sunday paper. The picture was of the baby and me, but without the mom. To this day it is a source of embarrassment for me. A midwife should never take the credit from the mom.

After Diana's birth I was hungry for more births. I did get to do some labor support for friends. One was a woman having a VBAC (vaginal birth after cesarean), which ended up, pun intended, being a breech. She had a c-section with her first because of a diagnosis of cephalopelvic disproportion (CPD), but this next baby, the breech, was a pound and a half bigger and born vaginally.

But during this time of my life, it was mainly the animals that filled in my education. One day on my way to the clothesline, I saw something digging in the dirt. I got closer and saw it was one of those beautiful box turtles with the orange on its shell. She was slowly, methodically pushing dirt behind her with one clawed foot, and swish went the sandy soil out behind her. Then she would do the same with the other foot. All of a sudden she spotted me standing there staring at her. Ms. Turtle froze and eyed me. I got down on the ground next to her. I hardly breathed while waiting for her to assess me. Was I a threat? She must have decided I was ok, or the force in her to continue was so strong that she kept on hoping for the best. I was not sure what she was doing, but I knew I was supposed to stop and pay attention. The digging continued long enough to make a hole about as deep as she was long. Then an amazing thing happened. She began to lay eggs, slimy, bouncy, looking like tiny pearl onions. I was thrilled and felt the same feeling of being in a holy place that I had when Diana had her baby. I stayed there pressed against the ground until the turtle covered the eggs with soil. She then eyed me again and walked off deliberately, like only a turtle can do. I got up off the ground knowing that I had just been blessed and educated by this wonderful "woman" wearing a shell.

Another reptile showed me about birth during this time period. I saw our cat standing on its hind legs, trying to hold onto something in its paws, out by the little stream behind our house. I dropped what I was doing and ran out the door. When I got close to the cat, he ran along the water, so I followed him and saw that he was chasing a snake that was swimming in the stream. A two headed snake! No wait, the second head got longer and longer, until it was another snake! I was seeing a garden snake having babies right there in my stream! I had just witnessed another birth—my first "water birth!"

I took to carrying a shoelace in my glove compartment just in case I came upon a birth. But the next births I went to were two of my own. When I got pregnant with my next child, in 1977, I got the name of a local general practitioner who did "home deliveries." Dr. Childers was a rebel for sure. The most relaxed doctor I have ever met, he gave me the due date of simply "May." Well, on May 1st I went into labor. I woke up with my water popping and running down my legs as I jumped out of bed. "Yippee," I thought, "I'm in labor!" I got into the shower and the contractions got really close. By the time my husband Ron called the doctor, I was moaning. The doctor laughed and told Ron that he would never make it on time. He gave Ron some quick instructions and said he was on his way. I was on my hands and knees on our bed, which was a mattress on the floor. Feeling very centered and safe, I gave into the pushing sensation. The baby's head started to come through the vagina into my supporting hand. Slowly the head came. Then suddenly, swoosh, the body came quickly. The baby was underneath me, so I slung my leg over the cord and picked him up. I was in that quiet, timeless and holy place again. Ron and I stared at our new son, Mike, and talked to him. We were mom and dad, we loved him and we cried to see him. We had just had an unintentional, unassisted birth. The doctor showed up in time to get the placenta, and we planted it in our garden after I got to see it.

Feeling the birth from both sides was an amazing experience. I was my own midwife! But my three-year old, Jasmine, was upset that I hadn't woken her up to see the birth. At the time, my mind was so totally on the birth that all else fell away. The birth was all I could do in the here and now. Remembering this happening helps me to be aware to facilitate what the mom wants to have happen during her birth, as she reports it to me prenatally.

Such was the case when Janet who told us she did not want to have the baby in the bathroom, no matter what. Sure enough as the baby was starting to come, Janet was comfortable sitting on the toilet in the privacy of her bathroom. I reminded her of her desire not to have a bathroom birth. "Oh, my gosh!' she yelled! "What am I going to do?" I told her to get up and walk into the bedroom. She did, and with the baby's head in her vagina and legs open wide, she bounced from one side of the hall to the other, using her hands and outstretched arms to push herself off the wall. Reaching her bedroom, Janet had a beautiful birth in the company of her waiting family. Later she thanked me for reminding her. I was glad that I had remembered her wishes.

Being at a birth makes us all telepathic, or at least makes us aware of it. How many times I have reached to rub a back or take fetal heart tones just to have the other caregiver at the birth be reaching to do the same thing. Or we'll have the same thoughts and start to express them simultaneously. With all this connectedness going on, any fears that are in the hearts of the caregivers or family who are present are being shared through this telepathy. This is where the caregiver who has confidence in birth makes the difference. If the training and experiences of the midwife are negative and she is fearful, it can be hard for a birthing woman to overcome more than her own fears. This factor alone should be enough to make sure midwives are shown lots of natural births in their training.

Before becoming a midwife I had worked in retail clothing sales. But I got "conscious" and did the "tune in, turn on, drop out" thing. I saw that my retail profession was nothing more than a vanity peddler, making people think they needed to have the latest fashion to be whole. This, of course, meant that more of the world's resources would be paved over, eaten up and polluted by factories making all this stuff. When I quit my job, I had no idea what to do next. Soon after, I got married, had a huge organic garden, learned to can food, became a vegetarian and got pregnant! A lot of change, fast! This is when the idea of being a midwife showed itself to me in Ina May Gaskin's book, *Spiritual Midwifery*.

After I became a midwife, I had to do other jobs to stay financially afloat. The job that suited me best and that I did the longest was as a home health aide. The people I would serve were "shut ins;" newly injured or fresh from surgery, elderly or disabled and dying hospice patients. I had a brief training course in generally how to assist people with the "activities of daily living." So my job was to spend two hours a day at someone's house making sure he or she was personally clean, fed and that the house was in livable condition. I could do laundry, cook meals, go grocery shopping, give a shower, wash hair, vacuum the house and socialize in two hours flat! That's a lot! The way the system was set up, I would see my patients, mostly women, three times a week. I'd spend two hours and move on to the next, usually having three clients a day. Medicare and Medicaid allowed thirteen weeks of care. The rhythm of this rotation was one of both hope and desperation. I would get to know and love the ladies and gentlemen I took care of for those thirteen weeks. Being a midwife possessed of a tender heart helped me to love them right away. Knowing about being in someone else's house when they are vulnerable, like women in labor, helped me to reach them on their own terms. I gave them respect and was gentle. I must say my sense of humor did endear me to them and helped to get us over some embarrassing moments. I felt my soul was working, giving its all while I cared for these people. I did not want to judge their "status" in life or think ill of their family because they were not there. While I was actually doing this work, I felt good about it. During this time I was also taking classes to learn Reiki, which is a form of energy healing. I used it whenever I could, advancing my skills and bringing comfort. My patients all loved it.

Since most of the people I cared for were my parents' age or older, I heard a lot of history. While they talked, I cooked them breakfast, cleaned the tub, washed their backs, set their hair, but always I listened. I felt like the golden girl who was being given the history of the tribe to keep sacred. Serving the elderly and frail was an honor, but hard work. And can some people whine. As all midwives know, pain affects people differently. There were quite a few of my clients who were so miserable the first few weeks I knew them, I dreaded going to their homes. Maybe their pain was from surgery or an accident. But as time passed and they healed, it was as if they were different people! They were like the moaning mom who becomes the smiling diva after the birth. For me, this work was temporary, which was one of the reasons I could be so upbeat and high-minded about it. If I had to do it for years on end, I'm sure it would have worn me down.

During this time, 1995-1996, I did the aide work three days a week and did midwifery the other two weekdays. All my birthing clients knew the days I was working as a home health aide, and in two years I only had to leave an aide job three times for a birth. In the end, the people I cared for taught me much about humanity, and I learned how to be better at giving love with my caring actions. I am grateful for this experience.

Not having a midwifery license for most of the years I practiced midwifery changed and molded how I worked and lived my life. I first started working in Texas and had a license there. But upon moving back to New Jersey, there was no midwifery license available. Even though I was doing exactly what I was doing with a license in Texas, in New Jersey I became illegal.

I formed a partnership with Barbara Schelling in 1984. She was a labor and delivery nurse who was doing home birth "underground." Our personae meshed perfectly. I was an "out there doing it public" savvy midwife, and she was a guarded, secret midwife with nursing skills! We were both patient and had "the gift of gab." Most important, we believed in birth and the mother's innate ability to give birth. But the fact that direct-entry midwives were not legal in our state made me feel invisible. I could not say I was a midwife out loud. We were once interviewed on the local radio station, and she used the name Gladys and I, Laverne, to protect our anonymity! In the event that I had to transport a woman to the hospital, I was the "friend" or the "doula." We observed a rule that all first-time and VBAC moms had to have a backup plan or parallel care with a physician throughout the pregnancy, as these were our biggest transport candidates. Our rate for transport was low (about 12%), and I think part of that was that we learned everything we could do to stay at home. We tried homeopathy, herbs, Reiki, physical positioning, and anything we heard about. We went to seminars and educated ourselves. I became an EMT and rode the ambulance. We did 30 to 40 births a year and over time developed relationships with friendly doctors who would help us.

But I do have to say that being a rebel took its toll on me and my family. I felt like I was always hiding something. Yet, I know what I was doing was the right thing. Being underground made me more fearful of speaking out. On the one hand, I knew that serving women who birthed at home was the right thing, but on the other hand, society said I was dangerous. Every time I had to transport a woman to the hospital, fear went with me. Would they treat the woman well? Could we keep mom and baby together? And was I going to be reported? I wanted my family to be proud of me and not worried about what would happen to me if I got caught. I was doing the right thing for humankind and paying the price.

Along with this underground secrecy was the factor that there were hardly any home birth midwives around then. Ladies would drive two hours to get our care. Our fee was small but had to be paid out-of-pocket by our clients. Years later more CNMs (Certified Nurse-Midwives) decided to do home births, and they could accept insurance reimbursement. Nurse-midwifery was licensed in New

Jersey but direct-entry midwifery was not. A few of our clients called us and told us that they loved us and our care, but that the CNM services would cost them nothing, a big factor for a new family. It seemed so unfair to us, but it was a fact of life. Now, years later, many insurance companies do reimburse CPMs (Certified Professional Midwives), who are direct-entry midwives, for home birth.

Another factor that has changed the way I practice is that I live in one of the largest Orthodox Jewish communities in the United States. A huge rabbinical school draws students from all over the world to Lakewood. I have attended their births for about fifteen years and do about six births a year in the community. Though I am not Jewish, I have learned a lot about the faith and customs. Working with families who live a strict code of ethics is enriching. What's more, they have many children, so when its their sixth or tenth child, they can say things like "with all my girls" or "with my spring babies," unlike women who only have two or three children. These women are not connected to the mass media and so have not been fed that birth fear. Privacy is of the utmost importance. They are not openly affectionate with other adults due to religious laws about blood and appropriateness. I am an affectionate person; it's part of my care. But I go slowly and we are usually hugging by the end of our prenatal months. Then physically supporting them at the birth comes naturally. I am grateful to be where I can be of service to them, and we have a good time.

Learning to be a midwife came from many different sources. Mostly, I think I learned to be patient and "hear" what was needed at a birth from tuning into nature. Birth is a natural process that happens in a slightly different consciousness. I think being helpful to women in labor takes being able to accept the ebbs and flows of birth into your own being. Not being afraid of birth comes with trusting nature, God/Goddess, the higher power or universe, whatever you decide to call the intense energy that comes with birth. This power knows what it is doing. The first human birth, besides my own, that I witnessed was fast and unplanned. Going with the flow of the moment left no room for fear. It was joyous and exciting. Really paying attention to my own births and remembering how I felt gave me inside information.

The teachers I had over the years were wonderful, giving women. Ina May Gaskin was my first teacher. Although I did not know her, the things she wrote opened a door for me. Her books—*Spiritual Midwifery*, *Hey Beatnik*, and *Practicing Midwife*—gave me the hope that I could be a midwife. But The Farm midwives were so spiritual and larger than life, and I wasn't sure I could live up to that. I did read everything I could get my hands on, and one day in the library I came across

Raven Lang's *Birth Book*. It really gave me a visual through the stunning pictures of home births. Complete with blood and tears, Raven showed real home birth. Photos of women on their hands and knees with turned out rectums and flattened perineums were the connections most primal for me. Somehow seeing blood connected the earthiness of the birth event to my heart. My first "in person" teachers turned out to be the midwives who caught my third child, Katy, at home. That was in 1980. They were labor and delivery nurses and "underground" home birth midwives. Alice Werner and Janet Drewes were gifts from God to many of us in New Jersey. Not only did they attend home births, but they also had a study group for midwife hopefuls like me. They welcomed me into the group and told me to get *Williams Obstetrics*, the major obstetrical text at that time. Of course to be able to read it, I had to also purchase a *Tabor's Cyclopedic Medical Dictionary*. Before I knew it, I had my hands on placentas, was learning to practice suturing on chicken breasts and attending the occasional birth. I was thrilled! Then my husband was offered a job in Texas. At that time Texas was the best place to learn to be a midwife, complete with licensing, home births and birth centers. We moved there, and I made a connection with Helen Jolly through my midwife friends. She had a birth center in Grand Prairie and knew most of the midwives in the area. Helen had spoken with Fritzi Thornberg, and I apprenticed with her for a year. I was doing lots of prenatal appointments and births. During this time I decided to go to the community college and take Anatomy and Physiology classes. I loved it and did really well, which was a surprise to me. I am not the classroom type. I am a hands-on learner. I need to be moving and doing to get what is being taught. Midwifery care is personal. To learn this kind of care, it needs to be a process, not a book. How you learn something has a lot to do with how you will use that knowledge. So apprenticing was perfect for me.

Then I went to work with Helen Jolly and Judy Bordelon at the birth center. I loved it there. I got to teach birth classes to the parents and catch lots of babies. Teaching helped me to be a midwife with words. I can be a dramatic storyteller and sharing wonderful births with the couples made the classes fun. I got invited to a lot of births.

Starting my own practice in 1982 brought clients up close and personal. I am like a reporter getting the scoop. What do they eat? Why do they want a home birth? What are they reading? What are their expectations and dreams? So for about a year, I will educate, coddle and love, yes, love these women. Sometimes I see myself as the fluffy brown hen, clucking around the woman, making that low-pitched, long noise—kind of a lulling sound—fluffing her feathers with my beak trying to make her feel loved and comfortable. Allowing myself to care on a personal level for the moms makes me be a better midwife for them. I let each woman know who I am, sharing my life. Then the door is open for her to do the same. While I find that I can go to a birth of someone I don't know and bond with her immediately, it is not the same as the relationship that I make with prenatal care. It doesn't surprise me that bad care is what most pregnant and laboring women get from overworked OBs and labor and delivery nurses. They don't know the women they see; it's not personal. The birth is more about their job than the woman. Love and relationships are real. It's the basis of how people treat each other. If the caregiver knows the mother, it becomes personal for her as well. This creates a partnership, a feeling of being in this process together. When this happens, the mother and baby get better care. Getting to know someone takes time. This is the strength and advantage of the midwives' continuity of care.

I tell stories about good births to the moms I see. I show them how to palpate their own babies. I let the woman know that I believe she can birth, almost take it for granted. By setting the stage for a good birth experience, the mother plays it out in her head and readies herself. Seeing it before it happens makes it manifest real. I feel I have done my job well when the woman is laughing in early labor and knows that she is the only one who can do the work ahead.

I like to use Reiki to help the women I see. It is a form of healing touch and makes me sensitive to energy. I know that the Reiki helps her to relax, open and let things flow. The baby feels it, too. Sometimes I will put my hands on the mom's back in labor and I can "see" the baby. I send the baby a message, like "tuck your head." I just picture it in my own mind and try to send it to the baby.

Something that I feel helps me at births is that I actually do enjoy the labor and birth process and the passing of time with women. Staying in the here and now and focusing on the woman helps to keep me in the same realm of consciousness as the laboring woman. Of course, many births are very forthright, just starting and going right through, textbook style. These births make us all remember to respect the process and not take credit for it all going so well.

The politics of birth are the same as the politics for or against women in general. Through history women have had to struggle to be equal. While I must say I am not in favor of abortion, I am also not in favor of some governmental decision about what a woman can do with her own body. The Bush administration pushed for abstinence in sex education. As a result, the rate of pregnant teens and STDs skyrocketed under this oppressive action. Telling hormone-driven teens not to have sex is like telling the Mississippi not to flood!

So let's look at birth. Why have the obstetricians, who are predominately male, taken over women's work? It has not gone well, as anyone who has read about the history of birth in America knows. Moving birth into the hospitals and out of homes proved deadly at first. I think history is repeating itself and now it is deadly again. One in every three women in the United States has a cesarean section, and the death rate for women having surgical births is on the rise. Tons of money is spent to support interventions and the use of devices to monitor women and babies during labor. Many of these practices are not evidence-based. Research shows that the use of some interventions actually makes things worse in terms of optimal outcomes. If this money were spent on making pregnant women healthier, the United States would have better maternal and infant outcomes. Let's educate the women about what to eat, how to exercise, and healthy lifestyles. Let's teach women the truth about birth, which is that they were made to do it! Whenever there is real research to show that a routine OB practice that women do not like—such as continuous electronic fetal monitoring—could be altered or eliminated, it is ignored if it is something that the obstetricians want to use. The obstetrician's needs trump the woman's needs, even when the standard practice, like continuous electronic fetal monitoring, is not an evidence-based intervention. So the current thinking is that the potential liability suit the obstetrician might have to deal with is a more terrible thing than the unnecessary cesarean section the birthing woman might have to suffer, even though there is a risk she might possibly die. Mothers and babies are subjected to the electronic fetal monitor as a standard OB practice even though it sometimes gives inaccurate information leading to unnecessary interventions. Money is more valuable than women's lives. So the monitor stays, but only because there aren't enough nurses to do the periodic hands-on listening to fetal heart tones that even the American College of Obstetricians and Gynecologists agrees would be enough. Is it better to pay for more machines than nurses? Most nurses are women after all, so that is politics again. How can one of the richest countries in the world have such bad birth outcomes? It's because here in the United States it's about the money, not about the women!

One thing I know that I have accomplished in my life is that there are over a thousand babies out there that have been born well because their mother knew me! Another thing that has happened is that I believe that I have stretched the societal norm. Things don't change unless someone does something extreme. Artists and philosophers bring about needed changes through their visionary works. As a midwife, I am a visionary. I hope that in the near future women will demand good care. Society will realize that the sacredness of birth and the mother-baby connection is the most important human thing we have.

One of my accomplishments is that I remain optimistic after all these years. This has not always been easy to do when even other midwives put you down. How can one midwife belittle another? Here is how I see it. The Certified Nurse-Midwives are making a space within the medical establishment, serving women in hospitals, clinics and obstetricians' offices. Yes, there are some Certified Nurse-Midwives who are home birth midwives, but the majority of them are not. The direct-entry midwives are pushing the envelope, working mainly outside the hospital and outside of the established norms. They are trying to change the laws in women's favor. We've been working to open people's minds to a better way to birth. So we midwives need to appreciate each other. This is something I have worked on, especially as a representative for the Midwives Alliance of North America (MANA). I have found myself sometimes surprised at the comments of disrespect and meanness made about a "fellow" midwife. Too many wonderful Certified Nurse-Midwives practices have been shut down because they didn't make money for the hospital. When it was necessary for me to transport a client from home to hospital during labor, I have been totally grateful to transfer the care of a woman I had grown to love to a like-minded midwife. That is a clear example of needing each other. But in the spirit of reciprocity did that CNM know that I have been out here trying to change the culture? When birthing women say, "It's not about the money, it's about good birth," then we will know we are succeeding in changing the culture. I think many women have been influenced by the underground midwives, by the direct-entry midwives, by the CPMs who hold the space for a truly natural birth at home. I don't think we rebels have been getting any credit for that.

Something else I think I have accomplished is that I am among the folk legends of this great country of ours. That may sound egotistical to say, but it was just my place in life, my job, if you will. If you believe that we all have a responsibility in life, then how could I not speak out for something as real and human as birth? I know that how we are born makes a difference. If we become a culture of people who cannot birth as nature intended, our basic humanness will change. Will we still love our children and each other? So much is at stake. In John Steinbeck's novel, *The Grapes of Wrath*, the hero, Tom Jode, said to look for him in all the downtrodden of the day, and similarly the midwives who have fought to keep birth sacred and free can be seen as folk heroes. We are legendary! I say thank you to all my sisters, and I am proud to be part of this noble cause.

The child is the gem

SHAFIA MONROE

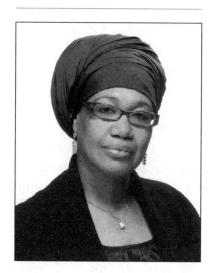

My life has been a blessing and a miracle. I am ever grateful to the universal spirit for birthing me in the physical form as a midwife. As I trace my steps from where I began and where I stand today, I am a midwife for life. It is spiritual because I can actually track the guidance from my Creator and my ancestors. When young women aspiring to become midwives ask me the famous question, "What made you want to become a midwife, or how did you know that you were supposed to be a midwife?" I sigh, smile and get excited, because it is such an amazing story. I am so happy to share my midwife journey, because for me it is truly a God-led experience; I was called to midwifery at the tender age of seven, was affirmed by the elders at age sixteen, began training at seventeen and completed it at twenty-four. I was an independent midwife at age twenty-six. Though I was practicing midwifery at age twenty-four, I was not yet a wise woman; this came later in my midwifery career. I believe everything we do is the reflection and the result of someone else's work, prayer and vision, mostly the spiritual vision.

My childhood was great and unique, just like a midwife's life. I come from a joyous family of nine immediate relatives: my wise and daring feminist mother, Yvonne Deliah Kenion Monroe; my fearless, religious, and environmentally conscious father, Thomas Walter Monroe; and my seven brothers and sisters. I fall somewhere in the middle. My dad was from Alabama and a rural southern Baptist who ate grits every morning. My Bostonian Catholic mother ate fish on Friday. My parents were African American, yet my home was bi-cultural with two languages: proper King James English and Ebonics with a Southern drawl. Both influenced how I embraced midwifery, but my love of nature and tradition (shaped into a traditional midwife) keeps me connected to my Southern roots. Though born in Boston, I claim Alabama as my home. My dad brought us home to Alabama every summer as long as I can remember. I love the South because of its oral history, the respect for the land, and the visible connection between my African ancestry and the Southern culture. This culture is evident in the food, greeting customs, songs, spiritual traditions and many other traditions. I rode horseback, walked barefoot, and learn about herbs and natural healing from my paternal grand-mother. The Southern culture helped me embrace the concept of natural living, thus natural childbirth. And most empowering is that the South is sacred ground, the birthplace of the African American midwife, the Grand Midwife, (referred to as granny midwife), and it embodies me. I was destined to be a midwife, but my Southern heritage gave me the cultural foundation to be proud as an African American midwife. I tell my audiences that the midwives of my generation—the Soul Sistah Midwives born between the 1950s-1960s—are the granddaughters of the Grand Midwives. We searched hard to capture their essence in order to pass it on to our daughters to protect the spirit of the Black midwife, and there is a difference. Every community had their midwife and we had ours. Since age seventeen, when I learned about the Grand Midwife in the South and in America, I have been on fire to get the word out to the Black community about our historical stake in the midwifery story in this country. Along with catching babies, I have served as a historian and traditionalist to preserve our history. Every organization that I have founded including the Traditional Childbearing Group (TCBG) in Boston—which joined the Childbirth Providers of African Descent (CPAD)—and the International Center for Traditional Childbearing (ICTC), has had a mission not only to reduce infant mortality, but in doing so, to also know our Black history as midwives, healers and wise women.

As a child I was very sensitive; my parents referred to me as gifted. I had strong intuition; I could read situations and I still do. I was uncomfortable seeing injustice and suffering. I always wanted to help those in need. I befriended the underdog, making friends with stray animals and unpopular kids. My inner spirit was growing my midwife spirit with sensitivity, leadership, and social justice awareness. I could feel the discomfort of others, (I feel the labor pains with the laboring mother). I was taught by both my parents to help people and find my purpose in life. It has been my gift to empower, uplift, and mentor women through pregnancy, labor, birth and parenting and to support aspiring midwives. These are the wise-women components that must be part of midwifery. Studying the lives of the Grand Midwives and learning from the elders, I learned that midwifery has always been more than just catching babies. It includes creating healthy communities and doing the political and social justice organizing to make it happen. A true midwife has a lot of power and responsibility.

I grew up listening to my elders reminisce while shelling peas, canning or sipping a cup of coffee; but I had never heard them mention the word midwife or discuss any birth stories in my presence. It wasn't until my late teens that I learned that my dad and all of my extended family had been birthed at home and with midwives, and that my grandmother had, on occasion, assisted their community midwife. I was elated and proud that my relatives knew the names of their midwives. My grandmother said, "Ms. Carrie just passed two years ago. I would have introduced you if I had known you wanted to midwife." But I felt empowered just knowing that I had ridden on horseback through the Alabama woods past the abandoned houses that had once been inhabited by practicing Black midwives.

So, in essence I grew up around midwives and women who birthed their own babies, but I didn't know it until later in life. As I matured I realized that my grandmother and elder relatives had emulated the culture described by the great Black midwives of ole, like Ms. Gladys Milton, Ms. Onnie Lee Logan, Ms. Maude Callen, Ms. Margaret Smith: it was in the way they carried themselves with dignity, always up with the sun, always so clean, their houses always so clean, how they used herbs and honey, how they dealt with babies, breastfeeding, nutrition and how they taught me to parent when I had my first child. It was how they worked with one another. I viewed the famous documentary, *Bringin' in Da Spirit* by Rhonda Haynes, which is a film history of African American midwives, and was moved because I remember those types of women in my childhood in rural Alabama. Witnessing again my connection to the circle of midwifery.

Midwifery includes maturity. Nowadays young women are midwives at early ages, straight out of midwifery school. Many don't have children and may never have been in a long-term relationship, but I learned that those experiences build your midwifery. Having clinical skills and evidence-based information are important, but having life skills is equally as important. As a young midwife at the age of twenty-four, I experienced rejection and sometimes disdain from older women. How could I counsel a thirty-two-year-old married woman having her third child? I couldn't. Sure, I could give good clinical prenatal care, but not "wise-woman" midwifery support. I wanted to emulate the lives of the Grand Midwives but couldn't do it until my late forties, and the more I gain years, of course, I become a better midwife. I have birthed seven children, had miscarriages, been divorced and re-married. I have lived life and can provide the emotional support, wisdom and evidenced-based life experiences to be a Grand Midwife. The Black midwives did more than just catch babies, they taught Motherwit, which was so important in empowering families and the community.

The second phase of my midwifery journey began when I was fifteen, after my mother died, two days after my birthday. Due to grief, I left home and moved into a Muslim community and converted from Christianity to Islam. When I arrived, I became acquainted with pregnant women. I hadn't much exposure to pregnant women; my prior experience was with animals and befriending children who were being harassed by their peers on the playground. Therefore, I was intrigued by these big stomachs that were holding babies inside. The women there were older; I was fifteen, and they were all in their twenties and older. Some were newly pregnant, and many already had children. All of them breastfed their infants. I had still never thought of being a midwife (having not heard the term yet), but I was amazed by these women and wanted to ask them many questions about how it felt to be pregnant and if I could feel their babies. Most found me amusing, but they were always kind, would answer my questions and sometimes would let me feel their babies moving. Later I moved in with a Muslim family, and the wife was pregnant with her fifth child. She was about thirty-seven years old and I was now sixteen. I informally served as her nanny, helping her with her younger children so she could rest. She didn't talk much to me about her pregnancy, but I learned about the normalcy of pregnancy in a very matter of fact way. I was fortunate to witness her in her daily activities, which remained the same, cooking, playing with her children, walking to the store, and so on. I would bring her water and help as needed. She would dress comfortably at home, so I was able to watch her uterus grow in size. I was always fascinated. I stayed, asking questions and always wanting to feel the baby. One day she said, "Shafia, you should be an obstetrician." I replied, "What's that?" I had never even heard of an obstetrician. She said, "That's a doctor who takes care of pregnant women and delivers their babies." I thought that sounded good, so I decided I would become one. She then gave me *Emergency Childbirth* to read, a book designed for fathers in case the baby was born before they made it to the hospital. I read it front to back and memorized it in a weekend.

When it was time to for me to register for college at seventeen, I entered as a pre-med student with the intention of going to medical school to become an obstetrician. I had not heard of midwifery. One day while visiting my uncle, I shared my career goals, and he asked me, "Why don't you become a midwife?" "What's the difference," I asked, and he told me what it was.

It was divine guidance, because *Our Bodies, Ourselves* was being published in Boston and *Spiritual Midwifery* had just been published by Ina May Gaskin. The entire birth movement was shifting back to women-led births and women being the directors using midwifery as the vehicle. It was indeed a very exciting time to be involved in the re-emergence of the midwife community.

So, at seventeen I was looking to find a place to be groomed as a midwife. There were several groups evolving in Boston, but they were void of Black women or Black women's contribution to midwifery in America. This void led me to organize Black women, to learn the history of Black midwifery, to become a midwife and to birth with midwives. There was an explosion in my spirit that midwifery was my platform to address the normalcy of birth, politics and racism. Once I learned the plight of Black infant mortality, the eradication of Black midwives from American history, and lack of inclusion of Black women in the midwifery movement, I was compelled to follow the footsteps of my predecessors and become a community activist using midwifery as the instrument. So midwifery was not just "Oh, I love seeing those babies born." It was deeper than that. I became convinced that if the Black community understood its political and spiritual connection to midwifery it would bring us closer, make us more active, improve our birth outcomes, support the Black family and support the Black man. Midwifery always included a connection to the Black man. In *A Midwife's Tale*, author and historian, Laurel Thatcher Ulrich, says that the Black midwife helped to protect Black beauty for its women and was successful in keeping the Black man connected to the birth.

My dad gave me the history of Black midwives in the South, saying "Oh, that's no big deal, your grandmother helped midwives. I was born at home. Everyone did that." I started researching midwifery and the African American experience, and I thought, *Oh, my God . . .* I was blown away. I had never learned about it in high school, never heard about it at the mosque, never heard about it at the church, and no one ever talked about Black midwives in this country during my era. Maybe they did in the early 1940s, but in my time no one talked about it. I was totally amazed, captivated and committed to letting the Black community know that we should re-embrace and re-empower that part of our history.

I searched for Black midwives to train me, and I was successful. I found midwives from Africa and the South to train me. In addition to taking pre-med classes in college I also took classes at Boston City Hospital to become a Certified Nurse's Aide (CNA). I was thinking, *Ok, how do I get this training?* I felt that there were no real acceptable programs for me, the African American Muslim Nationalist woman. Though I participated in the Massachusetts Midwives Alliance and other midwifery study groups in the dominant society, I wasn't able to get my training from them. So, I had to create my own educational track, which began by becoming a CNA. After I became a nurse's aide, I asked for placement on the delivery floor so I could get some experience. Instead I was placed on the postpartum floor, which I was very upset about, but I realized that again God was in control. It really worked out well. I worked the 11P.M. to 7A.M. shift. I was still able to see births, which were horrible back then, people lying on their backs and doctors silent, but I still saw the babies born and learned what not to do. And the postpartum floor was rich with birth stories from the mothers and I had exposure to breastfeeding. I understand now how blessed I was to have quiet time in the night at the bedside of newly delivered mothers, mostly Black and Hispanic. For over a year I heard their stories—everything from abortion stories to adoption and stillbirth stories. I was just eighteen, and I thank those women who shared with me their sad, powerful, and intimate stories. They shaped how I was going to practice my midwifery and made clear to me what I saw as the gaps in services for birthing mothers. As a CNA, I became efficient with the hundreds of postpartum blood pressures, temps, respirations, and pulses, seeing the bloody pads and women recovering with cesareans. Working in the nursery I learned to take care of the tiny newborns: bathing, swaddling, taking respirations and auxiliary temps, burping, removing extra digits and circumcision. It reinforced the need for women-led childbirth and home birth in the Black community. Of course, now we have birthing rooms and birth centers, but back then there wasn't even rooming-in. All babies were separated from their mothers unless they were breastfeeding. My job was to roll the baby to the mother and bottle-feed the babies in the nursery if they were not breastfed. It was a teaching hospital in the inner city that served poor patients, so it was a whole different type of experience. But it was a truly wonderful experience that also added to my midwifery experience and informed what I do today.

I grew up with an awareness of the power of women, but it didn't originate from the feminist or women's movements. I already felt like I came from a powerhouse. My mom, my grandma, my aunts, they just didn't take any mess. So I grew up with a voice. I went to Boston City Hospital, but that was just part of the clinical training. For me to actually learn to be a midwife, I had enrolled at the University of Massachusetts as a pre-med student. I remember standing on the campus almost every other day, asking any Black woman who walked by (especially those who were from Africa), "Are you a midwife?" I did that for I don't know how long until someone finally said, "Yes, I'm a midwife." And I said, "I need you. I know you don't know me but my name is Shafia, and I need to be a midwife and need you to help me." This lady didn't even know me, and she was kind of reluctant, but I kept calling her and eventually she met with me, providing more academics on the physiology of labor. I remember how hard it was for me to understand effacement, but I eventually grasped it. She was from the Congo, in central Africa. She also shared the birth traditions of her group.

At twenty-one, I gave birth to my first child, a 7 lb, 8 oz son. I had a home birth with a home birth friendly doc, and my husband and a friend were present. It was a pretty straightforward birth. I remember my last words during the crowning, "No matter what, don't cut me." I was the first Black woman in my community to have a home birth in 1976. I had wanted a Black midwife, but I did not know of any. In later months I heard of another Black woman who had just had a home birth with the same doc. I met with her, Majeeda Amaadeen, a registered nurse from Alabama. She was the daughter of a practicing home birth midwife. I was elated, another prayer answered, a Black midwife who wanted to organize with me. So, though I trained with international midwives—African, Pakistani and other midwives from Alabama—Majeeda brought everything to another level. We advertised and reached out to community women who wanted to become midwives, promoting home birth and advocating for the eradication of infant mortality in our communities. We formed the Traditional Childbearing Group (TCBG), doing home births and childbirth classes. I am grateful to Majeeda for having taught me midwifery from a Black Southern perspective. This was in

1978, during the movement of empowerment and self-identification, so it was all very timely and wonderful.

Majeeda was my midwife for my second birth—a daughter 7 lb, 6 oz. I was pregnant eleven more times with a total of seven live births, all at home with different Black midwives helping. Though my last birth (a planned home birth) became a hospital transport, I was still blessed to have a midwife in attendance.

I enjoyed all of my pregnancies and continued midwifing during each pregnancy. And at times I was catching babies with my own twelve-week-old baby tied to my back. Once I did a birth five days after my own birth, and when the assistant midwife came to help, she thought my newborn was the mother's baby. I mention that because there was not a lot of backup for me. Because my fees were so low I couldn't pay for a backup midwife, so I had to be present at all births.

I loved being pregnant, birthing and raising my children and, despite the challenges, it was part of life. People say, "Oh you have a lot of children because you are a midwife." That is not the case. I have a lot of children because they were meant to come to the world through me. I love my children beyond words, but they didn't empower me. I hear women say that birth changed their lives, but the births of my babies were matter of fact. I look at birth as normal. I'm not very mystical about birth. I don't feel like it made me into someone else; I never really had that experience. I'm kind of matter of fact about it. I just had my babies, took care of them, and raised them. I think what it did in terms of midwifery is it made me more sensitive to what women want because I knew what I wanted when I was pregnant and during and after my labors. I learned that it is very doable and that there is life after birth. For me, as a midwife, it's not so much about the birth. It's more about the prenatal part and the postnatal care.

I share with midwife students and pregnant couples that the actual birth takes minutes, but the raising of the baby takes your lifetime. As a traditional midwife, I know that there is a wise woman component that is not taught in classes, but the Grand Midwives taught parenting skills. As traditional midwives, we often leave out the parenting education and leave that for a parenting group, play group or the pediatrician. As my children have matured, so has my repertoire to give more to new parents. And they are hungry for those teachings. I think America is excited about birth, but not excited about raising children. And in the African tradition, they're excited about raising the child, not the birth. The child is the gem. So, I try to use midwifery to focus more on the continued celebration of the child. This form of midwifery support could help to identify parenting problems and reduce child neglect and abuse.

As a community-based, traditional home birth midwife, my understanding has evolved. I believe the power of being a community midwife is living, working, praying and shopping in the community that you serve. That allows me to midwife 24/7, which means I am able to educate throughout the life cycle. My responsibilities as a midwife do not end after the 6-12 weeks postpartum visit; it ends when I end, or when I am no longer in contact with the family. I enjoyed providing prenatal care in the woman's home; it gave me a chance to sit in her place and just feel what was strong and what needed assistance. When training midwives, I teach them to use all six senses to provide complete care. An example is going on a home visit: it's summer, the mother's hot, has edema, and has two or three elementary school age children at home. She has thought about a day camp in the area so that she can get some rest. Seeing her in her home tells me a lot more about her than her prenatal records do. Or when I move throughout the community, people stop me and say "I met you at my aunt's house when she was pregnant. Well, I am pregnant too. Can you help me?" Community midwifery is about creating long-term relationships for systemic change. Change happens best slowly and over a period of time; rarely is nine months sufficient. I always included a massage as part of my prenatal care because moms need a good rub. I bring herbal beverages to drink, literature to read and certain foods to eat. Home prenatal visits are great to get to know the dad and also the extended family.

There are risks associated with being a midwife; we all fear something happening to someone's baby and that person not liking us anymore. And now that I've gotten further into the profession, further into the world as it is today, we are looking at the fear of lawsuits. But midwifery is just pretty matter of fact. I feel like God wants me to do it and chose me to do it, so it's been a very easy, wonderful ride.

It is a fact that midwifery as a whole is still not recognized or respected. The United States is still very ignorant of what midwives have done historically around the world. As a birth professional, whether you are a nurse-midwife or direct-entry CPM (Certified Professional Midwife), regardless of how you function, it is still a male-dominated profession. And we are forced to compromise sometimes, depending on the setting, to do what we think is right. As midwives, we are not able to get third party reimbursement, and we are still being arrested for doing something "illegal." We still do not have a lot of schools that support our midwives, and midwives are polarizing themselves in terms of what credentials come after their names. First we were all just midwives. Then there were nurse-midwives, then lay midwives, then LMs (licensed midwives), then traditional midwives, then direct-entry midwives. Now we have the Certified Nurse-Midwife (CNM) who has to get a master's degree on top of that. So, we have all these levels of baggage that keep us saying, "Who is a better midwife?"

In fact, I always tell women that there's only one way they are going to have a baby, and that it will happen either by a vaginal birth or cesarean section. It doesn't matter what is behind your name—you still do the exact same thing with a PhD or a CPM. I understand the titles provide accountability, consumer protection, third-party reimbursement and customer safety. But as midwives we need to continue to support each other. Originally the midwife was the doula, but now you have someone else providing the support that the midwife historically gave. In the past the midwife provided the most comprehensive care. She was the doula, the midwife, the lactation consultant, the nanny, and the marriage counselor. I think, *My god, where is the continuity of care that we talked about? Where is the holistic approach?* It seems like we are not really doing it anymore.

One of the most important lessons that I learned from practicing midwifery is that it is one of the easiest jobs you can have. The mother does all the work. It's not rocket science to do this work. I know the medical profession wants to make it appear that way, but, historically, people have always done it themselves. It humbles me to think that even if I couldn't make it to assist a birthing mother, she could do it without me. That is very humbling. I provide support and reassurance, but I think that once women get to the point where they reclaim their intuition and self-confidence, more and more women will trust the normalcy of birth and seek women-supported births.

One of midwifery's goals is to reduce infant mortality, which is why I work as a midwife. I want to see a decrease in the deaths of babies before the age of one. That's common in America, regardless of race. We as a nation have one of the highest death rates in the world of babies dying before the age of one-year old. So as a midwife, the work that I do has helped women and men take better care of themselves so that their babies can live past the age of one. They can have a better birth experience, and then they can be empowered, not just in home birth, but also in whatever they do. They need to know that they have a right to be treated with dignity in any setting, whether they are birthing in or out of a hospital. And that is important to me because I want women to transform this experience of empowered birthing into their everyday lives. So, whether she is going to advocate for her child at daycare or going to buy a house, it strengthens the woman and her partner to have good self-esteem. When people feel good about themselves, they treat each other better and that makes a better world. And my goal as a midwife is to foster world peace. I've gone from infant mortality prevention to really seeing midwifery as a tool for world peace, as well as a sustainability movement. People who talk about sustainability in the Green Movement do not say that by breastfeeding we're reducing plastic and cans around the world. They don't say that by midwives promoting the use of cloth diapers we could reduce the amount of E.coli bacteria and feces and plastic diapers in landfills. Therefore, I think that we midwives are definitely part of the sustainability movement, as well as being peacemakers.

As a midwife, I have used my calling for community activism to address social justice issues, public health issues and discriminatory practices against Black women and their families. I'm extremely proud of the things that I have done. I became a midwife in a very difficult time, with minimal options for Black women on the East Coast to learn, and lack of outreach to Black women offering them home birth information and options. I created two non-profits. First, the Traditional Childbearing Group, which was historical by having outreached, lobbied, and challenged hospital administrations on their minimal birth options for pregnant women, provided a home birth service for Boston's Black community, and trained women as midwives. And now ICTC (International Center for Traditional Childbearing) has expanded the same mission around the nation. ICTC has launched blackmidwives.org in cyberspace, a Web site that talks about midwifery from spiritual and traditional perspectives, and hosts the annual national Black Midwives and Healers Conference that instills pride across the African Diaspora. The conferences have brought together Black midwives from around the world, from Canada, Africa, the Caribbean, Haiti, and Columbia. With our first conference only having begun in 2002, it has since become an important piece to keep Black midwives connected for support and professional development. The responses have included "wonderful" to "I didn't know that midwives still existed." So, the conferences have been a great promotional, educational, marketing tool to promote the agenda of several platforms for improving birth outcomes and organizing Black midwives and those interested in eliminating health inequities. I created the *Black Midwives and Healers Review*, the only one of its kind.

As a midwife I have been blessed to work full circle. And I always replay what the Grand Midwives did; I still want to be like them—I want their approval because they did it all. They were the midwife, the doula, the nanny, the marriage counselor, the entrepreneur and the wise woman. Rosa Parks said, "Memories of our lives, of our works and our deeds will continue in others." I will always hold the Grand Midwife in high esteem; they were the silent backbone of the Black community in an era when Blacks had zero birth options. I am driven by the work that I do because of what they did.

Midwifery is political work . . . very political, and so I'm always birthing the movement everywhere. My goal is to build capacity, to increase the number of Black midwives and the number of families who use midwives, to increase home birth, and ultimately to mobilize the Black community to address the health inequities that we experience. I believe our maternal and infant health disparities come from the eradication of midwifery and lack of national outreach in the Black community to encourage this calling, this profession, this work. Byllye Avery, keynote speaker at our first Black Midwives and Healers Conference, challenged us by saying, "I don't know how you're going to get them, but you need to get them, so this art (midwifery) doesn't become lost." We need more Black midwives. We need more women and families who know what midwives do and who will use our services. I love catching the baby—it is the ultimate experience—but I am also birthing a movement that will eradicate infant mortality, increase breastfeeding rates, and increase the number of Black midwives to improve community health.

I am pleased that with the help of all the sistahs and brothas, I have birthed ICTC, a Mecca for Black women to learn to become midwives and to be proud of their history. There are probably a lot of things that I won't get to see happen in my lifetime because life is always continuing. But right now I'm still living. I remain optimistic! As the Dalai Lama says, "Never give up."

So I tell younger midwives to never give up. If you are called, then this is your destiny. Walk it your way and you'll get there. I love being a midwife—I think it is the ultimate. I'm just blessed that I've been called to do this work.

Children came up to me to kiss my hands

SISTER ANGELA MURDAUGH

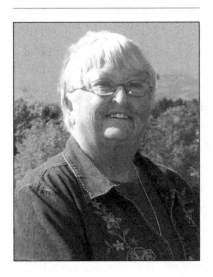

*W*hen *I remember what it felt like* when I first put my foot on the path to becoming a midwife, I find myself looking back and recalling what brought me to that moment, that life decision. My mother was definitely an influence because she was a labor and delivery nurse. I always sensed that she loved her work. She was proud of being a nurse, and all who encountered her knew that fact.

The decisive moment of influence occurred in 1967 on the first day I arrived with six of my college classmates on the maternity floor for the first clinical experience of our maternal and newborn rotation during our junior year. Our instructor for the day was Sister Mary Charitas Iffrig. She was well respected by her fellow professors in the School of Nursing of Saint Louis University and we students knew that. So, we were patient when, after twenty minutes of waiting, Sister Charitas had not yet appeared. When she stepped lightly into the conference room and gazed on us with her smiling face, I sensed that it was going to be a good day. Indeed it was. She announced that she had been with a couple who were one of five couples she had taught the Erna Wright Method of childbirth education. The big difference in this method was that the couple sang through transition. She was happy to tell us that this couple had agreed to allow us to observe the balance of labor and birth.

With that said, we trooped off behind her to the labor room. Sister shoved back the labor stretcher nearest the door and proceeded to take the chairs from all the other labor rooms, forming them into a semi-circle for us to sit and quietly observe. Sister then resumed her position of co-supporter with the husband.

In a few minutes, the couple burst out, singing "Oh, What a Beautiful Morning," followed quickly by a declaration from the mother that she needed to push. We all got out of the way as the labor and delivery nurses appeared and pulled the stretcher through the door, down the hall and through the swinging doors of the delivery suite. We all followed behind her like she was the Pied Piper. We lined up behind the obstetrician, who was respectful to Sister and pleasant with the couple.

It was 1967, so the mother was on a standard delivery table. The doctor sat on a stool between her legs, which had been placed in stirrups. He was gowned and masked, but it seemed not to dampen in any way the positive mood of that room. The baby slid out and announced her arrival. Then, the scene changed from the standard procedure of the era. The baby was not whisked off to the nursery, but the doctor placed the baby on the mother's lower abdomen and cut the cord. The baby was immediately passed to the mother who (with Sister Charitas' assistance) had the little one suckling at her breast right away. The husband beamed and repeatedly congratulated his wife.

I can only say that I was overcome by the emotion of a birth that was so family-centered and different from everything that I had read about up to that point. This first exposure will remain forever imprinted on my mind and heart. I went on to attend women in labor who were "not there" due to twilight sleep medication, and I was present in delivery rooms where mothers received anesthesia for delivery. The new mother would be awakened (or they were "brought up" as the expression went) after the birth with oxygen to make some nonsense statement of exclamation as the baby was held up momentarily for her to see, before being taken to the nursery. Then the facemask was again applied for the woman to go back to sleep for the repair of the routine episiotomy. But I had seen the best first, and that would make all the difference.

It was Sister Charitas who first told me about midwifery. Just prior to graduation, I was casually walking to the hospital cafeteria telling Sister my concerns regarding my future nursing practice. I did not want to be a floor or department supervisor, but rather a person who worked directly with the mothers. She suggested nurse-midwifery, which I had never heard of, but was totally open to that possibility. She obtained the information I needed for graduate school.

After graduating with my Bachelor's of Science in Nursing (BSN) degree in February 1969, I spent a year and a half rotating the various parts of hospital obstetrics and nursery with a few experiences on an outreach mobile clinic for prenatal care in the inner city of St. Louis. In the fall of 1970 I entered the graduate program in nurse-midwifery at Columbia University.

I was deeply influenced regarding where I wanted to practice by another of our Franciscan Sisters, Emeline Hitpas. She was a hospital administrator. I shared religious community life with her and eleven other Sisters during my years as a student nurse. She was the humblest person in authority I had ever met. She was totally approachable and had a driven desire to reach out to those who needed care. She easily enlisted the volunteer services of health care professionals to go to migrant farmworker camps or the inner city.

Sister Emeline was eventually elected to the governing group of our Franciscan Order. In that capacity she represented our Sisters in a group of Sisters from all over the United States who were interested in health care. That group had made it a priority to provide health care services to migrant farmworkers. Sister Emeline went to Texas to visit with the migrant families who called the Rio Grande Valley their home, and she would later share their stories with me. She sensed my interest and thus encouraged me to think about going to South Texas when my education was completed.

When I finished graduate school, I decided to do an internship in nurse-midwifery because I wanted to hone my midwifery skills prior to heading to what I perceived to be rural and isolated America. That was definitely a smart decision because I would find myself in a very small town twenty-five miles from the nearest hospital. I spent five months at St. Vincent's Home and Hospital for unwed mothers in Philadelphia. I followed that with a month of one-on-one tutoring from an obstetrician who had respect for women and their desires for obstetric (OB) care. I was finally ready to fulfill a long and satisfying "calling" to be a midwife.

Born from a local group of Hispanic farmworkers was a clinic, *Su Clinica Familiar*. The leaders of the community had elicited help from the Department of Health, Education and Welfare and from several communities of religious Sisters. There were two clinics twenty-five miles apart. Only the one in the smaller town of Raymondville, Texas, had the space to accommodate a maternity service. A wing was assigned to me in the old doctor's office building they had acquired. So, I found a small trailer to live in and set about starting a care program for pregnant women.

My first discovery was that the clinic was totally thrilled to have me, but they had not budgeted, hired or in any way provided for anyone to help me. Also, there was no salary allocated for me. I would have to make my own way. Fortunately, I had come with a rental trailer full of donated equipment from the maternity hospital in Philadelphia. A seventeen-year-old National Youth Corps member was assigned to help me after school. I used her as a translator and taught her to assist me in clinic. The Sisters who were nurses and a couple of hired practical nurses who worked in the general clinic would assist me during the deliveries. I did all the labor, postpartum and newborn care alone. In the 1970s, it was customary for mothers and babies delivered in the hospital to stay for three days afterward. My decision to keep them only twenty-four hours with a third and tenth day postpartum home visit was radical.

The closest obstetricians were twenty-five miles away in Harlingen, which also had the closest hospital for transfers. I made an appointment to see these doctors and was ushered into the office of the youngest one of a group of three. He was a kind man who agreed to be the consultant.

I saw my first mother for prenatal care on May 1, 1972. The general medical care part of the clinic had been providing some prenatal care with the local indigenous midwives doing the deliveries. So they turned over those charts to me. I made home visits to introduce myself to each mother and invite her to see me for her next visit. After establishing prenatal care with a woman, I would ask her to let me know when she delivered so I could make a home visit to check out both her and her newborn. Most did that by sending someone to the clinic because the vast majority of them had no phone. One of my most vivid memories was of a primipara (first-time mother) I was called to see five days after birth, who was burning up with fever. When I was ushered to her bedside, the odor was overwhelming. I pulled back the covers to discover an ordinary chicken egg on the bed between her legs. I asked about it and was explained the folklore that the fever would enter the egg, and then it would be broken in water. So here I was exposed to my first case of full blown puerperal fever, being treated by a local folk medicine custom. I said nothing about the egg (which was the right decision) and looked at her physically. She had purulent lochia coming from the vagina. On further examination I discovered she had an unrepaired fourth degree laceration through vaginal tissue, perineal skin, perineal muscles, and through the anal sphincter. She was terribly feverish. I consulted with the doctor, got her on antibiotics, and visited her daily. By God's grace, she survived. Over the next eight years she was to be my client for two more babies. I always watched her carefully because with the wide-open perineum her babies literally fell out when she got to complete dilation. Why was the fourth degree laceration never repaired? Very simple: she was too poor to afford to have it fixed.

I looked in the eyes of poverty over and over again. The first breech that presented in labor I transferred to the hospital. The labor and delivery personnel at the hospital put her in a bed and ignored her. She ended up precipitously delivering in the labor bed and was then faced with a hospital bill way beyond her means. Thus began my journey of delivering breeches. I decided to do only multiparous women who had previously given birth with a tried pelvis of at least a 7.5 lb baby. I was vigilant and did not take unnecessary risks, eventually becoming very adept at breech deliveries. At least I was with the woman in labor and not abandoning her because she was destitute.

Eventually, I procured enough furnishings to set up a birth unit. Everything was second-hand, but functional. My first delivery was a migrant woman having her tenth child. She was very entertaining during labor, telling stories about her life as a migrant. Her name was Maria de la Luz. She thought it was quite funny that when she went to a clinic in Michigan the nurse came to the waiting room and asked for Mary of the Light. She had an easy labor. She delivered a nice big boy she named José. After the delivery, the husband told me he wanted to pay me. The administrator of clinic had told me to charge twenty-five dollars. I took the father to my tiny office to tell him this. His reply was, "For you, thirty dollars!" and proceeded to lay three $10 bills on my desk. That was mid-July 1972.

The hardest part of my first midwifery practice was being tied to the phone. It would be two years before I got a full-time partner. By then I felt like the telephone cord was choking me. I was surprised how well the women accepted coming to the clinic to have their babies. I soon discovered that the local custom was for the indigenous midwives (*parteras*) to maintain a room in their houses or a small building separate from the house for the purpose of attending women in labor. Thus they did not expect the *partera* to come to their house. Coming to the clinic was for them like going into that special room at the *partera's* home.

It would be five years before my maternity section was allowed to hire enough practical nurses for someone to be in the birthing unit around the clock. So, before then I kept gloves and a fetoscope at my house so I could have the women come there to be checked to see if they were far enough in labor to be admitted. Some women came to our house for just about everything. One woman came with a small child severely burned, wrapped in a bedsheet. All I could do was give her twenty dollars to go to the emergency room twenty-five miles away. Another woman arrived after her husband hit her in her pregnant belly, worried that the baby might have been harmed. I listen to the fetal heart and assured her that it was ok. She went in front of my dresser mirror to examine her body to determine the number of bruises, all the while voicing threats to get back at him! Women would often knock at our door and give us carrots, onions or other vegetables, gleans of the fields they worked. One woman even gave me a pig.

From the beginning, I saw every mother and baby on the third and tenth days after birth to make sure breastfeeding was going well and to do a general examination of the mother and baby, as well as a newborn lab screen. I could also assess the home situation so I would not be asking mothers to do or obtain things that were impossible for them. I always had one of the clinic aides go with me on home visits mainly because they knew the area well and they could translate for me. These home visits were so important to me. Once, after the rain bans of a hurricane had flooded most of the towns in our county, I made home visits for the next week with my bag of supplies on my shoulder, wading through water with tadpoles swimming around my legs. More than once we slipped and slid on muddy roads where our families lived near the fields of the crops they worked. I barely missed being bitten by dogs. But I saw raw poverty and the strength of a hardworking people who honored me and called me "my midwife." I had children whom I delivered come up to me in the grocery store at the prodding of their mothers to kiss my hands. Mothers told me they pointed out my house to their children to tell them that "their other mother" lived there. I had a warm feeling from knowing I was the community midwife. I grew attached to those simple people who had gracious manners and unquestioning faith in my judgments. They were easy to love. How could I not love them when they loved me so much?

There was never a year of my practice that I did not make an effort to be a part of the American College of Nurse-Midwives (ACNM). I served on the Clinical Committee early on, but actually put the most years and efforts working on the Legislative Committee. When the ACNM determined that a minimum of five ACNM members could form an ACNM Chapter, I got together the three CNMs in the Rio Grande Valley along with one CNM in Corpus Christi and one in San Antonio to form the first independent chapter apart from statewide. I could probably count on one hand the number of times I missed a local chapter meeting during all of my thirty-five years. I was an actively practicing CNM. I have held all the offices in the chapter once or twice. I also was very active in the Consortium of Texas Certified Nurse-Midwives (CTCNM) on my return to Texas after being the ACNM President. There were representative CNMs from all over Texas who met quarterly. I served as treasurer, vice president, and twice as president of this organization. The Discipline Committee, which was appointed by the ACNM President, was the only national committee I served on after returning to Texas.

Though I did not like politics, I felt sure that only by being politically active could real change be made. I worked with other CNMs to get the first Attorney General opinion from Texas' Mark White that formed the basis for nurse-midwifery practice in Texas. The opinion basically said that the practice of midwifery was not the practice of medicine. The fascinating part was that he particularly said that midwifery also included doing episiotomies.

I received an opportunity in 1980 to go to Washington, D.C., to do an internship in political work at NETWORK, a national Catholic Social Justice Lobby. I did learn a few things, though it was not as good as I had hoped it would be. Mainly, I learned how to get around legislative offices on Capitol Hill. It was during this time, from October 1980 to April 1981, that I decided to run for the President of the ACNM at the urging of some of my colleagues. I pondered entering the race for the ACNM presidency for a long time. There were three CNMs running. I won by a very slim margin. I decided to stay in D.C. while I was president because there were some CNMs worried about how well the staff of the headquarters was doing our work. It was a good decision. I was sworn into office at the Annual ACNM convention in Denver, Colorado, in May 1981. I had gone to Helen Burst's home in New Haven, Connecticut, prior to that time to receive the presidential historical papers and get an orientation from her. It was during that Denver convention that I listened and took notes at an open-forum business meeting because I felt it was my responsibility to know the mind of the membership. The topic that year was Lay Midwifery vs. Nurse-Midwifery. There seemed to be an even split in those who came to the microphone on whether the true basis of nurse-midwifery was nursing or midwifery.

The one thing I remember frequently hearing repeated was, "We need to stay in dialogue with the lay midwives." At the time, I took that seriously. It was later that I was to learn that that phrase was like a potential employer saying to an applicant, "We will keep your application on file." In other words, those who said that, for the most part, did not intend to literally be in dialogue.

It led me to call five lay midwives who I considered to be leaders at that time and five nurse-midwives who had some connection with lay midwives or had been one prior to becoming a CNM. I invited them to the ACNM Office in October 1981 for a dialogue. A local CNM acted as the secretary, and the ACNM Representative from Region II also was present. This was the initial step that led the lay midwives to form the Midwives Alliance of North America. There were CNMs who became quite angry over this action of mine and, in fact, led some of them to discuss impeaching me. But for whatever reason, that never happened. I went through most of the 1982 annual convention in Lexington, Kentucky, oblivious to these rumblings. When someone approached me to tell me that it was going to happen, my response was that it would be all right because I really missed Texas and would be happy to return to my full midwifery practice there. I am not the type to worry about my personal name and reputation if I feel what I believe in is worth taking a stand for.

I have always fought for what I believed was right. In fact, for six years I fought for nurse-midwives to be recognized as Medicaid providers in Texas. It was through the Texas Rural Legal Aid organization that a young lawyer agreed to use some of my clients for a suit against the Texas Board of Human Resources. She sent the Board a letter describing the discrimination, which would provide the evidence to make it impossible for Medicaid clients to have the services of a nurse-midwife to care for them during their pregnancy and have it covered by Medicaid. Just a letter from this young lawyer changed their minds. I was awarded the first Medicaid number issued to a CNM in Texas.

I was featured in a film called *Daughters of Time*, made in late 1979, while I was at the birth center with *Su Clinica Familiar* in Raymondville, Texas. In March 1982 the ACNM Foundation used the film premier as a fundraiser. As I watched myself on film, I began to cry softly and wonder to myself why I had ever left Texas and the practice of midwifery among the sweet Mexican women. It stirred me to begin to think about returning there in the future. Actually, I formulated a strategy to return there. It began with asking the Sister who was the contact for my Franciscan Order of Sisters. She was visiting me in Washington, D.C. The morning after I had laid out my plan to return and start a freestanding birth center in Rio Grande Valley, Texas, she told me she had a dream that I was pregnant, and had to explain to the rest of the Sisters in Leadership how that had happened. I laughed and told her "Can you see? I am pregnant with a dream that could be thought of as impossible. It is your task to explain the possibility to the rest of the board."

I began to lay plans to return to Rio Grande Valley through correspondence with Sr. Marian Strohmeyer, the Catholic Diocese of Brownsville health care representative. Eventually, Sr. Marian secured the Bishop's permission to use some land the Diocese possessed just north of Weslaco, Texas, for the new birth center. It would be placed under the umbrella of Catholic Charities of the Diocese of Brownsville. This was very good as it gave us non-profit status so we could write grants.

While I was in Washington, D.C., I had been visiting with Sister Anne Darlene Wojtowicz, CNM, a Sister of Charity of Cincinnati, who was working in a clinic in the District. I had shared my dream with her. She was very interested and told me that if it came to fruition to let her know because she would love to join me. I had learned a hard lesson at *Su Clinica Familiar* that starting a birth center alone was too difficult, so I was determined that my next venture would begin with a CNM partner.

Thus, before my ACNM presidency was ended, I drove to Rio Grande Valley, arriving January 1, 1983, to begin to lay the foundation for building a freestanding birth center I named Holy Family Services. That name had a lot of significance for me. The Foundress of my Franciscan Order, Mother Odilia Burger, had begun her religious quest with the Poor Franciscan of the Holy Family in Pirmasens, Germany. "Holy Family" is the Catholic term for Jesus and his parents Mary and Joseph. The Rio Grande Valley is predominantly Catholic, and such a name would have meaning to the people I wished to serve. Besides, I was not going to remain under any government agency, but rather under the Catholic Diocese, so the birth center was openly Catholic and thus deserved a religious name. In fact, I was determined never to receive any government monies so that we could be free to care for any woman who came to our doors. Furthermore, no one could ever accuse us of using his or her tax dollars. I was able to maintain that policy up until I retired. Sister Anne D. Wojotowicz did join me, and we began to work together on September 13, 1983, which was considered the founding date of Holy Family Services Birth Center.

Wow! How fantastic that the birth center of my dreams was born. The foundation fulfilled many of my aspirations. First of all, I wanted to have a birth center service that was based on spiritual values. Those values would feed the way the staff would live. This included housing on the same complex so that a community could be formed. Living with others who shared the same values would, in turn, nourish us in the way we cared for the mothers. The health services we gave to those needy families would then enrich our community living.

Another value I wanted to incorporate was that the families who came to us would be expected to pay for their care. I had a strong belief that families were empowered and given dignity by paying for what they got. Thus, we set up a means for that to be done. The charge would be reasonable—only 10% over the actual cost. For those who did not have paper money, a contract would be set up so they could come and help on the four-and-a half-acre complex. Jobs like mowing the lawns, doing laundry, cooking, cleaning, and planting were assigned. Each person who came to give service would accrue $5.00 per hour toward reduction of the mother's bill. This lasted for many years until the INS (U.S. Immigration Service) decided that we were breaking the law for those families who were not American citizens. So, the practice did not stop. But it was now in the contract with each mother that she would pay a given amount and *volunteer* a given number of hours. There is a way around anything! I am of average intelligence, but I am definitely above average in cleverness and using what is at hand for creative solutions.

Building a chapel on the grounds of the birth center was important for me. So by the third year we had a small octagonal chapel that always remained open for the families or a passerby to enter and pray. Praying daily as a group was so uplifting for me. The very fact that a bell would ring to announce the prayer time was a bold reminder to me when I was in the birth room that even though I could not be physically present, I knew that all of us (mother, her family, me, the nurse) would be prayed for. Different members of the staff led the prayers, and the richness of their individual spirituality was a gift to me. Their needs or things weighing heavy on their minds were mentioned in the prayer time, which helped me to be sensitive to the concerns that the staff was facing.

I had always dreamed of having a midwifery service where I could roll out of bed and walk to the office to check a pregnant woman. If they were not in active labor or ready for admission to the birth room, they could be sent home, and then I could easily return to my bed. I had finally made that happen. Also, in the birth rooms there were double beds for a family member to rest with the laboring woman or for the midwife to lie down while actively consoling and attending her or resting if things were slow, such as when one is awaiting good labor contractions to get going when there was spontaneous rupture of membranes. I had known too many years of sheer exhaustion during my first eight years of practice due to a total lack of rest and unbelievably long hours on my feet. I was determined to remedy that.

The telephone is a story all its own. There is simply nothing that takes away the jar of being woken up in the night. The whole staff knew never to tell me before I went to bed if there was anyone in labor. I usually had the 3 A.M. shift. I slept better if I was ignorant of a high potential for being called. Impatience and irritation are probably my biggest sins. The telephone interruptions were responsible for bringing out those undesirable traits more than anything else. Perhaps, one of the wonderful rewards of heaven will be no telephone.

I was born at 6 A.M., and thus I think the hours around the dawn are very comforting for me. I also loved to be in the birth room when dawn occurred. It gave me renewed energy and a sense of optimism. A new day dawning and a new life about to emerge were kindred spirits.

Mentoring young midwives had been a strong desire of mine. So, a clinical fellowship of three months or more was established at Holy Family. The main purpose was to give new graduates extra experience under a senior CNM, but also to help with the staffing needs of the birth center. Occasionally, a CNM who needed some experience before returning to full practice was accepted for a clinical fellowship. I was also requested a few times by an educational director to take a new graduate to help heal them from trauma caused by a bad outcome or lack of self-confidence, or a bruised ego from accusations, or a hostile environment for clinical experiences. I found such challenges to be very rewarding. Absolutely every one of those "injured midwives" went back to practice quite productively. Generally, the clinical fellows I mentored left me with a feeling of satisfaction for having improved the profession.

Having student nurse-midwives was rewarding, as well. I accepted only students that were doing the last part of their education (usually called integration). I set high standards for clinical excellence and was myself considered a master clinician. Placement of students with us was a sought-after experience. I was so fortunate to have some students who would go on to be great midwives. During this time I began to be aware of certain attributes that separated those who are what I call "true midwives" from those who simply considered midwifery a profession for which they were educated and by which they could make a living.

I think the best attribute I noted for a midwife in training—who would go on to be a good practitioner of the art of midwifery—was eagerness. It was almost like the student got a high from being around pregnant women or at a birth. They never seemed to count numbers. I would look around and see them just "being present" even when they were not on call. They wanted to give of themselves. Frequently, they would ask for extra call or to help out when they observed that things were either very busy or hectic, but their eagerness never was in the way. Another important quality I observed was inquisitiveness. They asked deep, probing questions. If they observed a new or less frequent occurrence, then they wanted to learn everything they could about it. They seemed to have a keen sense of observation that led to their questions. I could always tell the sincerity of their questioning because they never seemed to be showing off. The most important observation I made is that they did not argue with a senior or experienced midwife. They could manifest a different opinion without being offensive. They did not want to stubbornly hold to a method that would block their ability to see another way by which a procedure, judgment or decision could be made.

In those with the potential to become very good midwives, I saw what I call "manifestations of the heart." These were the young midwives who knew when it was appropriate to cry, and in whose presence. They could show great joy or deep sorrow when such was called for. They could enter into the moment with the client. They knew how to unselfishly set aside themselves in the immediate situation so the client was the center of attention. They knew where to have their own needs for comforting or praise be met outside of the incident. Their most important quality was fearlessness with good judgment. They did not ask useless questions nor did they feel they had to run tests that would only tell them what they already knew. They were not afraid of birth, and it was manifested in their ability to instill confidence in the mother, family and nurses. If the unexpected presented itself, then they took care of whatever immediately required attention and asked for help appropriately. They were not reckless; they were quick thinkers. They were also cool and had a generally calm exterior. They had an innate sense of propriety.

I could spot what I knew would be good midwives by their ability to make decisions and their taking responsibility for the consequences. They would admit when they were wrong. They accepted their correct assessment with humility. I most often saw this when they would ask others around them to give advice or observations on a case. People who worked with them felt they were part of their team, and so their contributions were honored and utilized. A very important quality that gave me a clue to when I had a potentially good midwife before me was other-centeredness. They had a demeanor that was unselfish. They wanted to see happy families, well-cared-for babies and a smooth running team of providers without themselves grabbing the limelight. They seemed sincerely to be indifferent as to who got the credit.

Of course each of us has flaws and defects; we have good days and bad days. Nonetheless, outstanding traits can be nurtured by a good mentor. Those qualities that are the weakest have the potential to grow stronger with more experience. As a *Sage Femme,* I see my role to be one of taking the seed of hope in each new midwife and helping it to flower into a joyous person. The person who feels "called" will enjoy a good degree of self-fulfillment that will spill over to touch those they work beside and those who are the recipients of the labor of their hands, heads and hearts. These will be the midwives who can say with total sincerity, "I love being a midwife."

I was a sought-after speaker for professional conferences on a variety of topics. Requests to do a ceremonial Blessing of Hands for midwives held a reverence that was dear to me. Signing ACNM certificates while I was President was also one of those times when I felt a sense that I was passing on to the next generation of midwives a small piece of myself. Some of my speaking invitations were clinical, but the ones I most remember were the ones in which I motivated or inspired an audience of midwives to renew their call to their profession. Undoubtedly, the highlight talk of my career was the Teresa Dondero Lecture given at the ACNM Annual Meeting in Atlanta, Georgia, in May 2002. I realized that though I had received several prior honors with plaques and bowls, to be asked to give the Dondero Lecture was an honor itself. Hands down though, the greatest honor of my career was to be given the Hattie Hemschmeyer Award in May 1990. I keep a photo of the then-President of ACNM, Joyce Thompson, and I dancing on the stage to the tune of "The Yellow Rose of Texas" right after the presentation had been made. It was like getting an Academy Award! In 2002, I was appointed to the Texas Women Hall of Fame. I know that was fantastic, but it was more for the profession than for me that I am glad I am listed. To have a midwife featured in a hall with the likes of a woman governor, an astronaut, and a gold medal athlete is a boon for our profession.

My walls were lined with honors, yet I would reflect that somehow it seemed wrong to reward me for doing what I loved to do. I had a fulfilling life that encompassed so much of what I held dear. I consider myself as blessed beyond measure. So many people never have the opportunity to live and work in such an authentic manner as I was granted. It is amazing how days pass into weeks and then into months and years, leaving me wondering, *where did all that life go?* I am now retired, but I understand that I possess a wisdom born of joys, hard work, disappointments, accomplishments and failures, friendships made and kept, prayer in good times and in bad, loss and sorrow, countless hours of skin-to-skin touch on mothers and soft newborns, blessings given on countless foreheads, advice and teaching doled out to my disciples—all of which wove their way through my life.

My rewards were smiles, hugs, seeing new life begin again, an email of thanks from a student or a nurse. All of those are human contacts that can never be hung on a wall, but which have a distinct place in my heart. All I can say is how blessed am I to have lived, with fullness and zest, a meaningful life. God is good all the time!

A very fine line

CAROL NELSON

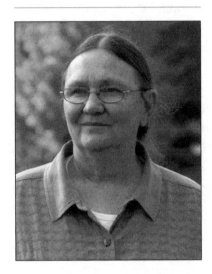

I grew up in the small town of Midlothian, Illinois. Midlothian is about halfway between Chicago and Joliet. It was on the Rock Island train line. The trains passed through, frequently blowing their whistles as they approached the crossings on the main road that went through the middle of town. At that time Midlothian was a rural area. It was situated in flat farming country, forest preserves were on the edge of town, and the streets were lined with large Maple and Oak trees. It was a beautiful sight in the fall.

I was the fifth child of Margaret (Vanderwall) and Herman Mayes. Herman's family was from farm country in Canada, and Margaret's family was from

Holland a generation before. I had four older brothers: Carl, Arthur, Edward and Thomas. It was helpful growing up with four brothers, an experience learning to get along with people who think differently than you do. My brothers taught me many things, including how to respect each person as an individual and always trying to see things from someone else's viewpoint, even if you don't agree with that viewpoint. My family helped me develop into a strong, independent woman.

Our father was a building contractor and a volunteer fireman. Hermie, as most folks called him, helped create the volunteer fire department in our small town. He dedicated many hours to fighting fires, rescuing people, building the physical building of the firehouse, and training other fire fighters. People always said if you were in trouble, Hermie was the one you wanted to call. He was a very special person to many people. He was a hero of our small town. He was a role model for our family and the greater community. He was a loving, caring, gentle person who always made people feel like they were his friends and important to him and his life.

My mother was a homemaker. Margaret (Margie) kept busy with keeping the house clean, raising a garden, canning, and keeping the meals coming for my dad and usually five or more hungry children. She was a very kind and loving person, not just in outward physical love, but in everything she did. She also volunteered at our church and the Midlothian Woman's Club. She served as president of the Women's Club for many years. This was a service organization that helped people in need. I can remember many holidays, including Thanksgiving, Christmas and Easter, when we delivered food baskets and gifts to the underserved people of the area. She was my Brownie Scout and Girl Scout leader, Sunday school teacher, and youth group leader.

We had many people living with us who were not our immediate family. Our house was open to many in need. Mom made sure we had a good education; she encouraged us in life and wanted a better life for us than she had growing up. I don't think that anything I have done in my life would have been possible without my mother. My mother gave me a safe place and that sense that she would be there no matter what happened, whether I succeeded or failed. She let me know that I could aim for the stars and that if I didn't reach them, she would love me anyway. She helped me understand that failure was a part of any life and that I should never be afraid to take risks. This gave me a lot of strength going forward in my life.

I graduated from our local Bremen Community High School in 1966. I worked in downtown Chicago for about a year at an insurance company. I tried to be grateful for the job, but it didn't seem right for me. One day I looked around, looked at my boss and thought, *Gee, if I am really successful, I could eventually have his job.* That night at home I was looking through the newspaper and saw an ad for our local nursing school. That sounded like it might be hard, but I thought I would like it much better than the commute and my job on the twenty-second floor of the Insurance Exchange Building in downtown Chicago. I talked to my parents and they agreed to help me.

The next day I was off to Oak Forest Hospital School of Nursing. I enrolled, gave my notice at work and started nursing school a few weeks later. It was 1967. Ours was a hands-on program, so we started working with patients after the first six weeks. I loved it, loved learning about the body and how it worked. I loved working with people, helping people and "fixing them up" the best I could, getting to know many families, helping them get through their crisis, whatever it was.

When we began our obstetrical (OB) rotation, I had never seen a birth before. But I was not at all afraid of birth. Although my mother really didn't talk much about it, she had a very positive attitude. She had all of us naturally, as had all the women in my family. Mom and Gramma didn't think childbirth was "so bad," just part of life. My Mom had successfully breastfed all of us. Birth and breastfeeding were natural events in her eyes. In nursing school we saw natural births, medicated births and cesarean sections. I noticed the difference in the medicated mothers and babies and the mothers and babies who had natural birth. There was a big difference. I couldn't understand why someone would want to be medicated and to medicate their babies like that—to start their baby's life out by being drugged. It didn't make sense to me. The medicated babies had a much harder time "starting" (to breathe), took extra nursing care, slept more, were hard to wake up, and seemed to be in a stupor. They frequently had trouble feeding. The mothers who had cesarean birth were put to sleep and the baby was taken from them. Sometimes the mothers didn't get to hold their babies for twenty-four hours or more. Many mothers at that time had drugs and were "asleep" for their births. I didn't know a lot about bonding at that time, but it was very obvious that the mothers who had natural birth had a much easier time with bonding and breastfeeding and getting up by themselves. In the 1960s the average hospital stay was three days, unless there were complications. The average cost of an uncomplicated birth was about $150.00 for the hospital stay. The doctor's fee was around $100.00.

I graduated from Nursing School in 1968, and my first job was working in our local hospital on the obstetrics (OB) floor. I was the floating staff person that filled in for the other nurses who had worked there longer. It was good because I got to work in labor and delivery, the nursery and on the postpartum floor. It was a very diverse job, and I learned a lot about all aspects of birth. Again, it became obvious that the doctors who did natural birth had much better outcomes than the those doctors who medicated their birthing mothers.

At that time the medication routine for women in labor was that when you arrived at the hospital you got your "prep." The prep included having your perineal area shaved, a large soapsuds enema, an IV, and then if you didn't have a doctor that did natural birth, you got Scopolamine (a drug that causes amnesia and dried secretions but also rearranged your thought patterns so it was hard to focus), and Demerol for pain. We also did what was called "buccal" Pitocin. Buccal is the mucous membrane area in the oral cavity where the drugs are given. We would put a drop of Pitocin in the woman's nose. Sometimes we would do this every fifteen minutes to get contractions going strong. In the late '60s in our hospital, no one was allowed into the labor or delivery room with the patient. So, mothers had to labor by themselves. I noticed that the mothers who had natural births did so much better if someone was in the room with them. So, when I wasn't busy I would go in and hold their hands, breathe with them, rub their backs, and give them any type of touch that seemed to help. The doctors loved it. However, the other nurses I worked with did not. Most of the other nurses were older and had worked at the hospital for many years. They actually yelled at me and told me not to spend so much time with the patients. They told me, "You are going to spoil the patients, and word will get around and people will expect that kind of treatment!" I did it anyway, instead of sitting in the lounge gossiping and knitting. As far as the nurses were concerned, the medicated mothers were less work, as the drugs kept them quiet; you just had to go in every so often and put drops of Pitocin in the IV. At the time of delivery, these mothers would be put to sleep, given a huge episiotomy, and the babies would be taken out by forceps. The babies were not alert and often needed assistance in taking their first breath.

In the nursery my observations were similar. The babies born from mothers who had natural childbirth were awake, alert, and had good APGAR scores. When they were brought to feed, if they were breastfed they would latch on easily. If they were bottle-fed they did well. However, if their mothers had been heavily medicated, often times at the birth they had trouble taking their first breaths, were lethargic and had trouble feeding, and had a hard time waking up, sometimes for over twenty-four hours or longer, until the drugs were out of their systems.

The postpartum mothers were obvious. The natural birth mothers were easy to get up and take care of. They rarely had trouble breastfeeding. They had fewer complications and usually went home earlier. The medicated mothers had trouble getting up the first few times. Often they would get dizzy and feel like they were going to pass out. They usually lost more blood at the birth and were the ones who had more trouble with postpartum hemorrhage after the birth. It seemed like their bodies and uteruses were also asleep.

I had many other adventures before I moved to The Farm in 1972. Ina May Gaskin heard I was a nurse and that I had worked in labor and delivery. I was only on The Farm a few weeks when Ina May called and asked if I wanted to go to a birth. Of course, I did. I hadn't ever been to a home birth and was looking forward to that. It was the mother's fifth baby. She was beautiful, peaceful, and pushed the baby out with such grace. Her husband was there at her side being so supportive. I was amazed at how beautiful and natural the whole process was. The baby was put right up onto her body. We never would have done that in the hospital; no one would ever mess up a "sterile field." Not long after the baby came out the placenta came, but then the mother started to hemorrhage. Before Ina May had a chance to ask for Pitocin (to help control hemorrhaging) I had already drawn it up into the syringe and was handing it to her. She and I were very telepathic from that time on. We laugh at our telepathy some times. Ina May put me on the midwife crew and started training me right after that birth. At that time (1973), we lived in tents and school buses, not many of us on The Farm lived in houses, so birth at home made so much more sense to me. It was so natural, peaceful, and loving. The wonderful vibrations and the beautiful visual colors made for such a spiritual experience. It was an awesome experience to see a woman changing through the process of birth, seeing the goddess come alive in every woman, seeing the new spirits come into the world, so mind-blown, so aware and absorbing of everything around them. I was in love with birth.

I met my husband Don on The Farm, actually at the Laundromat. He offered to carry in my big load of household laundry. I lived in a "single-mothers" house with about fifteen other single mothers and their children. Don helped me that day with our laundry, and he also chopped our wood and hauled our water in five gallon buckets. He would come over on cool mornings and start the fire in our woodstove before we got up in the mornings. These were very impressive tasks to single mothers who would have otherwise had to do those chores themselves. It didn't take very long for Don and me to decide we wanted to be together for the rest of our lives. My daughter Kimberly Ann was seven at the time. He loved her a lot and was a good father figure for her. But she wasn't real impressed with Don, and it wasn't until later in life that she acknowledged the positive influence he had in her life. Kim was a very sweet, open, sensitive and intelligent girl. She loved being on The Farm.

Kimberly's birth in 1965 was actually the beginning of my midwife career. I mentioned how the average woman gave birth at that time in the hospital setting. I was one of those Scopolamine/Demerol-drugged women. I ended up having a reaction to the Demerol. It made me very sick. The doctor gave it to me in my IV. Before he had it all in, I immediately got nauseous and threw up all over him, the nurse, the bed and the floor! It is one of the highlights of the whole experience I remember all these years later. After being put to sleep for the delivery, I was put in recovery flat on my back and left alone. It doesn't take a rocket scientist to know you don't leave people that have been vomiting flat on their back and alone. I threw up again and aspirated my dinner! Not a good thing. Fortunately, someone came back into the room and found me not breathing and turning blue.

I can vividly recall my out-of-body experience. I was above the room, looking down, wondering what was going on, and seeing all of the excitement—people rushing around and the cold, strange looking hospital room. I wondered, *What's happening? What is this about?* I looked closer and thought the poor young woman looked like me. *Oh Yes, Oh My Gosh, that is me! Why am I up here looking down! This is not good!* As they continued to perform CPR on me, my thoughts quickly went to the reason I was in the hospital—to have a baby . . . a baby. Where was my baby?

I floated over to the nursery and looked down and saw the beautiful baby. She looked sweet, soft, but not the best color, I could tell. *You look like you need to cry, my beautiful little baby girl. Take a good breath and cry for me.* She started crying and started looking a better color. *Good,* I thought. Then there were thoughts from my baby coming to me. 'Where is my mommy?' *I am your mommy,* I thought back to her. 'What is going on? What are we doing here?' her thoughts came to me. *I don't think we are really meant to be here right now, I think we should be down there,* I thought.

Then "boom" like a flash, down the dark tunnel, I was back in the bed with a bag mask pumping air into my lungs. Awful smelling black, dark mask. It hurt to breathe! "What are you guys doing to me?" I took my hand and pushed the bag mask away. I opened my eyes to about six doctors and nurses standing over me, very happy to see me breathing and coming back to consciousness. "Carol, how are you? How are you feeling?" they asked. I said, "You really want to know? I feel like SHIT, like I got run over by a truck and I'm still under the wheel. Why can't I breathe? Where's my baby girl?"

It was a horrible ordeal. I spent five days in the hospital with aspiration pneumonia. For the first several days, every time I tried to get out of bed I passed out. I nursed Kimberly; she was a hungry little one, hungry for nourishment, hungry for love and attention. After five days I recovered and finally got to go home.

Today Kimberly is a firefighter for the City of Miami, Florida. She was one of the first women hired by the City of Miami Fire Department in 1988. She was on the Miami Dade Search and Rescue team and helped at many disasters, hurricanes, floods, and was at the World Trade Center 9/11 disaster for the first three weeks after it happened. Kim has three children. I was her midwife for all of them, Samuel who was born in 1984, Megann in 1995, and Jennifer in 1996.

Shortly after I started going to births on The Farm, I got pregnant with my second child, Sally Kate, in 1975. My first-daughter Kimberly was ten years old at the time. I had an operation for endometriosis four years earlier and was told then I had such extensive damage that I would probably never get pregnant again. Sally proved the doctors wrong. I felt myself conceive with her. I could feel her spirit enter my body. It was a difficult pregnancy; I was very nauseous and threw up a lot. I lost eighteen pounds my first three months and only gained fifteen pounds back the rest of the pregnancy. But I was so glad to be having another baby that I didn't mind how awful I felt, just very grateful to be pregnant. I dilated quickly with Sally. My husband Don helped me through the labor; he really helped me stay relaxed. After about two and a half hours, I push her out. Sally weighed 9 lb, 9 oz. She was so beautiful, alert and aware. Sally's pregnancy and birth were a real learning experience for me as a mother and a midwife. I was so grateful to be at home, to have my loving husband with me for support, and to have midwives assist me. My dear friend Sharon Wells lived with us at the time Sally was born. Sharon is now a midwife and was very instrumental in forming the Certified Professional Midwife (CPM) certification. Sally's was the first birth Sharon ever witnessed. Sally now has three children—Lance, Emma and Bradley—all born at home with midwives. Sharon and I helped Sally have her babies.

I worked as a midwife in several different states. The Farm had a sister Farm in a rural community in Wisconsin. Midwifery was not regulated there, but we had the backup of a wonderful, caring, family practice doctor, Dr. Eugene Krohn of Black River Falls Hospital in Black River Falls, Wisconsin. Our Wisconsin Farm was outside the small town of Ettrick, very close to the Black River, and it was there I got pregnant with my son, Keif Oliver. I felt Keif's spirit enter my body during Sunday morning meditation. I thought from the beginning he was a boy.

When I was only six months pregnant (25 weeks) I went into labor with Keif. Don helped me relax and I got the labor to stop. I knew it was too soon to have him. At that time in 1977, babies that age did not survive. The next day we went to see our local doctor (since I was the midwife) and found out that my cervix was 50% thinned out and I had dilated to about two centimeters. Way too soon to have this baby! OK, bed rest for me. I had to get very unattached and get at peace with the idea that I might just go ahead and have the baby. I prayed a lot and felt very close with the Creator. I took Tributalene (to stop contractions) for several days and really didn't like the way it made me feel. So I took sips of alcohol to slow the contractions down and to keep my uterus relaxed. I didn't have to drink very much; just a few sips would do the trick. I realized that if I stayed flat and didn't get excited about anything, I could keep the contractions away. I had contractions on and off for ten weeks. I sewed, read, slept and wrote letters. I had a lot of help from Don and our twelve-year-old Kimberly, as well as the other Farm folks we lived with. I could not have done this without their help. Keif's birth was a very easy one. It felt so good to be able to relax and open up. Being early—I was 36 weeks—he was smaller than Sally had been, only 8 lb, and he came out easily. We were so grateful to have a beautiful, healthy boy. This was another great learning experience as a mother and midwife. It's so amazing what these newborns can teach you.

The Farm has a non-profit organization, PLENTY, an alternative Relief and Development Organization, affiliated with the United Nations Office of Public Information as a Non-Governmental Organization (NGO). PLENTY has managed projects in fifteen countries on four continents focused on support of the world's Native peoples, other disenfranchised people and our common environment. PLENTY promotes appropriate and sustainable technologies, such as small-scale agriculture, nutrition, primary health care, clean water, alternative energy, and more. I have served on the PLENTY Board of Directors since 1994. PLENTY started a project in the poverty-stricken area of the South Bronx, New York, in 1977. We were going through the red tape of New York City to get the much needed PLENTY Ambulance Service licensed. For a two year period (1977 through 1978), I delivered babies for our community and some of the local people in the South Bronx. We had informal backup by the nurse-midwives at North Central Bronx and by Therese Dondero, Certified Nurse-Midwife (CNM), and her future husband, Dr. Samuel (Sandy) Oberlander, a North Central Bronx/Montifiore obstetrician. This situation ended abruptly when PLENTY was informed that, off the record, the City of New York Health Department was aware that I was delivering babies, which was at the time and still is a felony for direct-entry midwives in the State of New York. The NYC Health Department said that if I did not quit delivering babies, they would not license the Ambulance

Service and would haul me off in handcuffs and put me in jail. So, I thought, *Well, OK then, if you put it that way, I guess I'll stop and go back to Tennessee where midwives are able to practice open and legally.* The ambulance service in NYC was licensed shortly after that.

Back in Tennessee the birth of our fourth child, Mariahna Margaret, who weighed 10 lb, 8 oz, was marked by shoulder dystocia (stuck shoulders). My water broke with Mari and I went right into labor. I dilated quickly, but I could tell she was my biggest baby so far. I had to really "stretch" to my limits to integrate the labor. When I became fully dilated, she moved down quickly with only a couple of pushes. I could feel her slip through my pelvic bones and head down the birth canal—such an intense but satisfying feeling. As she started to crown, I was trying to take it slowly so I wouldn't tear. Her head came out, and then the contractions went away! I tried to push but she wasn't coming. It was obvious her shoulders were stuck. Time was suspended at this point. Timelessness lets you see clearly what a very fine line there is between birth, life, and possibly death. After several pushes and different maneuvering with no results, one of the midwives there suggested I turn over on my hands and knees. I did this with a lot of assistance from everyone there. I felt the hands and knees position gave me more gravity and helped me ease her down. The position change saved her life. It took about two minutes to get her out. She was strong and started right up when she got out. She was so sweet, beautiful, alert, intelligent and fat! I was grateful we were at home with midwives who knew what to do in this emergency situation. We got a video of her birth that shows the hands-and-knees maneuver very well and is an excellent teaching tool for shoulder dystocia. Mariahna, now twenty-eight, has one child—a girl named Ajahna—born at home in 2000 with Sharon and me helping her.

In 1982 we moved to Florida to help care for my father who was dying of cancer. I received the last license Florida handed out under the old midwifery law that had been passed in 1931. Licensing midwives—what a great idea. It seemed so much better than the threat of being hauled off in handcuffs and taken to jail on a felony charge. Regulation of midwives makes so much sense. It is true that the midwives may have to give up a little, but for the trade-off of practicing openly and to be eligible to be reimbursed by insurance companies and Medicaid, it is well worth it.

I helped start the South Florida School of Midwifery in Miami, Florida. I was on the Board of Directors, along with Justine Clegg, Ricki Taylor, Margaret Hebson, Janice Heller, Cindy Ellis, Sara Pinkman, and Linda Wilson. A wonderful group of ladies (underground midwives), it was such a pleasure and honor to work with them to move midwifery forward in Florida. We all worked together on the rules and regulations for the newly passed licensing bill for Licensed Midwives in Florida. This model is based on the European midwifery model. I was also an instructor and main preceptor for all twenty-four students at the school. Seventeen of the students graduated and became licensed by the state of Florida. This was an incredible experience. I had a very active practice while in Florida.

We left Florida in 1988 to spend a few years in Dearborn, Michigan, helping to care for my husband's mother. While there, I didn't work much as a midwife because of our three growing children and my husband's mother. Rahima Baldwin Dancy and Valerie El Halta called me to help them at births occasionally, and some of the other local midwives did as well. I did not take on any of my own clients though. I volunteered at an organization called "World Medical Relief" (WMR). They were a non-profit that recycled medical supplies. It was a huge twelve-story warehouse that took up most of a city block. Most of the supplies were well sorted but there was one floor that had small boxes of things that were mixed items. The first day I volunteered, when I saw so many medical supplies just sitting there I decided I was going to make it my mission to move them out. We had just come from a month-long visit to Mexico and Belize, and I knew that there were many Third World countries that badly needed those supplies. I devised a sorting system for the items, and we sorted and packed the whole floor in the time I was there. In one year we sent out twenty-three semitrailer loads of supplies, and many other smaller shipments to over fifty countries.

At World Medical Relief we used to have volunteers from local Lions Clubs, Rotary Charities, churches and many other organizations to help us pack things. While with WMR, I had the great opportunity to travel with some of the shipments. I went to the Philippines, El Salvador, Mexico and Belize. In the Philippines, Corazon Aquino had become the president shortly before our visit. I had the opportunity to meet her and have breakfast and a luncheon with her. It was one of the highlights of my life. The Michigan doctors who accompanied me on the trip were childhood friends of Nanoi Aquino, Corazon's husband. We got to visit all of the clinics and hospitals which were awaiting our medical shipments.

In El Salvador the war was really still going on. I felt that this was one of the scariest places I had ever been in my life. There were soldiers everywhere, and the scariest part was that everyone acted like they weren't there. You didn't want to catch the eyes of the soldiers. Many of the guns they had came from the "Iran Contra Affair." Many people were "disappearing" at that time. We visited the clinics and hospitals that received the medical equipment. El Salvador is a very poor Third World country. We had lunch with the President's wife and had so much "security" around us it was frightening. I did not feel safe at all. In the hotel at night there were attacks on the city. I could see the mortars going off like fireworks, they were so close, and hear the machine guns.

I also took a trip to the Soviet Union with Ina May Gaskin and seventeen other midwives. We traveled the country, meeting with midwives and visiting birthing hospitals and other health care facilities. One of my strongest memories is of our arrival in Moscow. After having been told from childhood about the "Russians," I was so surprised to see these soldiers (young men) at the airport looking sweet and looking just like they could have been my brothers or cousins. They were not at all scary, and there were no weapons in sight. The Russian people were so sweet and welcoming. We went to several cities and took tours. It was surprising to see how the effects of World War II were still so evident. War is such a horrible thing for all involved.

We moved back to The Farm in 1991 and have been here since. I have been very involved in the development of the "Certified Professional Midwife" (CPM) credential. Many midwives were involved in the creation of the CPM: Sharon Wells, Alice Sammon, Ruth Walsh, Shannon Anton, Sharon Evans, Pam Weaver, Ida Darragh, Debbie Pulley and our consumer representative, Robbie Davis-Floyd, to mention just a few. Pam Maurath is a consultant who came into our lives as an angel in the mid-1990s. Pam helped us get funding and advised us on how to move midwifery forward in this country. She has been such a help and inspiration to me, as well as to the midwifery movement. The CPM would not be where it is today without her help and advice. Currently we have over eighteen hundred CPMs, and the number is growing. We have twenty-six states that regulate direct-entry midwifery with many more working on legislation. Last year there were eleven states that put forth legislation using the CPM as the basis for the regulation of midwifery.

Since 1997 I have acted as the Midwifery Education and Advocacy (MEA) Chair for the Midwives Alliance of North America (MANA), helping to unite all midwives, promoting the profession of midwifery and midwifery educators, and moving midwifery forward in the United States. I help create brochures and fact sheets and coordinate our professional educational booth that we exhibit at many different national conferences, such as the American College of Nurse Midwives, the American Public Health Association (APHA), the National Conference for State Legislatures, and others. I have been on the North American Registry of Midwives (NARM) Board of Directors, serving as the Treasurer since 1997 and as Director of Applications since 2003. I am the co-author of the APHA position paper entitled "Increasing Access to Out-of-Hospital Maternity Care Services through State-Regulated and Nationally-Certified Direct-Entry Midwives," which was adopted in 2001. I am also the co-author of the APHA position paper entitled "Safe Motherhood in the United States: Reducing Maternal Mortality and Morbidity." This was adopted in 2003. I am currently active in the Maternal Child Health Section of APHA, representing the profession of Midwifery and Midwifery Educators. I was the program chair for the Maternal Child Health Section of APHA for their Annual meetings for the past six years, and am currently the Co-Chair of the Innovations in Maternity Health Services Committee of the Maternal Child Health Section of APHA. I am also on the Tennessee Council of Certified Professional Midwives and work as a pro-bono lobbyist for the Tennessee Midwives Association in their legislative efforts.

About half of the births I attend these days are for the Old Order Amish community that is located close to us. Old Order Amish use no electricity or motorized vehicles. They get around on horse and buggy, use kerosene lamps, usually don't have running water in their houses and don't have indoor toilets. Their belief is everything is "God's Will," good or bad. When a woman goes into labor, the husband goes to a neighbor's house and has the neighbor make the phone call for us to come. The grandmothers deliver a lot of the babies but have us for the first baby and any "special cases." This year I helped an Amish woman have her eighteenth baby. Many of the women have fourteen or more babies and more pregnancies than that. We find with good care these women do fine; they don't really have a lot of complications, unlike what the medical profession would expect.

My words of wisdom in closing: Birth works. Believe in it! If it's not working, something is up, pay attention and check things out. You aren't doing anyone any favors if it's not happening by keeping someone home too long; if necessary, transport her.

I think that women as a group are so powerful. Yet, I don't think we are able to embrace our power well enough. I think women understand the bigger picture. We understand our impact on the environment, on the world. We understand the generations that will come after us because we gave birth to them, and in the case of midwives, we help other women to give birth to them. I think we women are still forming politically and spiritually—we don't realize how much power we have. I wish that we could come together more as a spiritual and political force. If women ran the world, I believe there would not be war.

I love spirit and how different people express it in relation to each other and to their communities. Finding spiritual meaning in your life is essential. It is part of the way we imagine, hope and explore. We cannot live without it. I believe that you have a much better chance of changing the world for the better if you start with yourself. I feel if everyone could look inward and realize all the enlightened wisdom, love and compassion in their hearts and express this love in the moment, World Peace would be possible. I am blown away by my life so far. I feel incredibly lucky to have had the adventures I have had and to have had the love in my life, my parents and grandparents, brothers, husband, children, grandchildren and so many wonderful friends. When the power of love overcomes the love of power, there will be peace on earth.

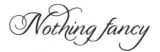

Nothing fancy

YESHI NEUMANN

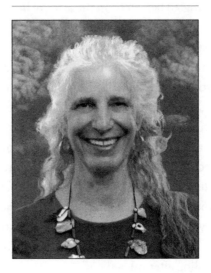

On my way to becoming a Certified Nurse-Midwife, I attended home births with a physician in Mill Valley, California. Sarah came in for a prenatal visit, nine months full of baby and having lots of contractions. After my hands lowered to her huge round belly, I traced the smooth curve of the baby's back on her right side. The baby's head was very high, not yet near her pelvic rim. We were having a leisurely discussion about how she would know she was in labor. Without warning, a large gush of wetness turned her beige pants dark brown. As she lifted her leg to remove her pants and soaking underwear, I saw something I had read about and prepared for but had not yet encountered in the hundred births I had attended. A two-inch loop of thick, shiny, twisted, pulsing umbilical cord protruded from her vagina.

I helped turn her on her hands and knees, chest on the exam table, butt in the air, to bring the baby's head further away from her pelvis. I put my index and middle fingers through the sea anemone of her cervix, now open four centimeters wide, and pushed the hard baby's head up and off the cord, so that the cord could continue to flow with the oxygen-filled lifeblood the baby needed. I told Sarah what I was doing and then told her husband to "get someone to call an ambulance. Now!"

Within minutes, the EMTs tugged and shoved until they managed to place a stretcher underneath Sarah. I kept my hand in place as they loaded us into the flashing ambulance. Soon we were at the hospital, greeted by the staff shouting instructions. Sarah untangled herself from the arms of her husband and was then hoisted onto a gurney. I stumbled along with her, making sure my hand didn't lose contact with the baby's slippery head.

Somehow this cumbersome many-limbed, rattling apparition that Sarah and I had become hurtled down the hallway to the operating room. Once there, no-nonsense, blue-masked nurses turned Sarah on her back. I rotated around my arm in order to continue upward pressure on the baby's head to preserve the pulse in the cord. My arm was inside Sarah halfway to my elbow. Sterile trays of instruments gleamed in the surgical lights. The blue drape was put up as the obstetrician prepared to cut Sarah open and remove her baby. Someone shouted in my direction, "Remove your hand!" I did, stood up for the first time since I had reached to feel the baby's head. Then I felt a firm thrust at the back of my neck. I found myself suddenly outside of the operating room with the words "We don't need you anymore," trailing after me.

I stood under the bright lights in the hallway and watched doctors, nurses, orderlies, patients and visitors go about their assigned roles, striding by me as if I wasn't there. I made my way to a women's bathroom, turned on the faucet with my left hand, and watched the warm water wash away the blood and amniotic fluid from my right.

Soon, with the legitimacy of a visitor, I was able to go see Sarah on the third floor. The postpartum nurse greeted me cheerily. Yes, she pointed, "Ms. Rowen is in that room." There Sarah was, propped up in bed, her head bent down, nose buried in the folds of her baby's neck. "She's perfect," she said as she raised her head to look at me, her face radiating love. "We named her Yeshi."

I knew from the moment my eldest daughter was born on December 31, 1970, that I was going to be a midwife. As I lay naked, entwined in my husband's arms the whole long candlelit night of my labor, Helen—the nurse whom the doctor had brought with him—stayed by my side. It didn't bother me that, because this was her first home birth, she took my blood pressure every fifteen minutes, even though it was completely normal. What mattered was her unfailing presence. Whenever I looked up, her dark black eyes reflected back to me that all was well. When my baby girl burst forth—a red, blue, yellow, purple, and green bundle of life and its secretions—I named her Rainbow. Gazing into the deep teal blue lake of her eyes, the words came to me, "I am going to be a midwife." I was as sure of that as I was certain of the very new sensation I felt as my newborn daughter sucked out the sweet, yellow colostrum from my breast.

I believe the seed of my becoming a midwife was planted when I myself was born. What follows is the story my mother told me. On the evening of October 14, 1940, my mother, Alice, noticed some bloody mucous in her underwear and that her pains were getting stronger and closer together. Before she could go to the hospital to have her second baby, she needed to roast the lamb with the potatoes and shell and boil the green beans for her husband's dinner. She wanted to make him a special dinner on this special night. My mother had been upset about her husband's harsh estrangement during the pregnancy. Although she adored her two-year-old daughter, she believed her husband might not stay with her if she birthed another girl. She hoped this baby was a boy.

Once she got to the hospital, my mother was immediately put on the delivery table, a mask thrust over her nose and mouth, as a huge breathtaking quake filled her body. My mother awoke into an ice-cold room with polished metal and bright light. She smelled disinfectant. Something was missing. A nurse told her that the dark, hairy, squalling being in the bassinet beside her was her daughter. My mother said, "That can't be my baby; it looks like a monkey." She turned her head away.

Alone that night, without her husband, her belly no longer full, and her arms empty, my mother was unable to sleep. In the morning she pulled on her pink, quilted, silk bed-jacket and ate her breakfast of oatmeal and coffee. Then a Baby Nurse came in carrying a bundled up baby. The nurse moved the breakfast tray out of the way, unwrapped one of the blankets and put me in my mother's lap. "She's a good baby," she said, as a simple fact. "Take good care of her," she instructed my mother firmly. The nurse lingered for a moment before she left the room. My mother felt blood fill her heart and then her cheeks. She reached out her middle finger and stroked my velvet baby forehead.

Like many women all over the world, my mother turned away from her baby in fear that there would be drastic consequences because I was a baby girl. Perhaps she also turned away because the dark, hairy monkey baby looked unmistakably

Jewish. My mother often told me that she hid behind her glamorous blond hair to claim she was not Jewish, although in fact she was. In 1940, when Jews in Europe were being herded into concentration camps, my mother could easily have felt that her survival depended on passing as a Gentile.

I heard the story countless times of the Baby Nurse declaring I was "a good baby" as she put me in my mother's arms. The story took on much more significance for me once I became a midwife and had been in the presence of many newborn babies. I felt I remembered my own birth. I had a memory of my cells shrinking away from the edges of my skin when I came out and no one welcomed me. Though just a newborn, I believe I made a vow, the kind of vow that only a very young baby makes about things some people do not believe a baby can understand. I vowed: I will keep babies together with their mothers.

This baby-made vow germinated and grew in the deep earth of my heart, and found its way to my voice the morning I birthed Rainbow: I will become a midwife. I will keep babies together with their mothers. The midwife is the one who, by helping the mother birth and sometimes literally by cutting the cord, detaches the baby from the mother. But the midwife, like the Baby Nurse who brought me to my mother, is also the one who can kindly but firmly help reconnect a mother and baby who have been separated.

In 1948 when I was seven years old my mother moved to New York City from Mexico City so she could work and support herself, my sister and me. When my father left, our little family became desolate and poor. My grandmother, Bele, moved in to help take care of us. As a teenager, Bele had been sent alone from Russia to America because her mother hoped she would have a better chance of surviving her chronic bouts of near-death pneumonia. She worked as a cleaning lady in a fancy hotel and endlessly studied the writings of Mary Baker Eddy, the founder of Christian Science, by a dim lamp in her small room on the dark side of our apartment. It was Bele who introduced me to *the wise woman*, the one who sits beside a woman in need and holds her hand in the night.

One evening in our first winter in New York City, my throat was burning and my damp body strangling with constricting coils of sheets. The cold wind off Riverside Drive rattled windows and lurked along the edges of my room. My mother's black work pumps clacked on the wooden floor as she went to call the doctor. Dr. Smith was a pale, flabby old man who smelled like boiled cabbage. In his office I had to strip down to my white cotton underpants, sit alone, shivering on a steel table covered with white paper and wait for him to press the icy, hard stethoscope against my chest, poke in my ears and gag me with a flat wooden stick.

I pulled the sheet over my head to dull the bright electric light and the sound of my mother's voice talking to Dr. Smith on the telephone in the next room. Suddenly I felt the gentle firm pressure of a hand on the back of my shoulder. My grandmother, Bele, had slipped between the sheets in her stocking feet. She too was talking to a strange man someone she called "our father" or sometimes "our heavenly father." I didn't know whom she was talking to, but gradually I felt myself begin to float on the wave of my grandmother's touch and her murmurings. The twisted sheets loosened their grip, my legs began to sway like ocean kelp and my breath glided free. The windy gusts became a gentle sigh that lapped at the windows of my room and sent me off to sleep.

I startled awake to the sound of my mother announcing the news from Dr. Smith. I was to sit up right now and swallow a big spoonful of bitter syrup. My grandmother was no longer with me in my bed; she had slipped out as silently as she had slipped in. Yet her scent, faint but clear as lemon, lingered.

As a seven year old, I could not explain what it was about my grandmother's healing visit with me that was a kind of forbidden secret. But now I understand that this quality of concealment has been a thread in my own life as a midwife and also in the history of midwives in the Western World. We have become adept at hiding the low moans and high-pitched wails of labor, the clean crisp smell of amniotic fluid, and the feel of a mother's smooth, oiled back against our hand. Keeping secret what we do has been our survival strategy in the face of threats of losing our licenses and hospital privileges, going to jail, or, in earlier times, being denounced as a witch and burned at the stake. Doing our work invisibly has also been the way we have protected the mothers and babies in our care. When Pharaoh decreed that Puah and Shifrah, the ancient Hebrew midwives, must kill all firstborn male babies, their ingenious response was to say, "Jewish women give birth so fast we can't possibly get there in time." And thus the babies were saved.

As a young midwife in the '70s, I read about Puah and Shifrah. I wanted to claim them as my own blood ancestors. Many of my sister midwives were getting arrested, fined and falsely accused of killing babies. I wanted to believe that I was the direct descendent of a lineage of courageous midwives, that I too had the guts and ingenuity that the path of a midwife required.

Although I knew immediately after giving birth that I was going to be a midwife, I didn't know how soon it would become a reality. In March of 1971, at thirty-one years old, I moved, with my three month-old daughter, Rainbow, and my husband Osha, to Black Bear Ranch, a hippie commune without electricity or telephones, deep in Northern California's Klamath National Forest. At last, the New York City kid got to put her own hands into the dark brown earth.

Among the sixty people who greeted us at the commune were nine pregnant women. They intended to have their babies right there in the mountains, three hours from the nearest hospital and snowed-in during the winter. What a wonderful opportunity to begin my life's work! Along with my friend, Geba, I read ravenously everything I could find about birth. I attended the births of our goats. Goat-by-goat, baby-by-baby, Geba and I became the midwives of that mountain and Salmon River community.

At Black Bear, we were midwifing not just the babies, but ourselves as a community. Although we certainly wore tie-dyed skirts and even flowers in our wild long hair, we weren't just sitting around. We didn't have a guru, but we had a collective vision. We believed that if we put our hearts and souls into what we were doing and came up with the right blueprint, we could reinvent our world. We already believed that Love, Peace, Justice, and Freedom were possible. And from our neighbors, the Karuk people, whose ancestors had lived in peace with the land for centuries, we learned that Love, Peace, Justice and Freedom were inseparable from honoring and taking care of our Mother the Earth. We also learned, not perfectly, but sincerely, how to get along with each other. We called ourselves a family.

River was one of the first human babies whose birth I attended. Lena birthed him in the warm-weather home David had built under a maple tree in the meadow. Her bed was the earth covered with a tarp and a few patchwork cotton quilts. As Lena began her labor that clear-sky July morning, we made a little fire in a makeshift fire pit nearby so we could heat water to wash our hands. As her contractions got stronger and closer together, the clouds gathered and a brief thunderstorm erupted. Lena's bag of water released. River bounced out into the world as the clouds cleared and the late afternoon sun brightened the valley. I discovered the miracle of easy birth. Once my clean hands were ready, there was almost nothing for me to do but sit quietly. This mother, baby and father needed hardly more from me than the wind needed to blow through the trees or the clouds needed to move across the sky.

Some of the births Geba and I attended required more active midwifery. One crisp fall afternoon Carla and her redheaded boyfriend came down the dusty Black Bear road in a battered green Chevy pick-up. She said she was due any day now and had heard there were midwives up here who could help her have her baby. We set her up in one of our little cabins. She went into labor at dawn the next day. Geba and I found Carla walking around nonchalantly. Although her belly tightened as hard as granite river rock every four minutes, she said she felt no pain. After many hours I put my hand inside her vagina and, much to my surprise, felt that the baby's head had already passed through the cervix. We expected the baby to be born soon. Eight hours later she still had no baby in her arms and also no more contractions. We brought Cedartree, a baby boy who had been born up the road a month before, to suck on Carla's breasts hoping to bring on contractions. But still Carla had no urge to push her baby out.

It took about half an hour for me to drive to the nearest phone. I called Dr. Gavin, a kindly General Practitioner in Yreka, the city with the closest hospital three hours away, and asked for his advice. "Is the baby's heart beating?" he asked calmly. "Yes," I said. "The baby will come," he said, "Just have the mother keep pushing."

When I got back it was dark. Carla was leaning against a willow tree by the river. Her contractions had started to come again. With each one, she reached up, held on to a branch and grunted her baby down. Her daughter Rose was born two hours later, looking up at us as she came out from under Carla's pubic bone. Dr. Gavin had put into words what I learned from this baby and her mother. Babies will come—and come in their own time. Just like the apples in our mountain meadow had their own time to turn lusciously red ripe and fall to the ground. My task was to be patient, fully present and trust the process of birth as it unfolded, each time differently.

After four years of attending births in the mountains, I was eager to learn more. I moved to the San Francisco Bay Area, and I apprenticed with Carole Hagin, a mother of seven and an experienced home birth midwife. Carole, with her constant curiosity, lightness and humor, was my midwife for my second daughter, Emma, born November 30, 1978 at home. This time I was blessed from the very beginning of my pregnancy with the delicious knowledge that a trusted and familiar companion on my journey would be there when I gave birth.

When Emma was one year old, I went to the University of California Nurse-Midwifery Program to become a nurse-midwife. Every day I received a cornucopia of useful information about pregnancy and birth. In 1982, a year later, I went to Austin, Texas, for the inaugural meeting of the Midwives Alliance of North America. Midwives came out of the shadows from all over the United States bubbling over with excitement to share our stories, our songs and our dreams in the light of day. I was ecstatic to be part of such a tribe. Like my sister midwives, I had a dream that one day midwifery care would be universally respected, that it would be an option all women could choose and that midwives would be fully incorporated into our health care system.

I didn't have a sense of what this dream could possibly look like until I went to Nicaragua in 1983 to teach traditional midwives in the first U.S.-Nicaraguan Health Colloquium. In an effort to address the serious health problems of its people, the revolutionary Sandinista government recognized the wisdom and the important position held by the "grandmothers of the umbilical cord" (*las abuelitas del ombligo*) at the core of their communities, incorporating them into the new national health care system. At the formal closing of the colloquium, in the brightly lit government auditorium filled with thousands of people, the Minister of the Interior, Tomás Borge, asked the *parteras* to stand and be honored. I wept as I watched twelve grey-haired, wrinkled-faced midwives, representing hundreds of others, rise from their seats.

I returned to the United States inspired to organize all of us midwives, licensed and unlicensed, home and hospital—to stand and take our rightful place in the health care system. In reality it was all I could do to work full-time as a hospital staff nurse-midwife, be a single mother of two young daughters and care for my beloved sister, Ricky, who had just been diagnosed with breast cancer.

My life changed in December 1988 when Ricky died. I was forty-eight years old. One way I felt I could keep my sister alive was to step into her shoes and continue her social justice work. She had created Unlearning Racism Workshops, which she presented all over the country and the world. Her shoes felt huge; yet once I stepped into them I felt certain that I was supposed to walk in them.

Although I continued to work per diem as a hospital staff midwife and occasionally attended home births during the 1990s, mostly I facilitated diversity work in health care and educational institutions. As I witnessed the participants in my workshops breathe the fresh air of becoming free from imprisoning misinformation about other people and themselves, I felt as though I was doing the work of a midwife in another realm.

In 1998 I went on the Interfaith Pilgrimage of the Middle Passage. The monks and nuns of the *Nipponzan Myhoji* Japanese Buddhist Order believed that retracing the route of the Middle Passage could contribute to healing the legacy of slavery, the racism that continues to plague us to the present day. I and about one hundred other pilgrims—descendents of slaves, slave owners, witting and unwitting colluders, and abolitionists—walked twenty miles a day for six months from Levittown, Massachusetts, until we reached New Orleans, Louisiana. Step-by-step, my heart opened to a deeper humility, an acceptance of more personal responsibility as a White person and also as a human being for the enslavement of African people. By the time we got to New Orleans I had also somehow retraced my own steps inside myself back to the work I felt I was put on Earth to do. Before coming back home, I gave the little blue embroidered silk bag containing my sister, Ricky's, ashes to Avila, my friend who was going with the Pilgrimage all the way to Africa.

It was time for me to work with my hands again and to plunge back into the river of midwifery, the amniotic fluid, sweat, tears, and inevitably the meconium. One sunny afternoon in May of 2000, Amrit, a home birth midwife with whom I had partnered when I returned to California, and I were sitting on my couch hashing and rehashing the latest birth. We started fantasizing about how to bring some of the essential elements from our home birth practice into the hospital. This was our vision: we would see pregnant women and their families in their own homes for prenatal care. We would spend enough time to build a relationship of trust, enough time to explore the answers to all their questions together, and enough time to encourage the women to trust their own wisdom as they made choices about their birth. We would be with them during their labor at home until they were ready to go to the hospital. Then we would stay with them throughout their labor and birth at the hospital. At the hospital we would create a birthing sanctuary. We would turn down the lights, move the bed out of the way, put a large futon on the floor so the birthing woman could move freely about, or be in an intimate embrace with a loved one. We would provide a birth tub so a woman could immerse herself in water and float, rock or glide to help herself open to the coming of her baby. We would remain with the mother for several hours after she birthed to make sure her baby stayed with her, help the mother and baby breastfeed if they needed help, and tuck them in for the night. Amrit and I continued imagining how we would mother the mother during her postpartum time. It was basic midwifery, nothing fancy. Just unhurried, soul-satisfying, woman-to-woman care with the birth itself taking place in the hospital, where the overwhelming majority of women in the United States give birth. We named our dream Homestyle Midwifery.

By April 2007, over 400 women had given birth with Homestyle Midwifery. We had gone from one to sixteen births a month, from being a private practice with hospital privileges to being employees hired to carry out the Homestyle Midwifery program at the hospital. We had become a site for the University of California nurse-midwife interns and had the privilege of mentoring totally dedicated future midwives who worked by our side. Our outcome statistics clearly demonstrated that our care promoted the health of both mother and baby.

Our success was hard won. Homestyle was at its third hospital within four years. Getting Homestyle in the first two hospitals required banging on closed doors that grudgingly opened and then at the slightest excuse slammed shut. But St. Luke's Hospital, a small community hospital in San Francisco, had a CEO with unabashed enthusiasm for thinking outside the box and a Chief of Obstetrics who was an open supporter of midwives. They both believed in our model and wanted Homestyle to be part of the Women's Center at St. Luke's. In addition, because Homestyle attracted many privately insured clients, our practice had the potential to generate income for the hospital, the majority of whose other patients were uninsured. It was wonderful to finally feel welcome! Homestyle flourished. In October 2006 we received a certificate of honor from San Francisco Mayor Gavin Newsom, and in 2007 we were voted "Best Place to Have a Baby" by *San Francisco* magazine.

Because Amrit was a direct-entry midwife, not a Certified Nurse-Midwife (CNM), she couldn't be hired by the hospital. I had lost her as a partner. However, I had hired three amazing CNMs—Cynthia, Hokhmah and Michelle—who shared the vision of Homestyle with me, as well as the long sleepless nights.

A challenge for Homestyle was how to partner with the other hospital care providers to support the desires of our clients for Homestyle births. For example, our protocol was to summon a pediatrician to attend the birth if there were any potential risk factors for the baby. Even if the baby was vigorous at birth, the pediatrician's customary practice was to take the baby over to the warmer on the other side of the room to do their initial exam. I found myself repeatedly heartbroken, agitated and in confrontation with the pediatrician when the baby was taken away.

Carrying out my deep-seated vow that I would keep babies together with their mothers required changing my style of communication. By listening more and talking less, I found out that the main reason one of the pediatricians wanted to take these apparently healthy babies away from their mothers for their initial exam was because she couldn't see well enough in the dim light at the bedside to make sure the baby was OK, which was her primary responsibility. She wasn't used to assessing babies in the near darkness as we midwives had learned to do. She and I worked out an agreement: If I would move out of the way, bring over a light and hold it for her, then she would examine the baby on the mother's chest. Everyone was happy. The Homestyle way was becoming viably embedded into the hospital structure.

Many of the women who came to Homestyle were very healthy. However, one of the reasons we had created Homestyle Midwifery was to be able to provide midwifery care that honored a birthing woman's own choices to women who had health challenges and clearly needed obstetrical care. Marta was one of those women.

Marta had moved to the San Francisco Bay area from Miami, Florida, where her planned home birth of her first baby had ended in a c-section. She came to Homestyle because she wanted full support to have a vaginal birth with her second baby. Her pregnancy was completely normal. At the thirty-six week home visit, Cynthia, one of the Homestyle midwives, did not hear a fetal heartbeat. Soon the ultrasound showed that Marta's baby had died inside the womb. A few days later, I sat with Marta while she gave birth, vaginally, as she had wanted. She and Michael took as much time as they needed to anoint their baby with flowered water and somehow maneuver her decaying, fragile, fluid-filled body—barely contained inside her skin—into a little, yellow, terry cloth onesie suit. There was no obvious reason for their baby's death, and Marta and her husband didn't want an autopsy to try to find one. When Marta came to see me for her final postpartum visit, a tiny light of joy flickered amidst the torrents of grief that still cascaded through her. She was pregnant again.

Marta wanted another vaginal birth and she wanted Homestyle Midwifery care. At thirty weeks she was diagnosed with diabetes and needed insulin. Given her stillbirth and the current diabetes, together with Homestyle's collaborative OBs, we agreed she needed to give birth by forty weeks. In spite of acupuncture, evening primrose oil, lots of sex and other natural labor encouragement, forty weeks came and went, but Marta was not in labor. Our collaborating physician was adamant about not using the usual induction medications to induce her because of the greater risk of a ruptured uterus with a prior c-section. Now, at forty weeks and twelve hours, a c-section loomed imminently.

As a Homestyle midwife, I usually negotiated with the OB to do whatever was possible to hold off using Pitocin, but this situation was different. I wanted to try Pitocin because Marta really wanted a vaginal birth, and yet I felt uneasy. I was in uncharted waters. Another woman in Marta's situation might have decided at that point or even earlier to go for a c-section while her baby was healthy and alive inside her. The OB came in and calmly explained the risks of using Pitocin to bring on labor versus getting her baby out immediately with a c-section. "Let's go ahead and try the Pitocin," Marta said quietly but confidently. She trusted her intuition that she and her baby would be healthier if she waited and gave birth vaginally. Her courage encouraged me and the whole team caring for her. The OB and I discussed various research studies and what was being done in other local practices, and finally we used half the usual dose of Pitocin to try and get Marta's labor going. Gradually it worked. I set up the turquoise blue, plastic, four-foot deep birthing tub, and Marta rode the tumultuous waves of her labor, her cries of "no" turning into moans of "yes." When her earth-shaking rumble signaled her baby was ready to come, Marta climbed out of the tub onto the futon on the floor, curled up against Michael and birthed her breathing, crying, perfectly rosy baby boy, Tito.

I went to Miami to celebrate Tito's first birthday. Marta's welcome was loud and bubbly as she picked Tito up and put him in my arms. "Tito, this is one of your grandmothers," she said. Michael's greeting embrace was wordless, tender and serious. It reminded me, perhaps more than words could have, what we shared together.

On April 16, 2007, the new owners of the hospital laid off Homestyle Midwifery. The official reason was that the mission of the Women's Health Center was redefined as the provision of basic primary care to the medically underserved. Homestyle midwives were "giving too much care." It's true our care was way beyond basic, as basic is defined by the for-profit health care industry. On the other hand, the families we served felt it was just the right amount. And I wouldn't have wanted to spend one minute less than I did with Marta or any of the other women in our care.

During the time since the lay-off, I spent hundreds upon hours trying to transform Homestyle into an independent private practice. A Homestyle Community Collective consisting of about two hundred former clients, as well as midwives, doulas, nurses, and physicians in the community, arose to support our continued existence in a new form. However, the current health care system presented insurmountable obstacles to a midwife-directed private practice. For example, even though none of the Homestyle midwives had ever been sued, no reputable malpractice company would give our consulting physician a malpractice insurance policy because Homestyle was a *midwife-owned*, not a *physician-owned* practice.

Even if we could have overcome this hurdle through a complex legal arrangement whereby our consulting physician nominally owned the practice, another factor was ultimately the crucial reason we decided not to pursue Homestyle as a private practice: Given the projected huge malpractice premium and the need to account for Homestyle services not reimbursable by insurance companies, we would have had to charge our clients a significant fee. We were not willing to abandon our original vision that Homestyle Midwifery care should be accessible to all childbearing families who wanted it, not just to the ones who had the ability to pay for it.

Now that I am in my late sixties, with the dream of Homestyle Midwifery not realizable at least for now, I wonder how I will ride the wave of working as a midwife to shore. My foremothers who kept the faith that it matters how babies are born, and my sister midwives who keep that faith now, have inspired me to continue this work. Perhaps one night, like one of the Nicaraguan "grandmothers of the umbilical cord" that I heard about, I will just keel over at the foot of a laboring woman's bed.

One day last August when I was sitting again by the Salmon River, I looked around and realized I had received into my hands most of the mothers whose babies were now playing in the sand, and some of those babies, too. From baby River, to Sarah's baby Yeshi, to Tito I have been blessed to have midwifed more babies than I have counted. I am filled with boundless gratitude to have been in the presence of magnificent women giving birth to sacred new life. My connection with all the families whose lives have touched mine has deeply satisfied my soul.

In the face of the miracle of birth, in the face of the myriad of unknown causes and conditions that contribute to the outcome of a particular birth, in the face of so much that is not in my own midwife's hands, I feel more and more humility. And yet my hope is that we midwives, the ones like me on our way out, and those on their way in, can step boldly out of the shadows that we have been relegated to and step bravely into the bright light of leading our communities.

As we use our hands to comfort a laboring woman or receive a new baby, let us reach out to each other and to the people who do not understand what we care about and who seem to be on the other side. May we remember what we have learned in the past about kindness, and may we learn what we don't already know.

No two are the same

DEBBIE PULLEY

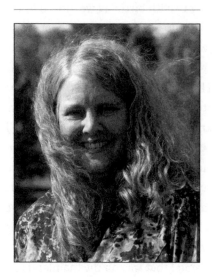

$\mathcal{M}$y roots are Swedish on my father's side and Scotch-Irish on my mother's side. Dad was one of eight children. They lived in Rochester, Indiana. Mom was one of two children. She and her sister were raised by their grandmother in Indiana and by her aunt, father, and four uncles in Michigan. I was born in Indianapolis, Indiana, on March 25, 1954. My dad was a salesman for Gillette, so we ended up moving on a fairly regular basis.

Before I was one year old, we had already moved to Parkridge, Illinois, and before my second birthday we lived in Jacksonville, Florida. Jacksonville is where my memories start. My middle sister, Kathy, was born there. My mother loved to act and was a beautiful singer. She was in quite a few musicals and operas. When my dad was traveling, she would take us with her to rehearsals where we would sleep in sleeping bags in the lobby. As I got a little older I got to be in the shows too.

Shortly after my sixth birthday, we moved to Atlanta, Georgia. Not long after we moved, my youngest sister, Tricia, was born. For years I thought I raised her, playing with her all the time, changing diapers, feeding her, and just totally being in love with her. I had to laugh once I had my own children, how off that really was. Sorry Mom, I guess you did have a hand in it too, like getting up with her at night, watching her while I was at school and outside playing, while I went to the skating rink every weekend and when she was sick.

The summer after my twelfth birthday we moved to Hong Kong. At the time it was a British Crown Colony. The five years we spent there were my most formative years. Hong Kong was crowded, but a very safe place to live. It was a wonderful life. We had a live-in *amah* (maid), cook and driver. I attended Hong Kong International School (HKIS) the first year it began in an apartment building. The next year we moved into the main campus in Repulse Bay. There was a beach at the bottom of the hill and a great place to hang out during lunch or after school.

My life was basically unrestricted during those years. Maybe there were some restrictions, but anyone who knows me knows I never really pay attention to those. As long as I went to school and was home by a certain time I was free to do as I pleased. I went to movies, the beach, hung out at the American Club, and on the weekend nights I would spend time at discotheques. We traveled around on buses or took a *pak pai* (taxi).

I found a British hospital that was on the mainland and would go over there and volunteer. I also found another hospital and volunteered there in the pediatric unit. One baby I was working with had severe burns all over his body. His blind grandfather took care of him while the mother and father were out working in the fields. The grandfather accidentally knocked over a kerosene lamp and the baby was burnt. I spent all my waking hours, except when at school, taking care of him. Of course I fell in love and wanted to adopt him so he could live in a real home instead of a cardboard squatter. Mom and Dad were great about listening to me and letting me know how having a baby at thirteen or fourteen probably wasn't the best thing for either one of us. I don't even remember discussing the fact that the baby already had parents. I spent all my free time in Hong Kong volunteering for this cause or that. Most of my spare time was spent at hospitals, but I also got involved with local charities.

I think I always wanted to be a midwife. I started babysitting at age ten for the neighbors and would skip church services to go help in the nursery. My idea of heaven was to be holding and cuddling babies. Shortly after moving to Hong Kong, I started volunteering at the local hospital in the pediatric unit. I spent every weekend and most holidays there. At school I would spend free time working in the clinic. Our school nurse realized there were a few of us who had a "nursing" bent, so she set up a nursing assistant training program. We met every day after school and did our clinical rotations at a local hospital. By this time I was fifteen. A woman I babysat for had been a midwife in England. That was the first time I had heard about midwifery and, needless to say, I wanted all the details. I would spend hours listening to her talk about her experiences. I decided that I wanted to move on to labor and delivery. I put in my request, and that basically blew everyone away. The hospital administration decided that I was too young to work in that unit. I asked them how old I had to be and was told sixteen. In the meantime I assisted in surgery. On my sixteenth birthday I walked into the hospital, went to the administrator's office, showed them my ID, and said "I am sixteen now. Can I go up to labor and delivery?" That day I witnessed three births and knew that was where I wanted to be. I continued to assist in labor and delivery on weekends and holidays until I moved back to the States in 1971.

One of the best things about living in Hong Kong was that we were able to come back to the United States every year to visit relatives. We saw them more when we lived out of the country than we did when we lived Stateside. We would leave every summer in June and spend a couple days each in different countries. I visited much of the Orient, Middle East and most of Europe during our travels. We even got to spend time with relatives in Sweden. It was tradition from the time I was six years old to spend a week at Callaway Gardens, in Pine Mountain, Georgia. We made the trip every year, even though we resided in Hong Kong, until I was twenty-years old. The rest of the time in the United States would be spent with various relatives, mainly in Indiana and Michigan, and attending the family reunion before heading back to Hong Kong in late August.

In 1972, the summer of my seventeenth year, when I was an incoming high school senior, we moved back to Atlanta. I felt like a fish out of water trying to get through my senior year. Living in the United States was so strange. I had all the credits I needed to graduate going into my senior year, so high school was a pain. The one positive thing was our senior trip to the Bahamas. It was there that I met Don. We were married a year later, March 17, 1973. Our son Chris arrived in October 1975. I cried for hours after that birth, tears of joy that I finally had a baby of my own. Michelle arrived four years later in September 1979. Now in 2009, Don and I have three beautiful grandchildren that we dote on.

In my senior year of high school I applied to nursing school and was accepted to start in the fall. In the meantime I started working on weekends at the hospital where I would be going to school. Unfortunately there were no openings in labor and delivery or in pediatrics. Instead, they had me working in geriatrics, which I soon learned was not my gift. I stuck that out for about six months before leaving. What kept going through my mind was if this was what I had to do as a nurse, then nursing definitely wasn't the path for me. I decided that working for a pediatrician might be more of what I was looking for. I answered ad after ad but kept hitting brick walls. They all wanted a trained medical assistant. So my next step was to go back to school and train as a medical assistant, which I did. I got a job with a pediatrician as soon as I graduated. It was the perfect job for me. The doctor was older and left most of the daily work to his other medical assistant and me. He took me with him to the hospital and taught me about doing newborn exams. Is the baby pink, nursing, peeing and pooping? If so we are probably OK. I learned so much in the two years before he retired. When he retired, I basically did too. My husband and I were thinking we would start our family soon.

When I was pregnant with my son, I got very involved with La Leche League. By the time Chris was born I had almost completed the requirements to be a leader. But I ended up not following through and becoming certified because they told me I might have to take calls in the middle of the night. I just wasn't so sure that would work for me. What irony, taking call. At least with La Leche League I would have been able to stay home while I counseled the woman.

During my "training," I volunteered at the county teaching hospital downtown. This was in the late '70s and early '80s. At that time it had the most deliveries because it was one of the few hospitals that accepted Medicaid. I worked there twice a week and assisted in at least ten births a week. It was a wonderful learning experience for me. Many of the mothers were high risk. I was able to see the complications and how they were handled, not something we deal with that often in a home birth practice.

I realized shortly after our son Chris's birth how paternalistic my doctor was. That was the norm in the '70s. I had a rough pregnancy and long induction for postdates. The good thing is he agreed to let my husband be with me, which was not always the case back then. As soon as Chris was born, I reached down to touch him. The doctor slapped my hand and yelled at me for contaminating the sterile field. I knew then that women deserved so much better.

By the time I got pregnant with our second child, Michelle, I knew more of what I wanted. I had been at a few home births. Unfortunately there was only one midwife in the area. In order to have an assisted home birth, her backup doctor had to give clearance. They felt, due to the complications with my first birth, I should deliver at the birth center. Home birth wasn't my main goal at the time, so I agreed with their recommendations. The only change I made was finding another obstetric (OB) group closer to where I lived who was willing to support me with a natural birth. I guess I was pretty firm in what I wanted for the birth because one of the docs asked me if it was OK if he was there. I told him as long as he didn't do anything he was welcome. Michelle's birth was perfect. We delivered in the "birthing room" at the hospital. This was rare, and they had to rush to clean it up when they heard I was coming in. The room was mainly used for storage. My husband was with me, my mother was taking pictures, and my sister and her friends were there, too. The nurse was fantastic. She asked me what I wanted for my birth. I told her to be at home. She said say no more! When Michelle was born, the doc ran in the room, tucked his tie into his shirt and caught her. She was never taken away from me. The pediatrician came over about an hour later, checked her out and OK'd her release. We stayed for about twelve hours before going home. I was able to sleep in my bed with no interruptions. What a stark contrast it was from my first birth where I signed out of the hospital AMA (Against Medical Advice) after five days.

What my births showed me is that the best place to have your baby is where you are most comfortable. There is not one right place for everyone. Mothers should have all the options available to them.

I first started going to births like many of the older midwives did. Friends were having their babies at home and asked me to attend. I had minimal experience having assisted in labor and delivery in hospitals and working for the pediatrician, but I really was just smart enough to be dangerous.

Chris was just over a year old when I attended my first home birth. My dear friend was pregnant with her fourth baby and didn't feel comfortable with the local midwife. She asked if I would help. It was a wonderful experience. In spite of all our help the baby turned out just fine. Soon other friends were asking me to "help." I realized after a while I was really there because I had some knowledge. I knew I needed to learn more if this was going to continue.

There was one local midwife in town. I tried to develop a relationship with her, hoping she would take me to births and train me. She held weekly study groups in her home and monthly Home Oriented Maternity Experience (HOME) meetings that I attended. I watched her children, folded her laundry, did her dishes, and cleaned her kitchen all to no avail. Our personalities never clicked, and it was soon evident my training was not going to be with her. As a matter of fact she told me and several others that I just didn't have what it takes to be a midwife.

As I was realizing that training with this midwife would never work out, God sent Barbara Lahey to Atlanta. She and I hit it off immediately. Where the other midwife didn't do any prenatal care, Barbara did. Barbara and I complemented each other. She knew normal birth, where I had more experience in the hospital with interventions and complications. We worked together through a midwifery distance-learning program that covered most of our didactics. Barbara was the one who taught me to trust birth and to let it work. She taught me to stand back but still listen to my intuition, and move in when called for. In most cases it worked beautifully. She was very patient with me.

In the mid-1980s several of the local midwives would get together and hold study groups. Occasionally, we would have student nurse-midwives studying with us. When they joined us it had to be on the sly because if their instructors found out, they could be kicked out of the midwifery program. We had the occasional doctor or nurse-midwife come in and teach us things like pelvimetry, suturing, newborn assessments, newborn cardiology, lab work evaluation, and other specialty subjects. We did CPR training together and later neonatal resuscitation.

About this time, I started attending MANA (Midwives Alliance of North America) conferences, my first one in 1985 in Wheeling, West Virginia. I inhaled every bit of midwifery education that was available at the time and was so excited to be part of more workshops and spending time with other midwives. I have since attended every MANA conference with the exception of one in 1989, which was right in the middle of our move to a new house.

I have been truly blessed to have my family's support through all the years of practice. I will admit that it was a huge adjustment for my husband who was used to having a wife who took care of our children, kept the house clean and had nice meals on the table every night at 6:00 P.M. He couldn't understand when I was gone for twenty-four hours or longer. He definitely didn't like it when I didn't get paid and when he had to pay for other people's births. With a few adjustments we made it through those early years. He is a fantastic support now and has even learned how to make his own meals when I am gone.

No one can ever totally understand what it is like to be a direct-entry midwife unless you have been there or worked in a similar field. This is even more intense when you work in a state that doesn't provide licensure. The law in Georgia currently allows for midwifery practice, but the midwives must be certified by the state. No new midwifery certifications have been issued since 1973. Needless to say that has made it impossible to play by the rules.

The political fears are always there. I always wondered, *will this be the birth they come after me for?* My neighbors have been great. They not only opened their arms to my children who needed caring for while I was at a birth and my husband at work, they also opened their houses to store my midwifery files and supplies when I felt the powers-that-be might come bust me for practicing. Fortunately for the neighbors our children are now grown and my files would now take a moving van to get out of here. Everyone in this state including the medical board knows who I am now. I stopped hiding as a midwife many years ago. Oh what a life!

In 1991, cease and desist orders started being issued against local midwives. This was when I really started becoming active in the political arena. I met with the county attorneys asking how they thought the midwives could get certified when certifications weren't being issued. I took piles of paperwork including all my letters to the state asking for certification. The cease and desist orders stopped being issued, although that didn't help the midwives who had already received them. I started attending every government meeting where the discussion of "lay midwives" came up. I would receive anonymous phone calls letting me know where I should be next. Sometimes they came just an hour before a meeting was to start.

A Senate bill was also introduced which would have made it a felony to practice without certification. This led to the formation of Georgia Friends of Midwives. We were able to get almost a thousand names in the database. Families from all over Georgia called the capital voicing concern over the bill. It was tabled within two days.

We asked a friendly senator to get an opinion from the Attorney General about midwifery certification being denied. He strongly suggested that the Department of Health revisit the issue. A task force was put together to create new rules. I was one of the midwives on the task force. Unfortunately the Director of Health died and a new one was appointed. On the day he stepped into the position he put in emergency regulations stating that in order to be a "lay midwife" you must first become a certified nurse-midwife. Well now, that didn't work out well! We found a supportive Representative who introduced legislation. We spent all our spare time lobbying that bill. We had support in committee, but it never made it to the House Floor for a vote. Through the years we kept a bill introduced in case things heated up for the midwives.

I have always felt that what I am doing is right, and I have worked hard to make the process easier for all involved, both on the local and national level. In

1991, regulations in Georgia were changed that made it more difficult to get a birth certificate for home birthed babies. Susan Hodges, President of Citizens for Midwifery, and I worked with the State Vital Records Director and the Department of Health and Human Services to come up with a new process. I created worksheets that the state now uses for "Out-of-Institution Births" and act as liaison between families and the local registrars. This has made the process flow much more smoothly. Midwives here still don't sign birth certificates, but I am working with the state on a way to make that happen in the near future. The key is to figure out a process that will protect the midwives.

Finally in 2006 we had a resolution pass and a study committee actually appointed. I was part of the House Study Committee that released recommendations that the Department of Public Health (DPH) resume midwifery certification. I participated on the DPH Midwifery Task Force that met late in 2008. The Task Force made a recommendation to the DPH Director that a pilot project using CPMs (Certified Professional Midwives) be set up. I am hoping to see this process completed later this year.

2004 and 2005 had to be the hardest years in my entire midwifery career. My midwifery partners and dear friends, Gaye and Vickie, both died of breast cancer. Babies were still coming so there was no time to grieve. On top of all that was a mother who developed Post-Traumatic Stress Disorder (PTSD) after the birth of her first child that I attended in 2003. She was very unhappy with her birth and felt abused and abandoned. I spent hours each day talking with her, going to see doctors and counselors to no avail. Her version of what happened was posted all over the Internet. She filed a complaint with the state midwifery association, North American Registry of Midwives (NARM), the state medical board, and also filed a request to the district attorney that I be prosecuted for practicing medicine without a license. I went through review on the state and national levels, and fortunately the cases with the medical board and district attorney were closed. Both the culmination of losing my midwifery partners and dealing with this mother and the investigations sent me over the edge. I stopped taking births and buried myself in my office unless I was traveling. I felt at the time that if I was going to hurt mothers like she alleged I did, then I had no business being a midwife. I spent, ironically, nine months re-evaluating my midwifery and figuring out where I wanted to go from there. The wonderful part of the entire nightmare was all the support that came in from families with whom I had worked. I gradually started back when repeat clients called and wouldn't take "no" for an answer. New families were added a little at a time. Today my practice is back to where it was prior to the investigation. Unfortunately that experience will probably haunt me forever. What I learned from it is that being a midwife is not always easy, and no matter what kind of relationship we form with the mothers we are not always safe.

My national work is ongoing. Through my work with the Midwives Alliance of North America (MANA), I continue to assist midwives who are trying to work on state legislation as well as those midwives who face legal troubles. Building bridges between all midwives is another role that is important to me. I serve on the Liaison Committee between the American College of Nurse-Midwives (ACNM) and MANA. I am looking for the day when we can all work together, knowing our role is to serve mothers and keep their births as safe as possible in the environment in which they are most comfortable.

I was one of the initial ten midwives in the United States to receive certification as a Certified Professional Midwife (CPM). Once certified, I began volunteering for the organization helping to process applications. Currently I am the Director of Education and Advocacy for the North American Registry of Midwives (NARM) that issues this national credential for direct-entry midwives. I also serve as Secretary on the Board of Directors. My daily job with NARM includes answering the main contact phone number and emails from inquirers. It has been so wonderful to talk with midwives all over the country. I also get to travel and work at the Midwives Model of Care booth at conferences. I really enjoy it but, wow, do my feet hurt at the end of each day.

When I first started attending births, fathers were nowhere to be found during labor and delivery. When my son was born, the medical staff only let my husband attend because he had a card showing he had attended a childbirth class. Mothers labored in one room, birthed in another, recovered in the recovery room, and then stayed five days on the maternity floor. Through the years mothers have demanded more, including family and support teams being with them when they birth. Most hospitals in my area now have midwives, and mothers are able to keep their babies with them for the majority of the time. Unfortunately, cesarean sections have risen dramatically, mainly due to the litigious society we have become. Doctors have lost the art of delivering breeches. Patience is no longer the name of the game for many.

As direct-entry midwifery increases in recognition, the powers-that-be have realized we aren't going away. This is very evident as we work on legislation in various states. The midwives and other "mid-level" practitioners are winning. But now the American Medical Association is working in an organized way, through their Scope of Practice Partnership, to control mid-level practitioners and fight any increased legal and legislative recognition for them. I definitely feel like we are back to "David and Goliath" when it comes to passing legislation. The good news here is that now we not only have Citizens for Midwifery (CfM) but we also have The Big Push for Midwives initiative, which is made up of some incredibly brilliant and talented legislative activists from all over the country. These groups have been an incredible resource for those working on legislation.

Birth is a phenomenal event. No two are ever the same. Birthing women are incredible! In most cases I have found the process works beautifully when I listen to the mother while at the same time listen to my own instincts. Between the two they rarely fail me. One really hard lesson has been that not every mother is going to be happy with what I do or don't do. What is absolutely right for one mother might send another mother totally over the edge. It really does an emotional number on the midwife when a mother is unhappy with her birth. Fortunately, I can count on one hand the times this has happened, but it does stick with you.

There is nothing more special than working with repeat clients and seeing babies you helped birth growing up. One mother I work with doesn't tell the children she is pregnant. She just piles them in her van on her scheduled prenatal day and drives over. The children realize once they get in my neighborhood that this is the way to "Miss Debbie's." "Mom, are we having another baby?" It is too cute. They are so excited when they get here.

I really love watching mothers psychologically controlling their labors. I can remember one mother doing that very thing, whose husband was away on a business trip when he called to say he was on their street and almost home. What had been a slow labor instantly changed to transition. The baby arrived about fifteen minutes after the dad walked in the room.

I had another mother due with baby number five, who called me to come to the birth. I arrived around 4 A.M. She labored until the sun started coming up, then stopped. She told me I might as well go home because the children would be up soon, and there was no way she was going to be able to focus again until they went back to bed at night. I stayed for a while but finally got a clue she was serious. I went home and waited. She called me back about 10 P.M. that night. The baby arrived around midnight. Babies usually arrive when the time is right. Mothers who aren't feeling well normally don't go into labor. School exams are completed before the baby comes. Special events for the children are completed. It always amazes me how many babies arrive right before I leave town or right after I get home. They don't all wait, but a majority of them do.

I have worked very hard on both the local and national levels to promote home birth and direct-entry midwives as safe options for pregnant women. When I first started practicing, we weren't allowed to pass the nurses' station when we had a transport, let alone pass on any information to the hospital staff that had occurred during the pregnancy or labor. Now, in most cases, we can accompany moms into the hospital and our records are reviewed.

In a perfect world midwives would be part of a birth team. The midwife would be the primary caregiver for the mother, but she would have the availability of consultation should something go outside her scope of practice or comfort zone. This could be something as simple as sending a mom in for certain labs, ultrasounds (if necessary), or treatment of a condition that is not responding to alternative treatments, such as a urinary tract infection. I would love to see the day when midwives and mothers did not fear going to the hospital. The midwife would be part of the birth team once they arrived at the hospital and would be treated with respect. Everyone would be part of the decision-making process, including the mother and the midwife.

Fortunately, I have a wonderful and supportive doctor who gives me these things. He treats my mothers like queens when they come in. They don't have to fear being berated for planning a home birth. Thanks, Doc! Unfortunately it is rare to find a doctor willing to do this in my state or across the country. As long as the malpractice situation is such that it is I am not sure things will change.

Being a midwife is wonderful, but it's also an incredible amount of work. If you choose to become a midwife, do so because of the passion. If it is just a job for you, it won't work. Plan on being on call 24/7. That is the reality, unless you are one of the few who works in a scheduled practice.

Every midwife wants to be the perfect midwife. After all these years I am still trying to get there. I love being a midwife, being able to support mothers and their families through pregnancies and births. I feel honored to have been able to touch about 1,000 babies as they arrived in this world.

Keep learning! You will never know it all. Read all you can get your hands on. Join midwife email lists to learn how midwifery is done outside your local realm. They are a great resource for learning the tricks of the trade.

Be reliable! One thing that can ruin your reputation fast is when the mother can't get a hold of you when she is in labor or when you don't show up for prenatal or postpartum appointments. They totally understand if you are at a birth or an emergency comes up. Just let them know. Communication is the key. On a side note, ask any midwife how many times she has picked up the phone in the morning to double check whether it is really working, especially when she thought she might be headed out during the night when she went to bed. We have all done it more than once.

Act responsibly! As midwives, we all do things that might not be considered the norm in the medical community. When something comes up that is out of the norm, think it out. What are the risks? Does the mother really understand them? Is this a hill you are willing to die on? Remember there are other mothers counting on you. How will this impact your family, other midwives and mothers? It is really hard to tell a mother, "No, I'm not comfortable with the situation." Having a successful birth at home is very important to most of our clients. None of us want to disappoint them. Just think it all through before you decide what to do. There are many factors involved.

Get involved in your state and national midwifery organizations. They are there for you and can use all the help you have to offer. Join committees and follow through! Go out in the community and promote midwifery. Until mothers are educated, they won't know what options are available to them.

Get out of town! I can't impress how important this is, or you will burn out fast. Occasionally, let your family know they are important, too, and are really the most important part of your life. Let mothers know at consultation visits that there are times you will be off call, and inform them who will cover for you. Hopefully, you will have a support network set up with other midwives that makes this possible. In Atlanta most of the midwives cover for each other so everyone can have some time away. They are all wonderful support to me, and I appreciate it more than they will ever know. If you don't have that type of support system, block off six weeks every year to take your time off call.

Take time to find other interests. When our children were younger, there were many activities I was a part of both at their school and sports. I loved it! The great thing about being a self-employed direct-entry midwife is that you can schedule your hours around special events. Of course a birth would take priority, but it is rare that the births come when you have something special planned.

Once our children grew up and moved out, I had to find other avenues of interest. I became very involved with the Freecycle Network about four years ago. Freecycle is a grassroots and entirely nonprofit movement of people who are giving (and getting) stuff for free in their own towns. It's all about reuse and keeping good stuff out of landfills. I started a local group that has grown to almost 7000 members, and then went on to work with them on the national and international levels helping moderators who were starting new groups. For fun I play gin rummy every night in an online gaming league, Gin to Win. I am a tournament host. This is my place to escape.

Above all, make sure you enjoy it. I compare midwifery to motherhood. There are days I wonder why I ever started doing it. The countless sleepless nights, family events interrupted, hearing from mothers who felt I was less than the perfect midwife, and so on. But then I see that newborn baby—the tears in the parents' eyes—and realize that just like motherhood, I can't imagine my life without it.

Make medicine out of suffering

ARISIKA RAZAK

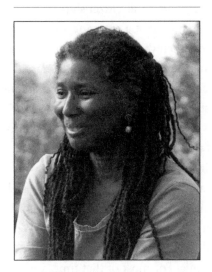

y involvement with midwifery came relatively late in my life, but my involvement with the needs and issues of women of color has been with me all of my life. My belief in the essential worthiness of all human beings and in the right of women to be treated with respect and dignity—especially when they are engaged in bearing the future of humanity—is at the core of my beliefs. I believe in the power of women to change the world, and this belief is grounded not only by my own experiences, but also by twenty-five years of listening to women from all over the world. I believe in women's ability to radically transform the social fabric because I have witnessed the struggles of women of every race and creed, women determined to make a better life for themselves and their children. In the birthing room, the sick room, the home and the marketplace, I have witnessed the power, love, and steadfast endurance of women who are rich, poor, educated or illiterate; I have experienced the brilliance of women who educate and teach, pastor and preach, found and head organizations, and offer leadership to their countries. In attending the births of women from over seventy countries I bow in homage to the awesome power of the womb, the brilliance of Spirit, and the Mystery of Life. May we be sheltered by all that is good; may we continue to heal; may we finally turn away from war and shelter and nurture the life of this planet! *Ashe!*

I am a sixty-year-old, mixed-class, African American woman who was deeply influenced by the civil rights struggles of the 1960s. I grew up during a time when African Americans were denied full citizenship rights in the country of their birth. It was taken for granted that a woman's ability, intelligence, and competence were absolutely less then those of men. This was doubly true for women of color, who were always judged against middle-class standards of femininity that they rarely could achieve. Struggles against racism and injustice, as well as struggles to provide just and equitable health care for poor and minority populations are essential parts of why I became a midwife, and my experiences in these struggles have dictated where and how I chose to practice.

My son's home birth was my first experience with midwifery. However, during the course of an unplanned but thoroughly welcomed pregnancy at the age of twenty-two, it was my experience in the Civil Rights Movement that helped me believe that I could have a home birth. While I read work about Grantly Dick-Reed and Dr. Lamaze, I understood that African people had been having babies for millennia. For most of that time, we had not had the support of modern western medicine—and we had not died off awaiting the arrival of contemporary biomedicine. My belief in the inherent capabilities of African Diasporic peoples led me to question the Euro-centric medical establishment. I passionately believed in my body's ability to meet the physical challenge of birth. And, while my sense of feminism was still new, I embraced the notion that a woman could do anything that was needed.

I had the sacred experience of having my first child at home with the support of my community. I had called the midwife late in labor; when she arrived she told me I would deliver in about an hour and a half. She never examined me, but her timing was impeccable. After about an hour and a half, I squeezed her hand as I felt the urge to push—and she told me that I needed to release her hand so she could catch the baby. I pushed three times, and for a moment I felt that I had a universe between my legs. An image of the Hindu Goddess Kali giving birth to the Universe—standing upright and ecstatic—flashed through my consciousness. In the next moment my son was born. The birth was safe, well-attended, and left me joyfully ecstatic. It changed my life forever.

However, my decision to become a midwife has a second, more difficult root. I witnessed one hospital birth during my obstetric rotation as a nursing student. This birth was so upsetting that the two nursing students with me said they didn't *ever* want to have babies. I couldn't believe that what I observed was related to the process I had experienced at home. The attending obstetrician was cruel and unsupportive. After waiting a half hour, he stormed out of the delivery room, snarling at the nurse, "Don't ever call me when one of those primips *thinks* she needs to push." During a prolonged episiotomy repair performed by the medical student, the patient complained of pain. The doctor denied her request for medication and stated: "That's what you Lamaze patients get for wanting to do it naturally." It was not the length of the labor or the woman's pain that made the birth difficult; the birth was horrendous because of the scorn of this provider who had total disdain for the birthing process.

The father of the baby was also not very supportive. After many hours of labor, the birthing woman stated that she wanted something for pain. "Oh no," said her husband, "we don't want any pain medicine." While I knew his job as a coach was to support an unmedicated birth, I instinctively knew that denying his wife's feelings was entirely inappropriate.

This woman's birth was so different from my own. Instead of being restricted to a hospital bed, I walked or sat whenever I wanted to, and my midwife later said I had danced through my labor. I rocked back and forth in "cat-cow" positions, and I crouched in a chair by the living room window. I never even sat on the bed my son was born in until five minutes before his emergence from my body. I had experienced strong back pains throughout my labor, and I instinctively responded by changing positions to make myself feel better. I know now that there isn't any magic position that makes labor pains stop, but just being able to move around alleviates some of the anxiety and fear that labor elicits in women.

Unlike me, my hospital patient was limited to the bed. We didn't have fetal monitors then, but walking around just wasn't allowed. Her options for moving or shifting were entirely limited. Lots of people came in and out of her room, but none of the staff was there to support her. No one offered her any real comfort: the medical students and nurses examined her; the nursing students observed. The husband responded to her pain and his fears in the classic way that men are taught to manage feelings: denial and stoicism. In witnessing this birth, I realized that the role of the coach—which at that time was modeled on the actions of male athletic coaches—was totally inappropriate for supporting women in labor.

My own experience of labor was very different. While much of my laboring time was alone, I was quite comfortable with this. Labor had started at midnight, but I didn't believe I was truly in labor. Early in pregnancy, I read an article on birth in the *New York Times*. It indicated that many doctors found normal deliveries quite boring. Obstetrics was no longer required in many medical schools, and doctors spoke scornfully of being called in to attend first-time mothers who were having "false labor." After reading this, I decided I wasn't going to be one of those women who called the doctor too early. So, I spent my first two hours of labor denying the pains that came like clockwork every fifteen minutes. At 2 A.M., still convinced I was having false labor, I got out of bed and began breathing exercises. An hour later, my breathing woke Star, my roommate. She sat and breathed with me, and told me I needed to call the midwife. I called the midwife, and in a way that was entirely organic, she validated my intuitive and instinctive knowledge. I had followed my body, and when the midwife came, she continued to encourage me to follow my body.

What I learned from these two birth experiences is that there is a huge difference between a birth grounded in respect for the body, and the body's intuitive knowing, and a birth grounded in the belief that the body is flawed, faulty, and potentially harmful. This difference is as palpable as the difference between pleasure and pain, or suffering and surrender. It is a difference to which our psyches are acutely attuned, and which is etched indelibly in the memories of birthing women.

I was afraid of dying, just as the woman I witnessed in the hospital was afraid of dying. I felt that the pain was more than I could bear. She felt this, too. I needed, just as she needed, the intimate and knowledgeable support of those who were skilled not only in the management of normal birth, but also in the management of the difficulties of birth. She, like me, deserved the support of people who respected and honored her emotional and physical struggles—and who deeply believed in her body's ability to birth safely and ecstatically.

I had this support, but she had only a piece of it: her support team only addressed the physical aspects of birth. They were unable or unwilling to address the emotional and psychological aspects or to offer her true understanding and respect. While both of our births encompassed fear and pain, in my case the ecstasy of giving birth in knowledge and power transcended my experience of pain and suffering. The doctor that came to my house gave me "two stitches" to repair a tear. He congratulated me and the midwife. The doctor that sewed her up took pleasure in making that experience difficult and more painful. He never acknowledged the power of her body and psyche, and the success of her labor. While she, like me, experienced the miraculous joy of giving birth to a healthy child, the attitudes of the staff diminished her knowledge of her own power and dimmed the radiant joy that accompanies a successful birth.

My understanding of the need for respectful and appropriate support in the labor and birthing room has deeply influenced my work as a midwife. Just before I entered midwifery school I performed a small anecdotal survey. I collected stories of women who found their first birth so traumatic that they chose to never have another baby. All the women I interviewed were women of color who had given birth in the hospital. They were middle and working class, college educated and/or college graduates. In a moment of utter vulnerability, they had all undergone a profoundly traumatizing experience at the hands of a cruel and uncaring medical institution.

In discussing their experience, these women never referred to the length of labor. They did not say that their birth was so painful that they thought they would die. Their birthing trauma did not arise from the experience of pain. What defined a traumatic birth was almost always the birthing staff's attitudes. Gender and race were not the cause of their negative treatment; the offending staff was often the same race or gender as the pregnant woman. What was most significant was the way in which boundaries between patients and providers provided a license for unthinking cruelty and lack of perception of a common humanity.

The women I interviewed said, "I came to the hospital, and when I asked for something for pain they told me I was a big strong country woman and I didn't need pain medicine." A common variant was, "When I was in pain, they told me to shut up; if it didn't hurt when I was making the baby, I should be quiet now." Being left alone in labor was especially traumatizing: "I came to the hospital and told them the baby was coming. They told me I was wrong—and they put me in a room by myself and I delivered all alone." A common variant was being put on a gurney in the hallway and delivering alone.

Women told me of nurses holding their legs closed when they tried to push because the doctor hadn't arrived. They told stories of doctors who laughed at their labor or their post-partal pain. One woman, a young African American medical student, had changed obstetricians so she could have natural childbirth in an Alternative Birthing Center. At her six-week check up, she told her physician that intercourse was still painful. "He grinned at me and told me that he had given me a couple of extra stitches. 'Your husband will love it,' he said."

These stories deeply influenced my subsequent work as a midwife. While I apprenticed with a direct-entry or "lay midwife" and was trained and certified as a nurse-midwife, the story of my own pregnancy and home birth, and the stories and experiences of other women of color who gave birth have been the greatest influence on my later work as a midwife. My midwifery care was also deeply impacted by notions of cultural sensitivity and social justice, for I grew up in New York as the daughter of a community activist. My mother believed that it was our social and spiritual duty to make the world we lived in a better place for everyone regardless of race or status. At the time I entered nursing school two years after my son's birth in 1972, I had no idea that I would become a midwife. However, I decided to apprentice with the woman who'd caught my baby in order to learn more about how and why my home birth experience had been so different from the hospital birth I witnessed.

June, the midwife with whom I apprenticed, provided home birth services and childbirth preparation classes. She didn't offer prenatal care, which had to be obtained from an obstetrician. While her clients were predominantly Euro American, I met African American, Jamaican, and African women who all planned to deliver at home with her. Some were having their first baby and others were former clients. About 25% of the births during my apprenticeship ended in the hospital. June later told me that if she had experienced as high of a transport rate in her first thirty births as I did in my apprenticeship, she wouldn't have become a midwife.

Since I had no expectations, I wasn't turned off by our high transport rate. In birth after birth I witnessed the power and strength of women as they moved through the birthing process. I offered my clients the comfort given to me: I rubbed backs and hands, walked with women in their homes, and verbally encouraged them. I saw husbands who were supportive and sensitive and/or fearful and inappropriate. While a woman might have decided that she wanted music, food, or particular friends around her, there was always a moment when she had to engage more deeply with the forces moving through her body. The world fell away and her energy turned inward; for a moment she was the equal of forces moving life from one side of the veil to the other. In that moment, I saw the face of God/dess creating the world—and my Spirit was touched with awe and wonder.

June taught me the power of patience—of waiting like the earth waits—of trusting in the moment and moving in harmony with the elemental power of the body. She didn't touch women as much as I did, but she didn't discourage my doing so. Early on, she said, "We're the oldest profession, not the hookers," and I've always remembered that comment. She told her prenatal class once that the reason men climbed Mt. Everest was that they didn't have babies, something I'd never thought about but with which I immediately resonated.

She was a solo practice midwife, and in the summer I worked with her, I was on call 24/7. While this worked for her, it did not work for me. I've learned since then that something in me doesn't relax when I'm on call: I'm always psychically "listening." In this era before beepers or cell phones, I could neither enjoy going to the movies nor relax enough to easily make love. I learned that summer that I couldn't be a solo practice midwife.

I also realized that I didn't want my role with the woman to end if she went to the hospital. Since we had such a high number of hospital transports, I experienced the hospital's contemptuous denial of a lay midwife's right to be with her clients when they entered the hospital. June or I often spent twelve to twenty hours with a woman before we decided to go to the hospital. We knew the woman intimately; we had seen her struggle with or against her body; we had seen her naked, sweaty, powerful and vulnerable as she danced with inner and outer demons of pain and fear. Sometimes we transported because we—and she—understood that there was a risk to the baby and that birth at home was no longer safe. But often that summer, we transported because the woman could not trust her own body, and had unconsciously decided birth was safer in the hospital.

When we arrived at the hospital, June and I were routinely barred from the room in which the woman was examined. The medical staff assumed that we knew nothing about labor and birth in general, and nothing about the particular woman we brought in. Our reports of cervical dilation, length of labor, rupture of membranes, and a host of other concerns were routinely ignored. In a few cases where our concerns were for the welfare of the mother and baby, valuable time was lost as medical personnel chose to ignore our diagnoses, simultaneously berating the mother for choosing a *dangerous* home birth and *ignorant* providers. Once the woman was admitted, June and I were excluded from the labor room because we were not personal family or next of kin.

During the early 1970s, if a woman deliberately or accidentally disclosed to her physician that she planned to have a home birth, the physician usually refused to continue her prenatal care. This is still true for many physicians. At that time in California, there were very few practicing nurse-midwives—and an even smaller number of them were delivering at home. It was obvious to me that this was an inhumane and dangerous way to treat patients, and my desire to become a nurse-midwife stems from my frustrations with this dangerous, fragmented and hierarchical care. I maintained a small home birth practice after finishing my apprenticeship with June in 1976. I also worked part-time with Sinem, a highly experienced direct-entry midwife who had a successful collaborative relationship with doctors at San Francisco General Hospital. Unlike my experience with June in Berkeley, the physicians at General regarded Sinem as an experienced and valued clinician. She was able to stay with clients she brought in from home, and she was able to manage uncomplicated labors in consultation with the attending obstetricians.

While I loved doing home births, I realized I wanted to attend women through the full spectrum of pregnancy and childbirth. I also wanted to work with women of color who were the most oppressed by the hospital system. Initially, I was concerned that my direct-entry colleagues would see my desire to pursue nurse-midwifery as an act of betrayal, but I was pleased to learn that they fully supported my decision to obtain nurse-midwifery certification. After receiving my Master's in Public Health (MPH) degree in 1978 I worked in a hospital for six months so that I could meet the prerequisites for applying to the UC San Francisco's Nurse-Midwifery Program.

While I've discussed my ecstatic experience of home birth in California, I also need to describe my prenatal care experience at a public clinic in New York City. This experience provided a standard against which I measured my own later role as a health care provider for indigent women. It taught me that we have at least two standards of health care in the United States. One is for the poor and the undocumented, and another is for people with private insurance. In 1971 when I was pregnant in New York, there were only two ways to receive public medical assistance. You either enrolled from your hospital bed or you came to *one* clinic in Manhattan. The waiting line was so long that if you didn't arrive by 7:30 A.M., you couldn't be seen that day. And the clinic didn't open till 9 A.M. Waiting in line on a cold, wet, January morning, I remember thinking, *I'm not sick; I'm just pregnant. Could I wait like this if I were really ill? Could I wait outside for public assistance?* I knew then that our health care system didn't care about the poor and that it was also a system that I could not trust.

During this pregnancy I was taking medical pre-requisite classes at the Old Westbury campus of the State University system. This new college had no residential dormitories so we were bussed in every day from another state institution. There was no cafeteria and lunchtime meals came from on-site vending machines, unless you had a car and could drive into town. I purchased a lot of yogurt from the vending machines during my pregnancy, but I knew I wasn't nourished in the way that I wanted. My prenatal care, which was my first encounter with the health care system, was impersonal, uncaring, bureaucratic and confusing. I experienced it as horrendous, and I later vowed never to give the kind of care I received. All the patients had block appointments, which meant that everyone came at the same time. Unlike today's group appointments, which provide health education and support patient interactions, our two- and three-hour waits were rarely broken up by interactions with others.

No one ever explained what was being done to my body, so the care I received never seemed important. It was fragmented and dehumanizing: one person weighed me, someone else collected my urine, and another person put his or her hand on my belly. There were no explanations: no one ever told me what was being measured, and no one ever talked about what the measurements indicated. The nutritionist lectured me about foods I should eat, but I had no way to acquire or cook them. I spent my whole pregnancy convinced that some part of my care was missing. Surely in private settings, middle-class doctors gave White middle-class clients the competent and personalized care that I was denied. My experience of being a poor client in a large, urban, indigent care setting is a critical part of my understanding of midwifery. It helps me understand why properly trained and culturally sensitive midwives are so successful in working with populations demographically at risk for infant mortality and preterm deliveries. My experience taught me that extending competent, loving, and individualized support is an integral part of being a good midwife. It taught me the importance of talking to patients, and embodied the idea that there is no substitute for cultural sensitivity and cultural awareness.

My experience of substandard, dehumanized care mandated that I always explained to women *what* I was doing and *why* it was significant; it meant that when I could not speak another's language that I always called a translator. In a birth, when a translator was not available, I used the human technologies of sound, touch, and soft tones to convey compassion and support the birthing woman. One of my most moving births was with a Cambodian woman who was positive for Hepatitis B. We could not speak each other's language, and I wore a mask since Hepatitis B is transmitted through blood and amniotic fluid. I knew that my mask and gown did not support patient comfort—but being splashed with birth fluids was quite common and I needed protection. Without a shared spoken language, I used humming to support this woman's labor, and after she delivered, she spontaneously reached out to stroke my cheek, acknowledging the loving care she knew I had felt for her.

What I learned over time was that physically competent care is not the only measure by which midwives are judged. Sensitive, caring, and respectful providers make a real difference to clients. While our clients didn't always know if our actions were competent, they were experts in recognizing—and evaluating—our sensitivity and compassion. If we provided empathetic and respectful care, they forgave our logistical problems: in spite of long waits, missing records, repeated labs, or occasional dirty rooms, our patients came faithfully to their appointments. Sometimes after waiting for hours, they declined the services of the physician, continuing instead, to wait for the midwife.

Today, I believe that many of the important things I know and understand about life were learned or tempered by my twenty-five years as a midwife. As I say to my students, you can't believe that women are the weaker sex and work with women having babies. Midwifery grounded my belief in feminism and in women's power and exposed me to the reality of a spirituality that is immanent, embodied, democratic and ubiquitous.

As an inner city midwife I learned all the good, bad and ugly ways that women get pregnant. I saw women who didn't trust their bodies and who didn't trust birth. But what I witnessed again and again, as women lay down on a primal bed of pain was their absolute willingness to suffer, to trust, to endure, and to triumph. I witnessed the ordinary and extraordinary heroism of women as they entered a ritual that brought them to their knees, and I witnessed the absolute uncompromised joy that suffused their body-minds as they held a living child in their arms.

While I came to midwifery because I deeply cared for those who are poor, helpless, female and alone, and since I have at one time in my life been a member of each of these groups, I learned, as a midwife, that courage, endurance, self-sacrifice and love are universal qualities that have been given to all races, classes, genders and nationalities. I learned in the deepest part of myself that to be poor and indigent is simply to be part of the human race. It does not mean that you are stupid, lazy or ignorant; it does not mean that you don't care about your children.

My midwifery practice has taught me that most women love their children. You can convince a pregnant woman to do many new things if she believes it's for her baby's health. I've learned that a little kindness goes a long way. Patients whose names and births I really don't remember have remembered me for decades, whether I attended them prenatally or had the joy of catching their babies. My name is not an easy one to say or remember, and White and Black clients have named their babies after me in order to honor the love and respect I offered them. I've also learned how competent and able working class women are. With so much less than what I've been given, they struggle everyday to make a better way for themselves and their children. They care for multiple offspring and other nuclear and extended family members—and they deal every day with a system that rejects them.

Letting women know that they have survived and triumphed in an incredible rite of passage is very important to me. One of our teens spent her whole pregnancy hiding the pregnancy from her parents. She came to us during a school strike so her prenatal visits could be hidden from the school. She planned to give the baby up for adoption; when she went into labor she called the labor coach to get a ride to the hospital. She scaled a fence, went to the hospital and delivered her child. She left the hospital a few hours after the delivery so that she could register in school for the day. When I saw her postpartum, I told her that she could do anything, for her ability to birth was a marker of her ability to do whatever was necessary in the course of her life.

Working in a hospital taught me that getting along with all sorts of people was key to our survival as a midwifery service. I was not only a hospital staff nurse-midwife, but for about the first four years of our service I was the Director. The first Obstetrics Chief I worked with told me that translation services for non-English speaking patients were totally unnecessary. After seeing a father leave "his place" at the shoulders of his wife in order to witness the child's arrival, this obstetrician concluded that "fathers had no place in the delivery room." In this setting, many of the long-time nurses had adopted the negative attitudes of the attending physicians. They laughed at Laotian patients who were unused to high beds and used our sheets to make a pallet on the floor. They were contemptuous of our addicted women patients, and rarely exhibited love or compassion for women in labor.

Working with these negative staff attitudes in the early years of the service was very challenging. As I was a subordinate in this system, I learned to work around these issues rather than to confront them directly. I spoke kindly to staff whose treatment of patients horrified me, and I sometimes remained silent rather than publicly disagree with doctors or nurses whose attitudes were inflexible. I recognized the value of saving face even when I felt that my backup OB was wrong. And I used humor and subtlety in my communications. I can't always speak with pride about this, but I do know that compromise was a good strategy for me.

Many of the midwives who confronted the doctors directly ended up leaving our service. Their births were watched; their management was questioned; their consulting doctors rejected collaboration in favor of physician control. I was regarded as a team player who accepted medical authority, so I was routinely left alone. I delivered women in alternate positions and in birthing chairs; I permitted my Native American patients to burn sage; I *covertly* worked around the ridiculous time limits that we were given by individual physicians. I never lost a patient; I never lost the respect of the nursing staff; and over time, some of the most difficult medical personnel became my partners in the loving dance of caring for women.

To be a midwife in this country is to take risks. In the early years of the service I secretly worked with community organizations that were trying to make obstetric services better for women and children in the local community. The midwives worked openly with the hospital's community advisory board and with progressive nurses and physicians. We demanded translators for non-English speaking patients. We also worked clandestinely with grassroots community groups lobbying for safe and adequate levels of staffing, and culturally sensitive, family-centered care for poor women of all ethnicities. We had political meetings with the Board of Supervisors and met with other elected officials to ask for funding to improve patient care and access.

Sometimes there were consequences for this. I have been yelled at so loudly by a hospital administrator (who was rumored to have thrown a chair at another woman in a meeting) that people in the cafeteria later asked what had happened. I have stood up to my physicians and demanded that they hire more midwives so that we could adequately serve women; and I have led a unionizing effort to make this happen. When I was the Director, I made sure that we hired midwives who wanted to work with the poor and the indigent. My efforts—in conjunction with the lobbying of others—helped change perinatal services at our hospital. The midwives used the Alternative Birth Center that had been unutilized for two years; we ended the requirement that childbirth classes be a prerequisite for birth center deliveries since there were no prenatal classes for our non-English speaking patients. Before our hospital engaged translators, midwives in my service located volunteer translators in the community. One of my staff created a program that allowed the midwives to provide intake services to drug-using women at their first point of entry; we examined them at their first Emergency Room visit, drew their blood, and ordered sonograms, which gave them a strong incentive to return.

I believe that it is our steadfast advocacy for patients that has led to our service's greatest success: thirty years later the midwifery service that I helped establish and shape still serves women in the county. And perhaps most importantly we have helped to change the local African American community's perceptions about midwifery.

When our service began, Latin American women familiar with *parteras* routinely chose midwives. New Southeast Asian immigrants who had delivered at home also wanted midwives. Counterculture Euro Americans sought alternative birth services and midwifery care. But African American women, whose mothers and grandmothers had been denied hospitals and obstetricians in the segregated South, were reluctant to have their daughters and granddaughters attended by midwives. They wanted a *"real doctor"* and were suspicious that midwifery was second-class care.

In addition, poor women of color in the United States have often been targeted for medical experimentation. This is especially true in the reproductive arena: enslaved African American women were subjected to surgeries without anesthesia by Dr. James Sims, the father of gynecology; and the American eugenics movement championed birth control as a way to limit immigrant working class populations.

While these issues are not usually linked to midwifery, the legacy of these issues was quite real for many of the women I attended. I was profoundly happy that our hospital enforced California's mandatory thirty-day waiting period for elective sterilization. In our hospital, the midwives and doctors worked really hard to make sure that we obtained appropriate adult translators so that sterilization procedures were competently explained to the women we served. Since the reproductive rights of Black women are often contested or denied, I am proud of the fact that our hospital service declined to forcibly impose Norplant on women who used drugs.

Twenty years later, many African American women in the county freely chose midwives. They know that we provide safe, empathetic and competent health care. Our drug-using women often lied and said they were midwife patients when they presented in labor. They wanted the support and understanding midwives provided.

We also made a difference in perinatal outcomes. While we delivered less than a thousand patients in our first three years, an early retrospective review documented that our clients had rates of preterm delivery, and low birth weight that approximated the state's averages for all women—indicating that we had successfully impacted the high infant mortality rates of young, indigent and African American populations.

In my twenty-five years of midwifery practice, I have personally impacted the health and self-esteem of hundreds of women. One story that I am especially proud of concerns a woman whose first birth I attended, but who had subsequent deliveries elsewhere. Several years later she spoke with a lawyer I knew and told him that she didn't let the doctors do certain things to her when she was in labor because of that first birth with me. She resisted because she believed in her body, and this empowered her to stand up for herself. For me this is a real success story, for I believe that our job as midwives is to empower women. It's not the birth site that does this; it's what we reflect back to the woman.

Over the course of fifteen years I have watched health care go from bad to worse. Long waits, short visits, and inadequate counseling times are the norms even in the private setting. The health care system is broken, and I don't think it will be fixed in my lifetime, although Obama's election gives me hope. Machine technology has also had a huge impact on birth. Symbolized by fetal monitors—which I believe are here to stay—our culture's emphasis on technology is symptomatic of disdain for the "natural" and increased preference for the mechanistic. The Alternative Birth Center in our hospital, called the "Little House" by our Laotian and Mien patients, was taken over by the doctors and became doctor sleep rooms—and this embodied a reminder of birth's utter normalcy that will not return soon. I am saddened that birth in the hospital and birth at home are more and more different and that normal births are increasingly difficult to obtain.

I grieve that young women accept the notions that birth is so inherently difficult and that every woman needs an epidural. Having studied Buddhist philosophy for over ten years, I accept that pain and suffering are fundamental parts of our physical human existence. I believe that progress through life's pain can be redeemed though our body's ability to surrender, our psyche's ability to make sacrifice, our mind's ability to understand, and our Spirit's ability to accept. For women, the pain of birth is often transcended by the experience of joy that accompanies new life and the empowerment we feel serving as the doorway to human existence.

I also believe that our progress towards a more evolved or spiritual state of being can be accelerated by our work with suffering. This can occur through our own suffering or through witnessing the suffering of others. After sitting with laboring women for over twenty years, I often found myself asking why women suffered in birth. I don't believe that birth is inherently painful, but since it often is, I now ask "what is it that we learn from pain?" Birth teaches me that pain is a universal life experience; it humbles and softens us, opening the gates of compassion, empathy and understanding in ourselves as well as others. Birth teaches me that I can transcend the limits of my physical body, and that it is my willingness to accept my pain and surrender to its force, that is my ally in moving through it. Finally, I believe that pain is redeemed by our ability to "make medicine" out of our suffering, and that this ability lies at the heart of a spiritual response to suffering. I am grateful to be a woman who learned this wisdom as a mother and midwife.

God walks in

GERADINE SIMKINS

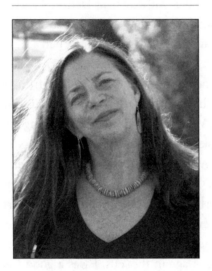

*M*y earliest memory is of being a two-year-old child, singing to my dying
grandmother. It was my job to make my grandmother laugh first thing
in the morning and throughout the day, so every morning my mother would lift
me out of my crib and carry me to my grandmother's room while I was still in my
pajamas. I wonder if I knew as a child that not only was I supposed to make her
laugh, I was also supposed to ease her pain. I did that faithfully until the morning
I woke up and she was no longer there.

As I got a little older, I loved to lie on my back in the deep moist grass and
watch the clouds turn into animal shapes. In the summer I would burst out of our

house and run across the street to the park to climb the big tree that grew on a slant into the leafy canopy of the forest. I broke my arm three different times from climbing and falling, but it never stopped me from running headlong into my wild adventures. In my early adolescence we would drive to our friend's house at the lake, and when we got there I jumped right in. I had become captivated with diving and swimming in deep water. It was scary down deep, and the water was a strange bluish-green color that had sparkles in it. The deeper I went, the more my ears buzzed and pounded with the pressure, and sometimes my feet got tangled in the underwater seaweed. The experience of being over my head in the subterranean kingdom was thrilling and sometimes frightening. But the secrets of the underwater realm called to me and left me utterly captivated.

I was born in the Upper Midwest near Detroit. I grew up in Motown during the height of the Motown era. What could be better for someone who loved to sing and dance? My parents, Margaret and Earl, had a variety of friends of many nationalities, religions, and political persuasions. And they invited travelers to rest awhile with us, including folks from India, Africa, Vietnam and Ireland. People from the neighborhood and all over the world would flock to our house for my parent's events. We gathered for political meetings, holiday parties, church get-togethers, and cookouts in the backyard. And while we might have been able to tell who was Black, White, Indian or Asian, a newcomer would be hard pressed to identify who was Democrat, Republican, Communist, Socialist, Jewish, Christian, Hindu, Muslim, or atheist. Of course, those parties also provided my brothers—Michael, Kevin and Eric—and me with ample opportunities to get into trouble. We especially liked the green beer on St. Patrick's Day.

As a teen coming of age in the '60s, I was a good Catholic girl, and I had planned to be a nun—until I met my first boyfriend, smoked pot, and grooved to the music of Janis Joplin and The Doors at the legendary Grande Ballroom in Detroit. Sex, drugs and rock 'n roll distracted me from my religious vocation. Nonetheless, I was eventually drawn towards a community of women who dedicated their lives to service just as the nuns did.

I was seventeen-years old in 1967 during the Summer of Love when the world was waking up to the hippie counterculture. This time marked the intersection of contemporary art and music, popular culture, civil unrest and moral upheaval in America. I was ripe for it and became cogent in the political conversations of the times. My parents became radicalized in the '60s. My mom and I spent a lot of time on the picket line. In 1968 I marched in solidarity with Dr. Martin Luther King, Jr.'s Poor Peoples Campaign as he crisscrossed the country to bring attention to racial and economic injustice. In 1968 I was kicked out of high school a few weeks before graduation because I skipped school to attend a rally where presidential candidate Robert Kennedy was speaking. I got "found out" because I ended up on the "Evening News," standing next to him on the dais in my school uniform. I had just wanted to get close to him. I was reinstated and graduated in May, and one month later Kennedy was assassinated; King had been assassinated two months earlier. 1968 has since been called, "The year that rocked the world." I went to Wayne State University in Detroit, and for two years I lived in an inner city commune and peace center in the heart of Motown. Eventually I dropped out of college to devote myself entirely to peace and social justice movements. When I narrowly escaped a jail sentence because of my non-violent civil disobedience and anti-war activities in Detroit, I hitchhiked across the United States and southern Canada to clear my head, stopping for a while in the hippie mecca of the San Francisco Bay area. Later I moved on to Cannon Beach, a small oceanside town in northern Oregon where I lived for most of the year in 1971 and "did art" while watching the migration of gray whales. As we would later realize, the 1960s and early 1970s were some of the most revolutionary, tumultuous and inventive periods of the twentieth century.

After returning to Detroit from the small paradise on the Oregon coast, I moved north to the tranquil terrain of the Grand Traverse region—the beautiful land of the indigenous Odawa and Ojibwa people along the shores of Lake Michigan. I have lived in Leelanau County—which in the Native language means "land of delight"—for the past thirty-five years and raised my family in this serene countryside. It was in the Grand Traverse Bay region that I was called to be a community midwife for thirty years.

Before I got married and had my first baby, I was an artist. I was a co-owner of a gallery, along with four other partners in Northern Michigan. In 1976 I married one of my business partners, and we had our first child, Maya, a year later. After I became a midwife, my artwork faded into the background. Primarily, I was a mom. Three years after we were married, my husband and I bought 20 acres in Leelanau County with a $3000 down payment from wedding money and savings. We had a 15-year land contract and monthly payments of $142. We only had enough money to buy land and not a house, so that first spring, summer and fall we lived in a tent with our two-year old daughter. We cobbled together our first little cabin by cutting and hauling cedar trees out of the swamp to use as foundation posts, gathering reclaimed barn wood for siding, and utilizing yard sale hardware and windows. We barely got into the cabin that autumn before the snow fell. We had to haul everything up the very long snow-covered driveway on toboggans, including 25-gallon water drums, propane tanks, groceries, kids and building supplies. We heated the cabin with a woodstove and had an outhouse for the first three years. The next summer I gave birth to my second baby, Leah, in our little cabin without water or a bathroom. We had a vegetable garden in the summer and gathered wild berries and herbs. We canned fruits, veggies, jams and baby food in the fall. We baked bread and made yogurt all winter. For several years we raised chickens and we ate wild game. A few years later I gave birth to my third baby, Sean. By that time we had a water-well and an old clawfoot bathtub that we filled with a hose. The "back to the land movement" was the kind of lifestyle that many young people were leaving the urban centers across the country to pursue. And although it was hard, it was also wonderful. I had a husband and three small children who I adored and a gorgeous place on the planet to live.

We were do-it-yourselfers, so "do it yourself birth" fit the ethic of our lifestyle. We were very active and I felt healthy and robust during my pregnancies. My three home births, quick and powerful, were hard work and the most stunning events of my life. It is true: Walking though the gateway of birth thrusts you into the depths of creation—messy and mysterious, wild and wonderful. My own births influenced me to become a midwife. Initially, I learned to be a midwife because I needed that skill, just as I needed carpentry skills to build a house and gardening skills to grow our food. But before long, I was inexorably drawn to birthing, as if a force of destiny had tapped me on the shoulder and asked me to follow, manifestly changing my life path.

I joined with other do-it-yourself women in my community, each of us helping the other to give birth, learning the craft empirically. After a year or so, we found that there were pockets of women in several parts of the state who were also acting as birth attendants in their respective urban and rural communities. Around 1978 we organized the first meeting of what was to become the Michigan Midwives Association (MMA), which we incorporated in 1982. A meeting was held in Detroit, hosted by the Motor City Midwives, and I became the first president of the MMA. From the beginning, we were dedicated to accountability and integrity in our practice of midwifery. Without any mentoring, but with a lot of background in grassroots community organizing around social justice and women's health issues, we designed a midwifery apprenticeship training program. We created a midwifery certification process and credential—the "Certified Midwife"—which preceded the current national certification called the Certified Professional Midwife or CPM. We implemented a peer review process and a means of gathering statistics on our pregnancy and birth outcomes. In 1982 I became the first MMA-certified midwife, or CM, in Michigan, and as such, I was one of the first certified direct-entry midwives in the country. Later we learned that there were a few other midwifery organizations in the United States that had simultaneously created a similar direct-entry midwifery credential just as we had in Michigan. And then several years later the national Certified Professional Midwife credential was created and patterned upon those regional models.

I cut my teeth in organizational management when we envisioned, designed, and launched our statewide professional midwifery organization in Michigan. But I put on my big girl panties when I became an active participant in our national (and international) midwifery organization—the Midwives Alliance of North America (MANA). The Midwives Alliance is definitely a child of the '60s and '70s in that its founding members were counterculture feminist-types who responded to the social ferment of the times. Primarily, they were women who had given birth at home as a reaction to the over-medicalization of birth in America, and then proceeded to help other women do the same. The founders of the Midwives Alliance were as dedicated to *process* as they were to *outcome*—not only in birth but also in business. They created an organization in which each woman's voice and each midwife's unique characteristics would be valued. This was, and remains, both a blessing and a curse. What MANA became is the sturdy basket woven together with an ethic large enough to hold all types of midwives—lay midwives, Grand Midwives, direct-entry midwives, nurse-midwives, traditional midwives, foreign-trained midwives, Christian midwives, radical midwives, lesbian midwives, midwives from Canada, Mexico, the United States, Latin America and the Caribbean—you name it. It is the only organization of its kind in North America. This all-inclusive paradigm promotes unity but subsequently has its limitations in terms of focus. It's a big-thinking, big-vision organization.

I was elected to the MANA board, first, as the Midwest Regional Representative, then as the Second Vice President, and finally in 2007 as the President. It has been an honor to work with such creative and brilliant women. I have never worked with people who are more fiercely passionate, generous and dedicated to their life's work. Being in MANA has satisfied the political animal in me. There is advocacy work to last a lifetime in making the midwifery model of maternity care accessible to all women in all communities.

The hardest part about being a midwife was being on call. I was always at the mercy of the moon phases and dramatic seasonal changes and thus the magic and mystery of women's gestating, laboring, birthing and lactating bodies. I have been interrupted while engaged in every mundane, special or intimate activity that I can think of to go to a birth—laundry, birthday parties, love-making, shopping, classes, sleeping (of course!), exercising, fighting, playing, traveling, cooking, and so on. But eventually I began to live in what author Mary Sojourner calls "animal time." I became keenly aware of the environment, I always knew what phase the moon was in, and I knew that the full and new moons drew babies out of the womb. I learned that May and June in the Midwest are busy months for births, and I knew that a drop in the barometric pressure was a signal to get my birth bags packed. Becoming attuned to the ebb and flow of nature in this way was one of the supreme gifts I gained. It is a way of walking through the world that has kept me connected to the natural cycles of the earth, the moon, the seas, and the heavens. I began to see why the ancients honored women's bodies as microcosms of Mother Earth.

The other gift is what happened to me after years of sitting with women in labor, observing and waiting. It is hard to explain to someone who has not done this time and time again, having the privilege of sitting with women during natural childbirth. It involves living in another dimension. It is a slowed down and exquisitely heightened sensory experience. Time takes on a different tenor. And it is in this elegantly altered place that one learns to listen very carefully to one's inner voices and at the same time respond to the instinctual behavior of women. I learned to sense when things were going well, when things were simply deviating from the norm, and when things were sliding into a dangerous zone. Of course, a midwife also utilizes her customary training, clinical expertise and professional skills. But I am talking about a different set of feminine skills of which midwives are master practitioners. These skills are part of the art of midwifery.

Early in my career I met an obstetrician (OB) who was doing some research on birth outcomes by local providers. He had a hard time believing that my statistics were as good as they were—like my c-section rate of only 3-5%. He was amazed that we had successful breech and twin births at home. He was intrigued by our maneuvers for managing shoulder dystocia when a baby's shoulder is stuck behind the mother's pubic bone in its descent outward. So we met for lunch to discuss and review my stats. He was rather stunned with my documents—I had a data form for every client kept in a three-ring binder—and he could see that they were solid. Afterwards he offered to provide me with a few consulting services. This doctor was not pro-home birth, pro-midwife; he was simply open-minded. He wanted his research to reflect the facts. He wanted women to have the best possible care. As an obstetrician, Michael Collins was a rarity. Most of the other OBs were covertly or openly hostile to us. Over the years I would call him when I had a client

I wanted him to see. I always told him exactly what the situation was: "She's thirty-four weeks pregnant, the baby is in a frank breech position with its back on the left and is about five and a half pounds." Without ultrasound at my disposal, he always wondered how I got everything right. But he was especially impressed one time when I transferred care of a woman to him at the end of pregnancy because I told him, "something did not feel right." In a recent exam neither he nor his ultrasound technology had detected any problems, and he had supported the woman's decision to birth at home. Two weeks later, when she did birth in the hospital the mother had placental problems and a severe hemorrhage, and they nearly lost both the mom and the baby. The baby was airlifted out because of birth defects that required immediate surgery. After the birth, Dr. Collins called me to ask, "How did you know?" I simply responded, "I just knew." Critics of midwifery might ask what would have happened if that birth had occurred at home. But the fact is that the birth did *not* occur at home. As a midwife I assessed the risk, transferred the client out of my care, and referred her into the care of a physician. And that's the point about intuition being a reliable skill. In scientific literature, medical anthropologists and sociologists describe intuition as "authoritative knowledge." This is the deep wisdom that midwives tap into regularly and use as guidance over and over again. Midwives who practice in out-of-hospital venues use appropriate basic technology—not ultra-sophisticated biotech equipment—and we depend on skills and knowledge that have been proven to be reliable and effective.

Being a midwife and witnessing the miracles of the childbearing year time and time again became a kind of spiritual practice for me. It satisfied several of the typical things we consider to be in the religious or spiritual realms—recognizing a purpose for our lives, giving service to humanity, honoring and cooperating with the Divine Plan within the Great Unknown, cultivating respectful and loving relationships with fellow Earthlings, transcending ego attachments, reconciling life and death issues, and bowing to the Great Mystery of creation. More than in any church, when I sit at the altar of birth, God walks in.

When people ask me about being a midwife, they always want to talk about that exquisite and transcendent moment of birth. But in actuality—as glorious as it is—that is only a minute in the childbearing year that we spend with a woman and her family. Pregnancy, postpartum and the interconceptional period is where we do two of the things midwives do best: we teach women about being healthy and strong, and we listen to their stories. We spend so much time with women at prenatal and postpartum visits that the relationships we develop are often like friends or even sisters. They may not remember exactly what we taught them, but they always remember how we made them feel. In a country where the medical system is often so unsatisfactory, there is no price tag that you can put on this one-on-one personalized care. Frankly, it is priceless and one reason why our clients are so loyal to us. And in many cases, their children grow up knowing us as part of the family.

The other thing that consumed much of my energy during my midwifery career was defending my profession. Plain and simple, midwifery is a threat to modern obstetrics. It is a clash in paradigms. And midwifery is also a threat to the modern, corporate, medical delivery business, especially out-of-hospital birth that allows women and revenue to escape the system. Maternity care is a multi-million-dollar operation for any hospital system, every year. When I remember my career I cannot forget how much we fought "the system" and how the system even hunted many of us down as criminals for practicing our art.

Although there were some ruggedly hard challenges, the first fifteen years of my journey as a community midwife were very satisfying. I loved the work, and the women and families of the communities that I served loved me. In 1990 I went through a sad and messy divorce. My children were four, nine and twelve-years old. And while it closed the door on many of my hopes, it opened a window on a new life for me. For one thing, I realized that it would be very hard for me to raise my three children alone on my income. The incomes of my former husband and I combined— we were both self-employed—were barely enough to meet our needs. In retrospect, it was a synchronistic moment when I walked down my long driveway to my mailbox and handed the postman my application to college on the same morning that he handed me a certified letter—the divorce papers from my husband. I was not sure at that time what academic degree I wanted to pursue, but I knew that direct-entry midwifery as it was practiced by many of us was not a sustainable career for me as a single woman, and that I needed more employment choices in order to support my children and myself. In addition, the physicians who were bugging me said, "Why don't you go get educated? Then maybe we can talk."

As it turns out, I pursued and received four degrees in eight years—registered nurse, bachelor's degree, certified nurse-midwife, and master's degree. It was a feat that even today I wonder how I accomplished, especially since I had to go to different schools in different towns and states for each degree. But I did it. And I also maintained my midwifery practice while struggling with single parenting. I was talking to my son Sean last night. He asked, "Mom, remember when you were working on one of your degrees and you took me to statistics class? Or when you would take us to the beach to study, and you and Marci and Kim had your anatomy and physiology books and quizzed each other while all of us nine kids played on the beach?" We laugh about it now, but at that time, much of it was utterly diffi-cult—for my kids and me. Thankfully, that was more than ten years ago.

When I finally did "get educated," I tried to get a job as a nurse-midwife at the hospital to supplement my home birth practice. I was even willing to try it full-time. By that time I was highly qualified—a nurse-midwife with a master's degree, with twenty years of experience, and a loyal following of clients. I approached every single obstetrician in town, but not one of them would sponsor me to get hospi-tal privileges. By that time in the mid-1990s, I had more experience in the field and was older than the majority of the doctors in town. One of them was even honest enough to say, "There's nothing more disconcerting to a physician than an educated midwife with ideas like yours." I had one more chance. A family practice doctor who was a friend said, "If you can't get any of those guys to back you, let me know and I'll help." I went to him as my last hope. As I stood before him he said, "I can't help you. The obstetricians are really fighting to take away delivery privileges of the family practice docs. I have my own battle to fight." My heart sank, my head dropped to my chest, and my tears began to fall onto his shiny shoes. But I didn't blame him. They locked me out of every opportunity to work as a midwife within the maternity care system. It was clearly restraint of trade, but by that time I was too worn down to challenge it. The obstetricians were fighting to take full control of maternity care. By then I knew for sure I did not want to work in that system. It was then that I discovered public health midwifery.

While home birth served one woman, one baby, one family at a time and caused a steady revolution, I began swimming in a bigger pond of maternal and child health care for underserved people. I began to work for a migrant farmworker clinic. The migratory lifestyle, language barriers, poor living conditions, and lack of sufficient financial resources make access to health care and continuity of care incredibly difficult for this population. For seven years I provided primary care in a bilingual, culturally congruent setting, focusing on women's health services. At the same time I continued my home birth practice, taking fewer clients while the migrant clinic season was in full swing. Working at the clinic was an exponential growth experience for me. It was a fast-track classroom. Not only did the scope of my midwifery skills expand because my clients had more chronic and acute illnesses and social stresses than my home birth clients, but I also learned about another culture, language and cosmovision. For once I was in the minority, one of only a few White people, and my native language was English amid a clinical staff and clientele who were Latinos speaking Spanish. I was thrust in the middle of a whole repertory of knowledge, customs and beliefs that were different from my own.

I found that I loved working with the migrant women and that I naturally gravitated towards working with underserved people in general. I had also begun working with American Indian tribes helping to design and implement maternal and child health care programs that were accessible, serviceable and culturally congruent. Once again I found myself to be a minority amid the diversity of tribal customs, languages and beliefs of the indigenous people. I have been working with Native American tribes for over ten years across several states in the Upper Midwest. For the Native American women with whom I work, theirs is a complex and multi-layered story. The women—primarily from the Odawa, Ojibwa, and Potawatomi tribes—have suffered the onslaughts of colonization and forced acculturation and yet they have survived. They have suffered poverty, loss of their lands, languages and lifestyles, including loss of their traditional diets and the daily activities that have kept the tribes healthy for untold generations. Yet throughout these changes in lifestyle, habitat and status, Native American women have endured. I was once giving a weeklong training for a group of maternal and child health care workers in the Northern Plains, mostly Native American. I was talking about the importance of good prenatal nutrition to keep a woman healthy and grow a healthy baby. I provided them with lots of handouts and strategies. When I finished one woman said, "That's all well and good, but where I live the only food within walking distance is at the gas station. And the only store within driving distance rarely has fresh fruits and vegetables. And, of course, the commodity food we get is all carbohydrates. What do you suggest we do?" Many of the women were also living in communities where crystal meth—the new poor people's drug—was prevalent, rates of tobacco smoking were very high, domestic violence was prominent, poverty was ubiquitous, and depression and mental illness were common. Fresh fruits and vegetables were not first on their "to do" list. Neither was "making a good birth plan." Survival was on top of the list.

Public health midwifery became a passion for me, just as home birth midwifery had been. Addressing disparities in maternal and child health was another social justice issue on the continuum. I began to devote my energies to helping make a difference in whole communities, in whole populations of people. I joined forces with folks who were working to improve the health status of all mothers and babies, in all communities, all races. I am always applying the midwifery model of care to everything I am doing. I am always trying to find ways to bring midwives back into Native communities. Native women have taught me a spectrum of lessons, from the ravages of intergenerational grief to the beauty of traditional pregnancy, birth and postpartum ceremonies, songs and stories. Their strength and resiliency humble me.

At the same time that I was working for the migrant farmworkers and indigenous communities in the United States, I was also traveling to many countries and learning about other indigenous people and cultures and what public health looks like worldwide. I first went to Guatemala to study Spanish so that I could better communicate with my farmworker clients and colleagues. Once there, I visited some Mayan midwives whom I had met stateside. I brought them some midwifery supplies, and in turn, I was invited to stay in their homes, cook and eat with their families and participate in community events. I have traveled to Mexico and several other Latin American countries, including Honduras, Colombia, Ecuador, Nicaragua, Costa Rica, as well as India, Nepal, Guinea West Africa, the Dominican Republic, Ireland, Scotland and the Caribbean. Having been a political activist since I was a young teen, I thought I was well informed about many of the civil wars and indigenous struggles of Latin America. But I wasn't. It was much worse than I had imagined and it was far worse for women. Everywhere, I observed women and how they lived. In the Himalayan Mountains in Nepal and India, I saw woman after woman making gravel out of huge boulders by striking them with a hammer. This was their work, their contribution to making roadways. In Nicaragua, I visited a school where several skinny kids, between eight- and twelve-years old, carried their even skinnier two-year-old siblings several miles to school to care for them while their mothers worked. Often, the fathers were gone. In Guatemala I heard stories of women losing their babies in childbirth and husbands kissing the hands of the midwives in gratitude because their wives did not die, too. Maternal mortality is very common. It is one thing to lose a baby—people expect that might happen—but it is devastating to lose the mother, and that too happens often enough. From my experiences here and abroad, I have learned that reproductive health exists within the context of a woman's overall health status and environment. As social scientists and epidemiologists alike are learning, the health and well-being of the family depends on the health and well-being of the mother. Midwives are, and have always been, women's health practitioners with a family-centered and community-based public health agenda. In all of the situations I observed, it was clear to me that women are the planets around which the constellation of their families circle. If their gravitational energy declines (health of body, mind and spirit), the others are in danger of being lost in space.

All of these vital experiences—working with the home birth moms, farmworkers, tribal cultures and other indigenous people—led me to an even deeper commitment to improving women's health care, preserving midwifery and focusing on maternal and child health. For me midwifery is not just a calling but also a call to action; not just catching babies, but transforming systems.

My story would not be complete without honoring the magnificent women with whom I have worked as midwife partners. In the beginning I had five partners. After two years and the need to get their first babies born were satisfied, four retired. Brenda and I worked together for many years, and she was a wonderfully patient, kind and smart midwife with whom I loved working. We trained several apprentices, all of whom had been our clients. Wendy became my partner when Brenda retired. She was a dedicated, good midwife with whom I shared some amazing experiences. I saved her life during a massive postpartum hemorrhage, and she helped my son breathe when he was born limp and blue with a cord wrapped three times around his neck. Wendy and I trained two more apprentices—Kim and Nancy—who not only became my partners but my soul sisters. I loved working with them more than I can express because we were not only dedicated to our clients but to each other, through good times and bad times. When I got divorced, Kim moved my three kids and me into her home until we could get reorganized. There were six kids altogether, and two midwife-moms on-call who also were in nursing school full-time. When I went to nurse-midwifery school, Nancy cared for my teenage daughter for five months while I was in another state doing my midwifery clinical integration. Without her generous assistance I could not have completed midwifery school. These women became the sisters I never had. Nancy Curley is the midwife with whom I worked the longest—about twenty-five years—and our friendship sustains me daily. When you spend as much time with each other as midwives do in an intense, demanding, and highly focused job, day after day, year after year, you develop a relationship that is not unlike a marriage. At births, Nancy and I moved together silently, impeccably and gracefully. We learned to play "good cop, bad cop" with clients when it was necessary. When we went to births, we always said a prayer together. We sat in the car, or stood outside under the stars and prayed that the mother would be strong, the baby would have a safe passage, the family would be supportive, and the midwives would be guided. Sometimes we sang our prayers. And after each birth we said prayers of gratitude together. If the birth was particularly challenging and we were very exhausted, the prayer would be simply, "Mother lived, baby lived, and midwives did not go to jail. We are grateful." If it was the right time of year we would drive directly to the Big Mother—Lake Michigan—our beloved inland sea, and pray on her shores. Often, we would peel off our clothes and jump straight in to be bathed in the cleansing sweet water, washing away any tension, soothing our weary bones. In 2003, I worked with Kip Kozlowski, Clarice Winkler, and Nancy to open a freestanding birth center that was wickedly hard to do but fabulous to operate. I have always said: hospitals are the domain of doctors;

homes are the domain of moms; and births centers are the domain of midwives. The Greenhouse Birth Center was an uptown gig for us though not without its challenges, and it was a joy to work with seasoned well-honed midwives.

Sometimes I wonder why I became a midwife and how being a midwife changed the course of my life. First, I was a midwife for *practical* reasons. My friends and I were in our childbearing years, and what was available in the contemporary health care system was unacceptable. I walked into midwifery out of practicality; I needed my babies to be born naturally and gently.

Second, I was a midwife because of *socio-political* reasons. Midwifery exposed a human rights issue to me. Modern obstetrics colluded with market forces to make maternity care big business, creating a lucrative market for the overuse of pharmacological, technological and surgical interventions. They did this by encouraging women to fear birth and mistrust their bodies, making birth an emergency rather than an emergence, and profiting by exploiting fears. Midwifery was the resistance movement that pushed back against the dominant medical paradigm.

Third, I was a midwife for *spiritual* reasons. Pregnancy and birth became the most sacred rites of passage that I had ever witnessed. Women needed to be given a safe haven as they walked through the sacrament of birth. Babies needed to be properly welcomed as they began their Earth Walk. And the ancestors needed to be honored by having their descendants sheltered at the vulnerable yet potent time when new members of the family lineage emerge from Spirit into flesh.

Fourth, I was a midwife for *psychological* reasons. Birth, more than anything I know, has the most amazing potential to instill a sense of power in a woman. I came to realize that if women could harness the internal resources to face the pain and stresses of labor and birth, they could do anything. It was a joy to be part of building that confidence in each woman, and seeing it provide a solid base for self-reliant parenting.

But ultimately, I was a midwife for *personal* reasons. The impetus to do this work was, and remains, the most potent and definitive call to service that I have ever felt. I was born to be a midwife. I was born to serve mothers, infants and families and help bring about a transformation in the maternity care system, and to remedy social injustices. In the process I learned undeniably that we humans are hard-wired to care.

Midwifery is like the deep-sea dive I learned to love as a teen. It has taken me to the subterranean realm of women's deepest emotions, secrets and longings, including my own. It has allowed me to get to know the strange and precious sea creatures that float in women's wombs before they become two-leggeds and walk on the Earth. It brought me in touch with the cycles of the moon and its effect on the earthly tides and womanly tides. It satisfied my longing to be immersed in life's great mysteries, even if there were moments when I felt like I was drowning.

I am heartened when I see what the young women and men of today are accomplishing, and yet we have so far to go. What I wish for each of my children—Maya, Leah and Sean—and their peers is that they know the magnificence of their bodies and be able to trust that they were created perfectly. I want my children to know this perfection not only in terms of pregnancy and childbirth—for they may choose not to have children—but in every way. I want them to become very familiar with the rhythms to which their bodies dance in response to the moon, like the ebb and flow of the tides, the surge and swell of their menses, the waxing and waning of their sexuality, and the changing seasons of their fluid emotions. I wish for them to be able to resist the marketing messages of modern media that tell them that their bodies are the wrong size, that they are not strong enough to withstand the rigors of childbirth, that they need drugs to cope with pain, that they need rescuing by medical interventions. These messages ultimately instill in them a profound fear of life itself. I wish for them to be able to distinguish between good pain and bad pain, between pain with a purpose and pain that causes harm. I want them to be able to experience the exhilaration that happens when they do something really hard, extraordinary and of their own volition—like climbing a mountain, running a marathon, or giving birth. Because in those moments they will come to know their unanticipated strength and innate power-fulness, and no one can take that ecstasy away. That knowledge lives deep in the bones like an embedded intercellular matrix. Those experiences form a solid foundation on which to stand. Those moments weave potent strands of resiliency and endurance, like silk, into the fabric of our lives.

A fundamental rite of passage

SARASWATHI VEDAM

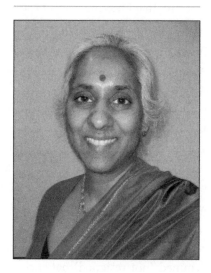

I am an Indian woman who grew up between India and the United States. I grew up in the United States at a time when there were very few Indian immigrants, but my mother kept a very Indian home and was strong in her message that it was fine for me to be "different." I dress like an Indian woman, I wear a *kumkum*, and I am a Hindu. Part of choosing an unconventional appearance, or unconventional profession like midwifery, is accepting the responsibility of answering questions and engaging people on a personal level, and dispelling stereotypes.

As a first generation child of an immigrant family, my life has been a series of encounters that challenge preconceived expectations of who I am, both within the Indian community and among members of the dominant culture. For the most part this has been an asset, not a hindrance. As a midwife in North America you have to explain yourself constantly, regardless of your education, licensure, or credentials. As a nurse-midwife who attends home births, I have had to defend and explain my practice choices to my nurse-midwife colleagues, and physicians. Curiously, I have simultaneously been held suspect by my direct-entry home birth midwife sisters, solely because of my nurse-midwifery credential. In Canada, as a U.S.-trained, academic nurse-midwife educator, I have had to defend my credibility as a clinician to practicing community midwives. I believe that a core comfort with a non-mainstream persona has sustained me through much of my personal and professional life.

The bi-cultural perspective that I was inevitably exposed to has also served me in countless ways in my service to the Diasporas of families. My mother, Nalini Vedam, mothered a growing Indian community at Penn State University that didn't have access to culturally appropriate postpartum support and prenatal education through family, because their families were halfway around the world. They would spend a lot of time in our home when they were pregnant. My mother would make special foods for them. When they delivered, often they would stay with us. My mother gave countless babies their first baths, helped countless women with breast-feeding, and gave me the attitude that birth and pregnancy and family-making was an exciting, positive, normal and important step in a woman's life. My mother began this caretaking work in 1956 and still does it in 2009 at age seventy-eight.

My commitments, like deferring judgment on others' personal choices and actions, promoting peaceful human interaction, accepting the gray and uncertainty in life, and determined (not resigned) patience, are fundamental values springing from my Hindu and Indian upbringing. My father, Dr. K. Vedam, taught me about peace, unconditional support and gentleness in all human contact. He was a student activist during Gandhi's non-violent resistance movement and has always modeled the spirit of that time. My brother, Subramanyam Vedam, has faced incredible injustice and isolation in his life. Despite this, he has maintained his calm, determined manner and has never wavered from his pursuit of knowledge and thoughtful attention to family and community. I credit my parents and my brother for my attitudes in my midwifery and family roles, for strength in the face of adversity, and for my ability to live with cultural congruency.

I have been observing and caring for women during and after pregnancy for over thirty-five years. As a child, during the summer holidays, I made rounds with my aunts and cousins—five obstetric providers in India. By the time I was a teenager, I was actually going "on district" with them, visiting women, sometimes in the Bombay slums, in rural villages, in tertiary care hospitals, emergency wards, and free-standing maternity centers. I was immersed in pregnancy as normalcy and exposed to women working with women. At the time it was not common in India to go to a man for obstetrical and gynecological (OB/GYN) care, so most of the providers were women. My aunt, Lieutenant Colonel Anasuya Subramaniam, was a teaching nurse-midwife for over thirty years. She epitomized unabashed, outspoken strength, and independent thought and absolute advocacy for women at a time in India when none of those things were fashionable. She served many thousands of families in the most adverse conditions, and believed completely in the wisdom of midwives as autonomous, full-scope providers at the core of all maternity care. Because the access to technology was varied and expensive, many of the births occurred without the benefits or risks of technology. Some of the cases had conditions that are more advanced than we would handle here without technology, but there was not always a choice. I was made aware early on that there are a variety of ways to handle complex perinatal events.

In 1975, I was one of the first women admitted to Amherst College. For the next three years I was the only student of Indian descent and one of two women of color on campus. Amherst had decided to phase in coeducation with transfer students, in hopes of providing wise and strong mentors in the upper classes when freshwomen were admitted in 1976. Indeed, many of the seventy-three women came from remarkable backgrounds of leadership, feminist work, and pioneering roles in the working world. Several were older than the typical college girl. I was an exception. For my freshman year at Penn State, I had lived at home. Moving to Amherst was my first experience away from the enclave of home. I had been raised to believe in dedication to studies, but also to see motherhood as a fundamental rite of passage. At the height of the feminist movement, those values were unpopular. The other women spoke of autonomy, equality and rights as being synonymous with independent career aspirations. I absorbed much of the dialogue with great interest, but learned to trust my own desires. Curiously, within my family and cultural context, the desire for motherhood was not in conflict with the concept of a strong independent female spirit. All of my nine aunts were formidable in intellect, manner, and achievement, and held pivotal roles within the family whether or not they had professions.

Aside from admitting us, Amherst had not anticipated the challenges and unique services that the transition would demand. We had no Women's Dean, no athletic facilities, limited washrooms, and no experienced gynecological or contraceptive medical providers. The faculty was 90% male, and not all were supportive of the change; but the recourse for sexist classroom dynamics was non-existent. The women students began to organize. I was introduced to women's health care advocacy when I helped to initiate a peer contraceptive and gynecological counseling service, and lobbied for a nurse-practitioner for the infirmary. It was a hot era for women's issues in health care and abortion rights. Scandals, such as with DES, the synthetic form of estrogen given to women and linked to cervical and vaginal cancer, and the recall of the intrauterine device, the Dalkon Shield, mushroomed in quick succession.

Ten years later, in 1985, I received a master of science in nursing and nurse-midwifery from Yale University. When I was at Yale, the dean was Donna Diers, famous for her views on feminism in nursing and autonomous practice for nurse clinicians and nurse-midwives. She was also an early leader in the evidence-based practice movement. I was fortunate to enlist her as my thesis advisor. Helen Varney Burst was head of the midwifery department. Her deep and abiding commitment to excellence in clinical midwifery education has inspired and sustained my own path. Helen intervened when, to my dismay and confusion, I encountered extreme cultural prejudice from two of the faculty. Throughout my career Helen has stood by me through the most challenging and exhilarating times. She assumed an additional supervision burden so that I could pursue home birth placement while I was still a student at Yale. Of course, her acumen and finesse in the world of midwifery politics and leadership is a source of many pearls.

My introduction to continuous primary care for the childbearing cycle was in India. All maternity providers were expected to be accessible on-call twenty-four hours a day—a necessity in a country with such a high volume of women in need. The expectation of the population for natural childbirth and "women caring for women" also dictated a shared philosophy of care. Imagine my distress when, while in midwifery school at Yale University, I only rarely witnessed midwives who offered continuous call coverage and consistent philosophy of care. Access to professional midwifery care in out-of-hospital settings was barely mentioned much less modeled. Fortunately, I discovered the inspirational words of Ina May Gaskin and Suzanne Arms. Many years later, I had the good fortune to become Suzanne's neighbor and Ina May's friend. Ina May has been a constant source of wisdom and loving support especially at times when I felt marooned on a desert island.

My rescue came serendipitously in my final year. I was seeking an internship site somewhere near my husband's home in Syracuse, New York. Someone highly recommended Pat Deibel, CNM, a midwife in Rochester, New York. She had her own private midwifery practice that offered home and hospital births, one-hour prenatal visits, continuous labor support, and a lot of postpartum and newborn care. Her clients chose the birth site. Pat had been a cardiac and neonatal intensive-care nurse, had her midwifery education in England, and was very skilled. Although Pat had been in practice for about six years, her essential humility made her feel that she wasn't seasoned enough. I had to coax her into taking me as a student. I asked her to try me for a summer rotation. She agreed, and I spent the next summer following her everywhere—in the office, on prenatal and postpartum home visits, and to births.

That summer my whole perspective and world was opened up to the concept of service. I learned about the value of a strong client/midwife relationship, and the differences among birth settings. I realized that birth setting and the autonomy of the midwife were directly related to the preservation of woman-centered, evidence-based care protocols. Pat is largely responsible for who I am today. Though I am years her junior, she has always treated me with deep respect and built my confidence through simply trusting me. She taught me how to listen, and how to teach, and she renewed my faith in normalcy. She was the first to introduce me to independent midwifery home birth practice and the truth and rewards that accompany unconditional love and service.

After leaving Yale, I sought a midwifery position in a city where there were only two midwives, one who delivered only in the hospital and one who delivered only in the home. There were two nurse-midwife positions available, one in a physician practice and one in a large Health Maintenance Organization (HMO) that wanted to start a midwifery program. I joined the HMO and worked on creating a midwifery practice that reflected Pat Deibel's practice as much as possible. As I was the only midwife on staff, in order to ensure that my clients were guaranteed continuity and midwifery philosophy of care, I was in clinic five days a week and on-call 24/7. Though the births were all in hospital, I offered both labor and postpartum support at home. It was a very busy practice. The first month I was there I attended eighteen births; but I was young and childless myself, my husband was immersed in medical school, and so I was able to devote myself to midwifery.

Many women I cared for at that HMO didn't know what a midwife was. They called me "Dr. Saras" and I kept correcting them. The physicians' productivity was measured on a standard of seven and a half minutes per prenatal visit. This assumed that a nurse had measured vital signs, the woman was undressed, and labs were completed when the doctor entered the exam room. I told the OB/GYN department head that if he wanted me to start a midwifery program,

I would have to be measured on a different level of productivity. I negotiated to get twenty-five minutes for a prenatal visit and forty minutes for an initial visit. The midwifery service grew rapidly because the women appreciated the continuity, their involvement in decision-making, and the preventative and supportive aspects of care. Still I believe that "time" was the single most important factor in the rapid growth of the midwifery service.

Despite, or perhaps as a result of, the huge success of the midwifery service, the road was not always smooth. Half of the physicians and most of the nurses had no idea what the philosophy and scope of midwifery practice was. One of the physicians in the group was apparently threatened by what I represented. He engaged in a subtle campaign of engendering doubt in the others. I was told I could no longer do home visits. I could not even offer postpartum breastfeeding assistance at home. I was young and idealistic, unrealistic and furious. Fortunately, the chief of service, a patient man who valued my service ethic, found he could not disagree with my interpretation of safe practice. He convinced me to stay and accept the limitations.

I had developed a warm relationship with the underground local home birth midwife, who was my age, very smart, and philosophically compatible. She occasionally invited me to accompany her to her own home births or visits, which fed my soul and reminded me of the gold standard of service to women. After a year in solo practice, I hired two additional midwives to cover the midwifery caseload, hoping they would share my philosophy and commitment to 24-hour coverage and service. I then took a one-year leave to have my own firstborn, Maya, and spent the following year attending a handful of home births and learning how to balance mothering with midwifery. In 1987, I joined my mentor Patricia Deibel, CNM, as a partner in her practice, Family Maternity Service, in Rochester, New York. Here we served families in homes and hospitals. We were assisted by the endorsement of a brilliant and kind physician, Bruce Iuppa, Chief of Obstetrics, at the community hospital. He himself had been mentored by his father who had practiced well into his eighties. Bruce passed on many of his hand skills and clinical pearls to us.

After four years and another child, Zoë, we moved to the San Francisco Bay area, where I thought the sensible thing for me to do was to get the kind of midwifery job that involved twelve hour shifts. I had two young children, my husband, Jeff, was a medical fellow, and mothering was my priority. However, when I interviewed at Kaiser Permanente, the midwife I interviewed with talked to me about the style of midwifery there. There was no continuity of care. The midwives were not involved in any prenatal or postpartum care. Moreover, the philosophy of care was one I could not share: One of the first interview questions was "How do you feel about intrauterine pressure catheters?" While I believe, as with all technologies, that there are appropriate indications and applications for IUPCs, I thought that the query indicated the culture of the practice, if not her own philosophy.

Meanwhile in California at the time, there were midwives who practiced in the hospital, and there were midwives who practiced in the home. There were no midwives who offered both as we had in Rochester. Underlying this split was a lack of access to hospital privileges and an absence of liability coverage for home birth providers. Two of the home birth nurse-midwives, Harriet Palmer and Yelena Kolodji, convinced me to open my own home birth practice. They practiced in adjacent communities and had to travel to serve women in the Palo Alto area. I was hesitant because until then I had always worked in someone else's practice. Organizing care, practice management, and billing were all new to me. Harriet and Yelena provided me with all of the support I needed to make the leap. One of them came over and painted my little room that I had behind my garage and created a perfect office. Harriet gave me a beautiful antique wooden exam table (which I still use), and Yelena taught me about billing. They just started sending me patients. So, I then discovered that I could maintain my philosophical core and still balance my family's needs by being my own boss.

When I had my third child, Lakshmi, I could schedule people around nursing and napping. Clients appreciated both the continuity and slow-paced care, and the modeling of how to integrate work and family. I provided 24-hour on-call coverage for my clients and occasionally cross-covered with Harriet and Yelena when we had more than one woman in labor or needed sick time or vacation relief. We advertised as a group and called ourselves South Bay Midwives. Over the next four years, Harriet taught me how to exude calm and to believe that flexibility can live alongside adherence to guidelines for safety in practice. Yelena modeled that rare person who can balance a pragmatic, entrepreneurial spirit with a willingness to suspend self in favor of service and advocacy.

When we moved to Indiana in 1995, I was able once again to purchase liability coverage, which allowed me to offer primary midwifery care in all settings. I became the sole licensed midwife offering home birth in the state. The other home birth midwives were Certified Professional Midwives (CPMs) who served women under the threat of a felony charge; yet they graciously invited me into their circle of support. By contrast, the nurse-midwives in the community maintained their distance and sometimes were openly competitive. Though most of these CNMs were less experienced, and all of them had less autonomy in their professional roles, several were suspicious and critical of my collaborative relationship with consultants. They viewed my co-management of complex cases as aberrant instead of a model of inter-professional care worth replicating. Others in the medical community assumed my model and philosophy of practice was rooted in "the old country." Once, when I raised a World Health Organization (WHO) standard in an effort to advocate for my client, a neonatologist told me that the WHO was for "where you came from, not for modern America." Fortunately, I found another soul-mate in Indiana. Sandy Countryman, my practice partner, was more loyal than a sister. She and I developed the ability to communicate without words and balance each other in a way that only longtime couples have perfected.

Along the way, I have been fortunate to work with some excellent physician consultants. One of them was John David Hoff, MD, PhD, and Chief of OB at one of the hospitals in Redwood City, California. He is a brilliant man and an eminently reasonable person. Even though I could not get privileges or liability coverage because I was attending home births, he understood the issues of access to care, and we developed a great collaborative relationship. My patients would meet him once during their pregnancy, and he was available to us as needed throughout the perinatal course. If I consulted with him prenatally or transferred someone to the hospital in labor, he fully acknowledged my role as primary provider and encouraged me to remain involved and present in both supportive and care roles. Later, in Indianapolis, I learned how to be steely underneath a charming smile from Patsy Webberhunt, MD. My most steady and influential consultant, though, was Dr. Mary Beth Soper. She is a no-nonsense woman with incredible integrity. She epitomizes living according to truth, respect for self-determination and common sense. These physicians respected the wisdom of equity and mutual respect in inter-professional relationships. They gave me the confidence to stick with my convictions and knowledge of effective care in the face of community standards that were neither evidence-based nor woman-centered.

All of these qualities—compassion, commitment to family-centered care, being able to listen to what women's agendas and priorities are, vigilance, and attention to details—are common grounds for us as midwives, whether we are women of color or not, home birth or hospital birth midwives, or nurse-midwives or direct-entry midwives. Over the years in several states, my practice was chosen as the preferred maternity provider for families from the observant Jewish community, the orthodox Black Muslim community, the Hmong community, the Amish community, the Central American Latino community, and the fundamental Christian community.

At our first meeting these women often doubted my ability, as a Hindu Indo American, to understand and respect their world at the most precious of moments. The beauty was that as we got to know each other we both discovered more and more our commonalities rather than differences. I was welcomed into homes in stratas of life and economics and cultures that, in another profession, I would never have had the privilege to understand on a personal level. These experiences helped me to appreciate the wholeness of the human fabric. You cannot discount people for the values they profess when they are at their most human—in their own homes. So it has been very much a growth opportunity for me, and these families have been my most important mentors.

There is a lot of overlap between cultural congruity and what we do as midwives. Midwifery advocacy for me means supporting clients who make choices about birth and parenting that are not common practice. But for me, advocacy in those cases must be placed in a historical and cultural context. In Indiana I worked a lot with young African American women, a population where few breastfed. Yet, my clients were almost universally successful and, as a result, reclaimed breastfeeding as normalcy across their community. Perhaps it was just appropriate prenatal education and postpartum care, but I believe that success also stemmed from being with them and trying to tap into their environmental resources. Maybe they didn't know the history of African American women sustaining the growth of an entire population through the tradition of wet nurses, and the power they gave and got from their own milk. Or perhaps, creating a sister-to-sister postpartum helpline and care network (as Black women have always enlisted the sisterhood) helped them sustain success.

In 2002, after nearly seven years of practice in Indiana, I was offered a midwifery faculty position at Yale. As a home birth midwife, I have had the privilege of having midwifery, medical, and nursing students seek me as preceptor in all of my practice settings over twenty-five years. Catherine Gilliss, Dean of Nursing at Yale University, invited me to model private practice midwifery and out-of-hospital midwifery by integrating theory and practice education into the core curriculum. It seemed like a unique opportunity to elevate the profile of home birth midwifery practice. In Connecticut, on top of being full faculty, starting a new practice again, building the practice, training the staff, hiring people, and seeing the patients themselves, my practice became an annual clinical site for all of the twenty students. Once again I survived because of a sister midwife. Vicki Nolan Marnin brought her superb organizational skills and incredible stamina to our practice, and our clients and students had the benefit of all worlds.

The concept of "service" has become synonymous with volunteer and faith-based community organizations, but historically service was integral to health care and professions of succor. Our students want to "serve women" but must witness that service to women can simply mean quietly standing by, in an active listening role, with the woman setting the agenda. Many clinical settings have become so busy that the pace of visits impedes both relationship-building and confidence-sharing. This has impact on both woman and provider.

I remember being with a client who had had two home births with my practice. I saw her in between births and knew her family well. Her husband became our favorite handyman. She was a wonderful gardener and potter and would bring us gifts of natural wonder. She was several months into her third pregnancy when I saw her for a regular appointment. We were forty-five minutes into her prenatal visit before she shared that they were having serious marital problems. Our mutual regard and trust still needed that prolonged engagement to inspire confidence. This situation had an impact on prevention, what kind of antenatal intervention was possible, what type of postpartum support she could expect, her risk for depression, and financial stress. This connection becomes even more critical for women who are exposed to social risks, such as physical or substance abuse and unsafe living conditions. Those are very value-laden subjects that people won't necessarily talk about. I had another client who outwardly appeared to be in the ideal situation. She and her partner were both yoga teachers, ate organic foods, and were highly educated, young and positive about the pregnancy. Unfortunately her husband was an alcoholic and very troubled by drug dependency. Both of them dealt with huge layers of shame and embarrassment, which prevented them from sharing their struggle and fears about their ability to maintain a family together. Close to delivery, they were able to believe that they would encounter a patient and non-judgmental ear in my office, and we began to unravel together the tangled web they had woven.

We live in an era when there is as much emphasis placed on personal gratification and growth of the individual as responsibility to the community and others. There is much talk of midwifery "burnout." We have the option as midwives now to share call with other people, to be in a larger practice where the demands on our time are not as great and the prevailing obstetric culture encourages diversification of care and active management. Some believe that this is the solution to avoiding provider exhaustion. I wonder, though, if more midwives are being burned out in settings where they must accommodate to a very fast pace. Midwives who work at a pace that does not encourage their personal investment may begin to resent another case, another problem, another demand. Our students place a lot of significance on the moment of birth and our role during labor and birth, but my message to them is consistent, "Catching the baby is only a tiny part of what we do as midwives. All of the anticipatory guidance, vigilance, and confidence-building that we provide in the antepartum and postpartum periods are the key to exemplary midwifery."

As home birth midwives, our commitment to our clients is to stay with them throughout labor, to stay with them in their homes after they deliver until they are stable, and to visit them daily and weekly postpartum. It is not just about clocking in, clocking out—it is not just about walking in to catch a baby. It is a significant time commitment for every client. My mentors were people who believed that service was about taking the "self" out even as we talk about listening to women and being with women and the art of doing nothing. If you take that one step further, it's about taking away your own agenda even if that means the balance between family time and work commitment. Even now, after over twenty-five years, my husband, who has always willingly expanded his parenting role at the beck and call of my practice, and supports, in principle, my perspective, still does not understand why I have to talk to a woman on the phone at dinnertime for an hour about a nursing problem. He says they would never expect to do so with a physician. Yet, I know that if I don't answer the question or support her through this moment of crisis, then not only am I de-elevating her, but also I could miss that window and she could give up. It can be a fragile thing. If you really believe that it's better for mother and baby, then you have to go that extra mile.

Research and informed practice is a two-way street in my practice. As emerging research presents itself in my academic role, I feel obligated to inform both students and clients as we strive for pregnancy and birth planning based on the best available data. As clients and students ask questions, raise issues, and discover alternative therapies, I am inspired to investigate and apply these ideas to my research theory development and data collection.

My interests in patient-centered, evidence-based care have naturally led me to study, speak and publish about home birth practice and aspects of care that are uniquely maintained by midwives. Donna Diers, Holly Powell Kennedy, and my scientist-husband, Jeff Miller, taught me about rigor and honesty in data analysis, but more importantly, gave me the blueprint of how to honor midwifery philosophy and wisdom through research. When autonomous midwives practice in homes or freestanding birth centers, they have unique opportunities to evaluate and apply the best available evidence towards the promotion of normal labor and birth.

My experiences in anticipating and managing antepartum, intrapartum and postpartum complications and variations from normal, like any experienced midwife, have included incidences of preterm labor and delivery, postpartum hemorrhage, prolonged labor, malpresentation, neonatal resuscitation, miscarriage, second and third trimester loss, abnormal bleeding, evidence of fetal distress, multiple births, breech delivery, pregnancy induced hypertension, shoulder dystocia, and caring for survivors of sexual abuse. Over the course of more than twenty-five years of practice in out-of-hospital settings, I have also had opportunities to examine, assess and manage the care and referral of newborns with a variety of variations from normal, including fetal anomalies, genetic conditions, failure to thrive, and many other conditions. I have responded to all of these situations in homes and in hospitals. Because of my in-depth and continuous involvement with these clients, each experience has been an opportunity to explore the research literature, engage in wide ranging clinical discussions and learn from the clients' sense and experience. Every time I think I want to return to the simplicity, flexibility, and familiarity of clinical practice, I am lured back to the shimmer and elusive promise of academic sirens. Fortunately, I have had like-minded partners on this path as well. Years ago Peggy Garland and I worked together with others to establish the North American home birth literature. Much later, and to my eternal gratitude, she invited me to join the new breed of professional midwives, research savvy and strong in their core values, as we elevated the profile and credibility of the evidence on birth site and midwifery magic.

Surprisingly, it is my research life that has brought me back to my other passion—the pursuit of peaceful human interaction. As we grow as midwives in this country we must find our collective power to speak and advocate on behalf of women and each other. Peace among midwives, among maternity providers across professions, and between providers and families is critical to our shared future. Diane Holzer and Kathy Camacho Carr came into my life at the same time and curiously renewed my faith in the collaborative spirit. As presidents of the Midwives Alliance of North America and the American College of Nurse Midwives, they worked to establish a harmonious relationship between MANA and ACNM.

I have four daughters. They are twenty-two, nineteen, sixteen, and fourteen years old. I have a husband, aging parents, students, and clients. I have a brother who has been wrongly incarcerated for twenty-seven years. His case requires my attention. I am a business owner. I have had my own practice for many years. In the last decade I have had faculty and university commitments, and national committee roles. I am not a newcomer to academic life because my father was a physics professor. I grew up with him going back to the lab in the evenings and watching him and my mother, who was an at-home mother, create balance.

Before coming back to Yale as a professor, I was balancing work and family mostly by being creative about the career path I chose. My being a home birth midwife lent itself to some flexibility; being my own boss also lent itself to some flexibility. My at-home offices have also allowed me to have some flexibility and integration of my various roles. I had various clients and friends through La Leche League and through my work, who helped to form a network of other adults who were available at the drop of a hat when I had to go to a birth, because my work life was not predictable and I couldn't have the kind of child care that most people can access.

When I returned to Yale, I was excited by the opportunity to speak and teach about the life that I live because I love my work. I love being a midwife. I love being a mother. I want my daughters to see that they can have those options for life. What I did not recognize when I came back was how much of an additional time commitment being full faculty meant, and how much more I would have to multi-task. I have taught midwifery for many, many years just by integrating students into my practice and doing occasional guest lectures. As full faculty, however, lecture preparation and clinical precepting, as well as course planning, updating, advising, grading, committee responsibilities, research, publishing and writing responsibilities are all dependent on being able to stay doing what I love.

In 2007, after five years at Yale, I was invited to be Director of the Division of Midwifery at the University of British Columbia. The model of midwifery in Canada truly is what it professes to be: autonomous midwives practice in small shared-care or solo practices offering both continuity for women and sanity for midwives. Midwives credential themselves at the hospital. All midwives are able to, and required to, practice in all settings, and all midwifery students are placed in home and hospital settings. Despite the scarcity of midwives, availability of medical consultation for midwives is provincially mandated, and collegiality and mutually respectful behavior is palpably growing across professions.

The challenges here in Canada are quite different. Many women in rural and remote areas of British Columbia cannot access any maternity provider within several hours of their homes. Most must leave their communities and families for weeks just to have an attended birth. The need to expand midwifery and access is obvious. Of course that means translating the benefits and cost effectiveness of the model to the Ministry of Health, the university and the public.

In May 2008, my favorite causes got a remarkable nod when I was awarded an Honorary Doctorate in Science from Amherst College. I was so honored to be in the company of such remarkable leaders as Mohammed El Baradei. When I first was notified, I thought that I must have been identified because of my alum status, or because I was one of the first woman grads, or diversity, but it turns out that the College and Trustees had done much research into our backgrounds and truly knew the tenor of my work. All of the kind words they said were about bringing science to the discussion around home birth, and putting mothers and babies at the center of the conversation instead of treating them like merely bystanders in a medical drama. I am stunned and thrilled that such a traditionally male institution has evolved enough to acknowledge a "woman's profession!" It gives me hope for my daughters.

When my youngest, Sophia, was eight, she said to me, "Amma, I've made my decision. I'm going to write to Yale University and tell them you don't need to work for them anymore." Even though I tried as much as possible to do the writing and the lecture preparation after she was in bed, she still sensed that when I read her a bedtime story, I felt rushed. Still my daughters seem to have accepted and integrated my midwifery presence into their own personal histories as evidenced by my eldest daughter's college essay which described her mother's kitchen table: conversations on feminism, birth rites, guests, including patients and colleagues, and a variety of cultures, economic backgrounds, and ages.

Indeed midwifery requires much giving, and in order to be able to give freely, you have to be filled up again. There is absolutely no question that my four daughters—Maya, Zoë, Lakshmi and Sophia—are the core of my life and the reason for continuing on this journey. The relationships I have been privileged to enjoy with my clients carry an abiding mutual regard and caring. The quality and depth of these friendships fill me up even when I am "on call" 24/7. My life partner, Jeff, and my midwife sisters and mentors walk the walk with me through dark days, and the students keep me honest and fresh and infuse me with purpose. Recently I named "Assertiveness with Grace" as a key aptitude we were seeking among our midwifery applicants. This quality is most striking when I work alongside midwifery leaders Geradine Simkins, Peggy Garland and midwifery researchers internationally. I have also learned of this remarkable quality from former students, Leslie Mosley, Tiffany Lundeen, Karen Mera, Amy Romano, Stacia Birdsall, and many, many others. These young women give me hope.

Along the path to my consciousness as a midwife, a home birth midwife, a midwife in autonomous private practice, a midwife educator and an academic midwife, the enduring threads have been service to women across birth settings and across cultures. My passions and convictions are met and nurtured, especially through planned home birth where I believe it is most possible to support empowerment for women and a peaceful transition for a growing family. Whether or not the birth is completed at home, or without intervention, exemplary midwifery prepares and supports the woman in preserving as much normalcy as is possible within her own cultural context and within the health care system.

Choice is a fashionable word and concept in both Canadian health care and women's health care advocacy in the United States today. However, my belief is that true choice can only be made in the context of informed decision-making. Advocacy on my part includes understanding and translating the best available evidence and current knowledge of perinatal physiology so that a woman can make informed choices about the details of her care. Ultimately, whether or not her choice is congruent with my philosophy, the medical evidence, the community standard, or her own cultural or religious beliefs, I can only provide loving and vigilant care to the degree that she is willing to accept my service. The quality of our mutual regard and confidence means everything when eliciting data, exploring options for care, reacting to unexpected events, or embracing the spirituality inherent in birth and in abiding friendships.

Afterword

As I finish crafting this anthology, I am filled with deep gratitude for the chance to offer you the life-stories of these amazing women. From my vantage point these memoirs have added tremendous richness, texture and dimension to the "herstory" of midwifery and women's health in contemporary America.

It is tricky to tease out the themes of the authors' stories without including themes about women in the childbearing years and beyond. The dynamically interdependent relationships that are shared between midwives and the women we serve are like a grapevine, a braiding of interlaced roots, branches and fruit that feed and support one another. So, it is probably fair to say that what matters to childbearing women matters to midwives. Some of the things that are fundamentally important to these authors are what you would expect from any health care provider; other things are specific characteristics that midwives bring to the table through the lens of the midwifery model. There are many themes that emerged in these memoirs, themes that cross lines of class, race, religion, age, geography, lifestyle, credentials and practice styles. Regardless of the differences, the thirteen themes that came to light over and over again are what matter to all of us.

Context Matters

Everything in life is experienced within a context. Therefore, context is not a neutral aspect of maternity care.[1-8] Everything imparts meaning—the physical locations involved in maternity care and birthing, the way that physical space is organized, the objects and people in that space, and who provides the care to mothers and babies. These all have a profound effect on everyone present. Context also determines who is in power, and it impacts a woman's sense of safety and trust. I once had a client who was deaf from infancy and who had been through years of medical and institutional health care that was not always satisfactory to her. When she walked into the birth center for the first time she went from room to room touching everything, opening cupboards, signing wildly to her mother, and finally just broke down crying and said, "I feel safe here." That feeling of safety within this context allowed her to give birth quickly and powerfully, and that empowerment built confidence in her ability to mother her child. The circumstances and people that surround a woman will significantly influence how she interprets her experiences and finds meaning in them.

Content Matters

The content of maternal and child health care—the substantive and fundamental features—is defined by the model of care. The midwifery model and the medical model each utilize different content—values, beliefs, perceptions, ethics, skills, tools, interventions, rules, rationalizations, practices, protocols, providers, relationships, politics, economics, and so on.[9-16] The enactment of childbirth has been remarkably stable and similar across time and cultures until the twentieth century. Over the past century in the United States, childbirth has been culturally transformed by the dominance of a model that emphasizes mechanization and separation (medical model) versus physicality and integration (midwifery model). The shift in our perceptions and our behaviors during pregnancy and childbirth has required women and infants to conform more to a series of mechanized routines in the birthplace than to the instinctual unfoldment of processes that involve body/mind/spirit. This transformation has resulted in a childbirth paradigm that focuses more on production than reproduction, more on emergency than emergence.

Holism Matters

In human history and across cultures, it has been unusual for birth to be defined and treated as if it were a mere physiological function.[17-18] Pregnancy and childbirth are complex and multi-layered experiences of tremendous importance to individuals and society. A holistic approach recognizes that what affects one part affects all parts because everything is intimately connected. Holistic health care is a model that incorporates working fully with the whole person, not just with single components of the physical body, or symptoms and syndromes. A holistic framework for maternity care integrates all aspects of care for a mother and her infant and addresses their needs within the context of family and culture. This includes not only her physical needs such as diet, exercise, lab work and "baby checks," but also social, emotional, intellectual and spiritual factors that affect her. It includes addressing her values, beliefs, environment, relationships, support systems, mental health, stress level, and safety. A holistic approach to maternity care—which can be utilized in any setting—promotes integration of a variety of complementary techniques, therapies and modalities. Holism encourages both client and provider to make use of their physical, mental, emotional and spiritual resources in an interactive exchange. The midwifery model is a holistic model that uses the least amount of intervention to achieve the optimal outcome for mother and baby, as well as utilizes advanced technology when appropriate.

A feature that defines the midwifery model is that the woman is the central player and is the primary care provider for her baby and herself. The midwife's role is to assist her in making good, informed and healthy choices—because each choice is connected to and affects every other choice and will impact the woman and her baby for a lifetime. The role of the midwife is to help empower each woman in seeing the big picture holistically and take responsibility for the unique choices she makes for herself, her baby and her family, and thus, for society.

Nature Matters

Contrary to the pervasive messages with which women are constantly bombarded, birth is a process that is meant to work well. The central theme of the midwifery model is a fundamental trust in the female body's innate ability for pregnancy, birthing, lactation and mothering. We have lost sight of the fact that, like animals, we are exquisitely designed to give birth naturally if we are given a safe space, privacy and support. Women's bodies know how to conceive, birth and nurture human infants. Babies know how to grow in utero and be born. Most women and infant dyads are capable of crossing the birth threshold together successfully. It is true that nature can make mistakes, things can go wrong, and not everyone is able to conceive, birth, breastfeed or thrive. But in most cases, nature has designed these elegantly complex processes to work innately, and no amount of tampering can improve them. The dependability of these processes working well has kept our species alive on the planet for millennia.

On so many levels, we humans are in a gridlock of culture versus nature. Culture encodes our shared learning through a system of customary perceptions, values and beliefs. This system is human-made. It is our cultural overlay in America that influences women to think of labor pain as unbearable, birth as horrifying, and breastfeeding as inconvenient. These are not the beliefs in every culture. Luckily, humans have a remarkable capacity to choose their destinies, to make choices both as individuals and as a collective body. By making collective choices we have changed the course of history time and time again. I share a fierce belief with each of these authors: if mothers were willing and allowed to birth and nurse their babies using their own innate wisdom rather than being drugged, medicalized, episiotomized and excised, the quality of life would be greatly enhanced for women and infants, and thus, for society. Working in concert with nature—rather than against it—may be our key to survival, not just in the realm of women's procreative lives, but in every realm.

Sacred Matters

Midwives have described "woman" in a way that the ancients once did, and many indigenous cultures still do. We see woman as a living environment, the first environment,[19] and the chalice in which all human life gestates. We honor woman as the sacred portal through which all human life emerges. We perceive woman to be the sustenance by which newborn human life thrives. We believe woman to be perfectly and elegantly designed for biological functions of mythic proportions. We believe that woman is a reflection of the divine. We believe there is an invisible domain of the soul through which our children must pass to enter a human body. We believe birth is not just physiological; it is a soul journey. The soul realm is not an idyllic fantasy; quantum physics has made this worldview not only completely possible, but probable.

Even though the contributing authors come from many different religious and spiritual traditions, our belief in the invisible sacred and its importance in the birthing process is one of the themes that connect us all. Sadly, the sacred is not intentionally incorporated into the dominant birthing model. It is well documented that our current maternity care system is not producing optimal experiences or optimal outcomes for mothers or infants.[20-25] And we suffer a profound loss when we sacrifice the mystery of birth to mechanization. Reclaiming the sacred in the ordinary miracle of birth is deeply satisfying to the souls of all whom the birth experience touches—those giving birth, those being born, and those supporting and celebrating the journey.

Relationship Matters

This is what the Gen Xers and Millennials tell us: Even though they are enthralled and comfortable with the technological wizardry of the contemporary American birthplace, it is the way they are treated that most impresses, pleases or disturbs them. It is essential in human nature to be in relationship with one another. When we talk about the shortcomings of the medical model we are talking about the "system" not about individual people who have generously dedicated their lives to it. But how a system is designed makes it more or less conducive to acting on the human instinct towards caring. What clients like and crave about working with midwives is a mutual investment in building relationships that involve time, energy and heart. Time is a precious commodity. Adequate time is rarely afforded women in conventional maternity care in which the average allotted office encounter with a physician is six minutes.[26] With midwives in almost all settings, office visits run between twenty and sixty minutes. Without an extended investment of time, trust is difficult to achieve, and building meaningful relationships is less likely to occur. Pregnant women—in the midst of a life-altering situation—need to be listened to. Their fears need to be addressed. Their questions need to be answered. Their intuitions need to be supported. Their requests for their births and others aspects of their health care need to be privileged. Their unique expressions of emotions need to be honored. Most midwives put mothers first and treat them as if they are the center of the universe.

Honoring relationships extends to newborn babies as well. They have an extraordinary capacity for social behavior right after birth. Mediated by the limbic brain, a mother and infant dyad continues their synchronistic relationship with one another after birth.[27] One need only observe an undisturbed mother and newborn who are lost in enchantment of one another to see the resonance built into the design of human relationships.

And finally for us, fostering relationships with other midwives is an essential part of surviving in the profession, and sometimes the depth of a midwifery partnership can feel like a marriage. In our memoirs we cannot tell our own stories without including the stories of our colleagues and partners, because our interdependent relationships are authentic, visceral and substantial.

Compassion Matters

Consider these problems. Widespread discrimination and racism are documented as causing disparities in perinatal outcomes and long-term detrimental effects for infants, mothers and families, particularly among African Americans and Native

Americans.[28-30] When a pregnant woman experiences ongoing exposure to stress, or is disregarded and abused, she will release stress hormones that impact her immune, nervous and cardiac systems, and thus her overall health status and that of her baby.[31] An emerging body of literature indicates that vulnerable women of all races who have traumatic birth experiences (including too many obstetrical interventions and too little social support) are at risk of suffering the effects of post-traumatic stress disorder (PTSD).[32-35] PTSD is a mental illness in which a person develops "characteristic symptoms following exposure to an extreme traumatic stressor," usually war, major accidents, rape and abuse, or catastrophic environmental occurrences.[36] For a growing number of women, trauma in the birthplace is causing not only postpartum depression but the more serious illness of post-traumatic stress disorder.

There is an antidote to these problems. What if it was widely understood that extending compassion to pregnant and birthing women would result in: reducing the rates of preterm birth, newborns with low birth weight, infant mortality, maternal mortality and morbidity, postpartum depression and mental illness; and increasing the rates of breastfeeding, mother-infant attachment and successful early parenting? Compassion, which is the capacity to feel what it is like to be inside another person's skin and respond with loving kindness, is the human quality that will bring us back to our humanity. The authors in this anthology eloquently describe how compassion extended to a woman throughout the childbearing year has a transformative quality that can impact her for a lifetime. Her infant will benefit as well. Compassionately welcoming a newly born infant who has just emerged from a quiet and individual place of dreaming into a world of sound, smell, touch, breath, light and people, and who is just beginning its Earth walk, is immeasurably important. This very first threshold contains the seeds of everything that follows. Anyone who has ever gazed into the eyes of a newborn knows that she or he expects to be greeted with kindness. As humans, our brains are hardwired to care about one another. Compassion is not a luxury. It is a biological imperative.

Self-Determination Matters

In health care, self-determination is encoded in the ethical principle of autonomy, which is considered a right of each client/patient. Autonomy, in the bioethical sense, refers to the right of individuals to hold views; the capacity to make knowledgeable, non-coerced, voluntary, and well-considered decisions; and the ability to take actions based on what they believe and value. For pregnant and birthing women, as with others, autonomy involves both informed consent and informed refusal. Yet typically, in the complicated world of modern obstetrics, women are not given enough information to make informed decisions. When they refuse certain standard interventions, they often encounter troublesome consequences, including coercion and even arrest. While women across a wide-spectrum of class, race and education have reported in a national survey that they have felt coerced by obstetrical care providers, [37] our most vulnerable women (low-income women, women of color, teenagers, drug users, women in prison and homeless women) are most at risk. These same vulnerable women have the most to gain when they are treated with dignity and are able to gain mastery of self-determination.

As legal scholars begin to address birthing issues as topics of academic research, and as court cases pop up across the country related to civil rights violations, we are becoming aware of how uncontested pregnant women's rights are. What is at the core of these issues is the right to self-determination: Are women in charge of their bodies, their births, their babies, their decisions, and their lives, or not?

Midwives—whose primary commitment is to their clients—advocate for women's ascendancy and right to take ownership of their pregnancies and births. Midwives affirm that women are the primary caretakers of their pregnancies and the primary actors in the childbirth drama—not health care providers, hospital administrators or any other agencies. Midwives encourage women to be informed, articulate and proactive regarding their individual needs—including the context and content of their care and every other decision related to their childbearing year. Midwives encourage women to become fully engaged in their health care, to take responsibility, and to work in collaboration with their care providers. Self-determination matters because life is more meaningful and satisfying when people have control over their activities and successfully conquer their challenges. This can lead to unanticipated collateral benefits for society.

Service Matters

In these troubled times, people are tired of all the bad news of the modern world and are yearning to do something that inspires their souls. Apathy and a sense of helplessness can be transformed when people become connected and contribute, even in small ways. The ethic of serving humanity and one's community is central to the work of midwives. Embodied in the ethos of service are the qualities of giving generously, working collaboratively, respecting and celebrating diversity, and nourishing a lifelong dedication to people, communities and the environment. In many places in the United States the ethic of service is at war with the urge for personal gain. And while many people long to do work that satisfies them, some of us sacrifice what would nourish our spirits for what is safe and dependable. It requires risk-taking to do what we are passionate about. Yet, following our passion feeds our hungry spirits in ways we cannot know until we become involved in giving of ourselves and serving others. Neuroscientists report that caring and serving actually improve our own immune, cardiac and endocrine systems. That is one reason why giving generously in service to others feels so good.[38]

Deep connection with a community, whether it is a geographic, professional, learning, social or spiritual community, creates an experience of belonging and purpose. Even though most Americans value being rugged individualists, human beings crave a sense of belonging. We are dependent on interconnection with one another for our daily existence and the necessities of life. Dr. Martin Luther King, Jr. called it "network of mutuality" [39] and within our communities, where the self meets the world, we discover who we are and what valuable contributions we can make.

Activism Matters

As midwives, we never intended to become so involved with navigating politics, crafting legislation, affecting civic decisions, developing policy, and organizing grassroots support just because we wanted to catch babies. But we had to because we held a big vision and were up against a big wall. At times we felt (and still feel) overwhelmed. What was the spark that took us from powerlessness to activism? It was a passionate commitment to creating something better, to effecting social change. We did not start out having knowledge or skills or advocacy acumen. We just simply started. We came of age at a time of major cultural change, and the poets, musicians and prophets of our time inspired us. We banded together and became fierce and courageous in our goals.

Why does activism matter? *Imagine* a world in which politicians and practitioners are engaged together in activities to address and promote the needs of women and their families across the lifespan. *Imagine* replacing unnecessary health care spending with cost-effective alternatives, regularly utilizing evidence-based practices, and institutionalizing a set of performance measures for all providers based on competency and outcomes. *Imagine* transforming our health care system within a social justice framework so that all people can experience the benefits of the system, and both providers of care and those receiving care feel satisfied, respected and valued. *Imagine* maternity care that offers high quality, accessible, affordable and culturally competent care to all and not just to those who can afford choices. *Imagine* a maternal and child health care system that has a diverse health care team of complementary practitioners working in collaboration to provide women and families with all of the services they choose. It sounds good, but it does not happen without changing our collective consciousness and the way business is done in the birthplace and the marketplace. Activism is about ordinary citizens taking charge of creating what we want and insisting that our leaders listen and respond to what we need. It's not idealistic; it's a practical way to live. And it is the way that many human cultures have functioned and still do function. We have learned that activism is a key ingredient in transforming a vision into reality.

Courage Matters

Courage underpins almost everything that midwives do. Of all the skills that midwives learn, courage may be the hardest quality to impart to our students. It is beyond boldness, it is beyond valor, and it is beyond daring. It is a hard quality to teach because courage is not a skill; it is a way of life. It is willingness, no matter how afraid we might be, to walk through life with an attitude of fearlessness. But there is no courage without fear, no courage without facing risks. Every midwife in this anthology has breathed through the frightening process of freeing a baby stuck in its mother's birthing canal, or worse, staring death in the face. Some of the authors in this book have opened their office doors to police, been charged with criminal activity for practicing midwifery, and sat in courtrooms while judges determined their fate. Our willingness to cultivate courage is grounded in our passionate belief in what we are doing. Over time, fearlessness became a way of walking in the world and a guiding light. We refused to let fear paralyze us into inaction. Courage may not be a virtue that we are born with, but it can be learned and cultivated. To be a midwife is to be willing to confront fear, pain, adversity and danger in the forms of professional challenges, political confrontations, oppressive attitudes, and medical dominance in order to live the kind of lives we were destined to live. Because courage has been woven into the fabric of our beings, we are able to model it. We mentor young women as they work to face the shadows and wade though the dangerous waters that birthing and midwifing can uncover, and help them find the courage to make it safely to the shore.

Lineage Matters

We stand on the shoulders of a lineage of ancestor midwives. They may be blood relatives or the family tree of midwives of the past—indigenous, traditional, immigrant or Grand Midwives. Their contributions to women's health care continue to inspire and impact us today. The image of the *Sankofa*, of the Akan people of Ghana, comes to mind. It is a mythical bird that flies forward while looking backwards over its shoulder, and holds an egg in its beak symbolizing the future. It implies, "One must return to the past in order to move forward." Looking backward and looking forward, we realize that we have inherited the legacy; we are becoming the elders in our lineage. We have accumulated knowledge, wisdom, savvy, and expertise, and are considered wise women in our communities and professional circles. Proudly, and humbly, we have begun to see our experiences as sources of nourishment for our colleagues, protégés and communities.

Our concern for lineage is not just about the past. We are dedicated to teaching and training younger students and apprentices in order to grow the ranks of the profession, but also out of a love of preserving our lineage. While we see ourselves as an unbroken link to the past, we have a genuine concern for the flesh-and-blood beings who will carry our hopes and contributions into the future. To us, our midwifery lineage grows like a grapevine—connected to a single root but dependent on the intertwining of every branch to produce fruit. The harvest of each generation produces its own varietal whose taste and texture enriches the inheritance of the entire lineage.

Midwives Matter

Our maternity care system is in crisis. Costs increase and outcomes remain poor while beneficial practices are underused and harmful or ineffective practices are overused.[40] Never before have we seen such intense debate around health care reform in the United States. Midwives hold the key to transforming a broken maternity care system into a health care model that is proven to work better, save government and taxpayers money, and satisfy clients. When we think globally, we find that the industrialized countries with the best perinatal outcomes rely on midwifery as the essential component of their maternity care systems.[41] When we look locally, we find that midwifery practices in the United States—regardless of whether services are provided in hospitals, birth centers, clinics, or families' homes—have excellent outcomes.[42-46] Numerous national and international organizations—World Health Organization, United Nations Population Fund, UNICEF, International Federation of Gynecology and Obstetrics, World Bank, Global Health Workforce Alliance, Johns Hopkins Program for International Education in Gynecology and Obstetrics, American Public Health Association, Pew Health Professions Commission—recommend that midwives be a central feature in any maternity care system.[47-49] In 2010, several of the organizations listed above partnered in calling for an investment in strengthening midwifery services globally to achieve United Nations Millennium Development Goals (MDGs), particularly MDGs 4, 5 and 6 that address maternal and child health and well-being.

Midwives, in this anthology and elsewhere, demonstrate that it is vital to facilitate a maternal and child health care system that is built on love, respect, justice and autonomy. Midwives demonstrate that integrated, holistic, accessible and affordable care is possible, and includes a balance of meeting the psychosocial needs of women and families while ensuring good pregnancy and birth outcomes. Midwives have shown that it is possible to dispel the myths that keep women disconnected from their bodies and deeply afraid of childbirth and return the soul-nourishing aspects of magic, mystery, ecstasy and joy to the experiences of giving birth and being born.

Not everyone chooses to be a mother, and we are grateful that contemporary women can make those choices. But today, many women who have chosen motherhood are impacted negatively by cultural norms, reproductive technologies, hormone-disrupting substances, and environmental contaminants that work against the natural instinctive processes of conception, spontaneous labor, normal birth and breastfeeding. And the aberrations are becoming more problematic every day. Even given these challenges, midwives believe that women are strong and capable whether they are women birthing, women catching babies, women mothering, or women carrying out any other activity. The essential analysis and assertion of these authors is that women are powerful, proficient, and intelligent enough to take control over their bodies, their work and their lives. Having midwives who will relentlessly advocate for women's ascendancy in their own lives, and who will continually take risks to do it, matters deeply.

The Last Word

Whether we enter it intentionally or unintentionally, happily or unhappily, prepared or unprepared, giving birth is a rite of passage like no other. And afterwards, birth is forever embedded in our memories and embodied in our flesh. The experience of giving birth is something that we remember deep in our bones and our souls our whole lives. Every midwife in this anthology has listened to thousands of birth stories. Women of all ages cannot resist the chance, once they learn we are midwives, to tell us their stories of giving birth. And if our children could remember their births (and some of them can) they too would tell us their stories of being born. Birth is that big, it is that important. I remember during her keynote speech at the Midwives Alliance Conference in 2001,[50] Alice Walker described a teaching given to her by Sonbonfu Somé from the Daraga tribe of

Burkina Faso in West Africa. Sonbonfu teaches that the most important thing in a person's life is that he or she be properly welcomed to the world at the moment of birth. She said that newborn babies "bring spirit home." [51] If we can grasp this wondrous concept and its immense significance for families and society— *bringing spirit home* with each new birth—we will be able to understand this one simple truth: how one is born, and how one gives birth, matters deeply. At its core, that is what this collection of memoirs is really about.

If you are a young person and you are still searching for a career path, consider becoming a midwife. Observe the joys and challenges inherent in walking in a midwife's shoes. Notice what it takes to dedicate your life to your passion. Explore the significance of ensuring health care choices for women or the value of moving the profession of midwifery forward.

If you are a parent-to-be, make an intentional birth plan. Actively participate in your own health care. Reclaim your body, repossess your rights and, above all, enjoy the astounding door that opens only a few times in your life. Being an active player in the dance between ancestry and eternity is yours to shape and mold. It is worth designing your birth with intention, surrounding yourself with the support you need and doing it your way.

If you are a midwife, tell the stories of your life and gather together the power that is generated by such storytelling. Don't let your wisdom die with you; share it with colleagues, friends, and students. Publish your memoir; leave a legacy of your life's work. At some point your life will cease, but the gift of your written words will remain.

If you are a critic of midwifery, notice if what you have read is unsettling to you, and be curious enough to investigate further. Be willing to evaluate the status quo in maternity care and decide who and what our current model is serving. Follow the money. But above all, be part of the solution that will help end the heartbreaking crisis of so many mothers and babies dying around the time of birth in this country, with disproportionate deaths among people of color. We can no longer afford to ignore this fact. Be aware that our infant and maternal mortality rates are among the highest of any nation in the industrialized world. Embrace the notion that the survival of our babies is everybody's business.

And if you are an everyday reader, remember that you got here through the body of a woman. Honor your mother, respect women's bodies and recognize the importance of welcoming newborns gently. Pay very close attention to the stories women tell you about their birth experiences. Do they talk mostly about pain and fear? Do they describe loss of dignity and loss of choices in labor and birth?

Or do they talk about feeling pushed, powerful, joyful and fulfilled by their birth experiences? Think about what contributes to women having vastly different experiences in an organic process that is fundamentally the same. I challenge you to be creative, fearless, and proactive in renewing your commitment to making your life meaningful and joyful on your own terms. Find at least one good way to serve the world.

It has been an honor to put together this collection of memoirs. My gratitude runs deep, and my respect is immense for each of the contributing authors. I offer blessings for the survival, health and well-being of all of our mothers, fathers, children, and families—as the Hopi Indians say—for seven generations to come. May we live lightly, and with profound gratitude, upon our Earth Mother and in peace with all living things. *Ashe.*

Marina Alzugaray, MS, CNM, CPM is internationally known as an innovative educator, water healer, dancer, midwifery consultant and women's reproductive health specialist. Marina is the developer of the American AquaNatal® method, a prenatal water exercise and educational program with over one hundred instructors currently teaching worldwide. She became a pioneer of water birth while swimming with dolphins in the ocean. Over the last two decades she has provided trainings on the use of water for labor, birth and beyond for midwives and doctors. She created *Birth Dance* for her master's thesis, which is based on eco-feminism, a theory she contributed to during its early articulation, which interlaces art and science. Marina's *Birth Dance* performance is what opened doors to her as an international speaker. She has presented in Japan, Philippines, Australia, Denmark, Germany, Austria, Hungary, France, England, Switzerland, Bolivia, Argentina, Chile, Mexico, Trinidad, Bahamas, Puerto Rico, Jamaica and the United States. Marina is the recipient of the UCSF Chancellor's Award for her research on maternal infant safety associated with second stage maternal positions. The current focus of Marina's work is teaching about reproductive health, the menstrual cycle, and women's sexuality. Marina created MyMoon Cards©, a colorful educational tool for understanding women's cycles. She is a founding mother of the Alliance of Latin American Midwives (ALAPAR). Marina is a midwife passionate about safekeeping traditional midwifery and the sacredness of birth for every mother and baby. She lives on the Gulf of Mexico not far from her homeland of Cuba, where she can see the dolphins.

Rondi Anderson, CNM, BSN, MS has worked as a midwife in many settings, including college towns working with hippies, the Arizona desert working with Navajo Indians, Lancaster County, Pennsylvania, working with Old Order Amish, and Salem, Massachusetts, working with both the urban poor and the very affluent. Her career has also taken her around the world. Rondi has worked in many different venues, including her own private home birth practice, the private sector primarily in hospitals and birth centers, government community health centers, and non-governmental organizations. In all these varied settings, the passion that has driven her work has been the realization that birth is profoundly important in the lives of women and therefore to all of humanity. She feels that this understanding has not been given the attention or priority that it deserves, either nationally or globally. Rondi recently returned from working with Doctors Without Borders in India. Previously, she worked in Sierra Leone, West Africa, and in eastern Africa in Somalia. Rondi observed that for the poorest of the world's women, pregnancy involves wading into the dangerous waters of life and death, and pregnancy-related complications are the leading cause of death. In these countries she provided support for reproductive health programs in the areas of antepartum, intrapartum, and postpartum care and obstetric emergencies. She also worked with programs for family planning, sexually-transmitted infections, and prevention of mother-to-child transmission of HIV. While working for Doctors Without Borders, Rondi had the opportunity to hike up exotic mountains and enjoy colorful aspects of different cultures.

Alice Bailes, CNM, MS, FACNM has been a birth activist, speaker, teacher and author, but she has spent most of the last thirty-five years serving families directly as their midwife. More than 1300 babies have come into her hands in the intimate, undisturbed environment of either her clients' home or at BirthCare birth center. In the late 1960s, fascinated by the mind-body interaction, Alice earned a Bachelor of Fine Arts degree in dance and theatre at New York University. Inspired by the birth of her daughter in 1970, she became a childbirth activist and educator. The home birth of her son in 1973 led her to a formal education in midwifery. In 1981 she earned a midwifery master's degree from Georgetown University and certification as a Nurse-Midwife. In

1987 she co-founded BirthCare & Women's Health. For the last twenty years BirthCare has served families that choose to give birth in their homes or at BirthCare's birth center. Alice believes that midwives need to own and manage their own businesses because this is the only way that they have control over their own employment and the principles that midwives know how to put into practice. In 2005 Alice co-authored a chapter in the seminal textbook for nurse-midwifery students, *Varney's Midwifery*, called "Birth in the Home and Birth Center." Currently, Alice lives on ten acres in the Shenandoah Valley in a place with a panoramic view of the western sky where she likes watching the sun set. She still enjoys dancing and making both folk music and liturgical music. Alice has two children and four grandchildren, with another one on the way.

Maggie Bennett, BFA, LM is a midwife, artist, activist and teacher who became involved with the midwifery movement as she prepared for the birth of her second child. During the 1970s Maggie became president of Birthcenter in Monterey, California, a place where she taught home birth classes, began to study midwifery as part of a small group, and helped design an apprenticeship program. Maggie has always been an ardent feminist. In the '60s her activism was centered on the issues confronting single mothers, and later her interest was in reproductive rights. Maggie considers reproductive freedom to be a continuum that includes not only freedom to choose when and if to be pregnant, but also how and with whom to give birth. In the early 1990s Maggie was Chairwoman of the California Association of Midwives when legislation was passed licensing direct-entry midwives. In 1993 Maggie was selected by the California Commission on the Status of Women as one of the Outstanding Women of the Year for her work in reproductive rights, childbirth advocacy and community service. Maggie served four terms on the Board of Directors of the Midwives Alliance of North America and was chosen MANA's *Sage Femme* in 2004. She is currently on the Board of the Foundation for the Advancement of Midwifery. Maggie is an accomplished artist who draws her main inspiration from pregnant women and their children. Maggie has two grown sons and a grandson who was born into her hands. She lives on the Monterey Peninsula.

Patrice Bobier, CPM is a midwife and an organic farmer. She was born into a medical family and throughout her youth Patrice wanted to become a nurse until she found out that women could become doctors. She graduated from high school at age sixteen and began pre-med studies, but countercultural life-changing experiences interrupted her college plans. She married young, and she and her husband started a family and an organic farm in western Michigan in the early 1970s. Although her childbearing experiences were typical for that era, Patrice had a passion for learning about pregnancy and natural birth, and it was to her that women turned when they had questions, even before she was a midwife. In 1977 friends invited Patrice to their unattended home birth. The seeds were planted, and in 1978 she began to study midwifery and started attending home births regularly. Patrice has had her own midwifery practice, Full Circle Midwifery Service, Inc., since 1982. Patrice has been a member of the Midwives Alliance of North America (MANA) since its beginning and has been the Treasurer of the Michigan Midwives Association for over two decades. She became a Certified Professional Midwife in 1997. Patrice and her husband farm 200 acres, growing food for themselves, their CSA (Community Supported Agriculture) members, and the Sweetwater Local Foods Market. They also raise beef, pork, chicken and eggs. Midwifery and farming have been completely intertwined in her life. Her son and daughter are grown, and she has three home-born grandchildren.

Kate Bowland, BFA, RN, CNM is one of the pioneer lay-midwives who rode on the first wave of the home birth movement. The advent of a strong feminist movement, a natural birth movement, and optimism in her generation that believed they could change anything if they just would "do it" were the combination of factors that supported her becoming a lay midwife. Kate earned a degree in art in 1968 from the San Francisco Art Institute, became a lay midwife in the early 1970s and earned a Certified Nurse-Midwife degree in 1984 from the University of California San Francisco. One of the sentinel events of Kate's life occurred on March 6, 1974 when the Santa Cruz Birth Center was raided, and Kate and two other midwives were arrested and charged with the practice of medicine without a license. The ensuing court battle, Bowland vs. California, bears her name. Over the past thirty-five years Kate has maintained a private home birth practice, spoken in schools and to the media, trained apprentices, written articles on midwifery, and lectured at midwifery workshops and medical, nursing and chiropractic schools. Kate was one of the founding mothers of the Santa Cruz Women's Health Collective, the California Association of Midwives (CAM), and the Bridge Club (a liaison group between ACNM and MANA). She has been honored with awards from: the City of Santa Cruz, including their Outstanding Woman of the Year, the California Nurse-Midwives Association as Midwife of the Year, and the Brazen Woman Award from California Midwives Association.

Katsi (guh jee) Cook, wolf clan Mohawk, is a healer, midwife, researcher and respected educator and elder in her community. For the past twenty-five years she has worked as a women's health advocate and activist for environmental restoration in her tribal community—the Mohawk Nation at Akwesasne on the St. Regis Reservation in northern New York State straddling the U.S.-Canada border. Katsi is the Field Coordinator of the First Environment Program of Running Strong for American Indian Youth'. Katsi has been involved extensively with research and writing about environmental reproductive justice issues in Native America. As a leader in the Mother's Milk Project, begun in 1984, she was instrumental in tracing the causes of contamination of the drinking water on her reservation. Katsi was the founding Aboriginal midwife of the Six Nations Birthing Centre in Ohsweken, Ontario, the first school of indigenous midwifery in Canada. She was also a co-founder of the National Aboriginal Council of Midwives (NACM), which was established under the umbrella of the Canadian Association of Midwives in 2008. Katsi was a recipient of a 2004-2005 Indigenous Knowledge Cultural Researcher Award from the Indigenous Health Research Development Program at the University of Toronto. She is Co-Chair of the Structure and Network Building Committee of the Women's Health and Environment Network. She currently works in Maternal and Child Health qualitative research for the Tribal Epidemiology Center at United South and Eastern Tribes. Katsi is the mother of six children and the grandmother of ten.

Ida Darragh, BA, CPM has been involved in childbirth and midwifery since the birth of her first child in 1974. The experience of being awake and unmedicated for that birth was a life-changing experience that led her to midwifery. Ida became a certified childbirth educator and attended many hospital births as a doula before becoming a midwife in the early 1980s. Early in her career Ida became involved in the politics of midwifery. After a midwife was served with a cease and desist order for opening a birth center in the poor, rural delta of Arkansas in 1982, Ida and a group of midwives lobbied successfully for a law to license midwives. In 1985 Ida received the first license to practice midwifery in the state of Arkansas. In 1986 Ida became an instrumental member of the MANA Legislative Committee, in 1996 she became a Certified Professional Midwife, and in1997 she joined the Board of Directors of the North American Registry of Midwives (NARM). Her work with NARM has primarily been in test development and administration as Director of Testing. When Ida became NARM Board Chair in 2003, her work with states seeking midwifery legislation increased, and she became a vocal, visible and authoritative advocate for the CPM credential. In 2005, she wrote a handbook on preparing for legislation. Ida developed a workshop for consumers and midwives planning to lobby for midwifery legislation and continues to speak at legislative hearings throughout the country. Ida has been married since 1971 to Kramer Darragh, and they have three children and three grandchildren.

Ina May Gaskin, CPM, BA, MA, PhD (Hon.) is a midwife, author, childbirth and reproductive rights activist, and national and international lecturer. Ina May, her husband Stephen, and 270 people founded the famous intentional community known as The Farm near Summertown, Tennessee. The Farm midwife partners created one of the country's first contemporary community-based midwifery services. At The Farm it became the community norm to give birth at home and to breastfeed. Ina May has written about pregnancy, birth, and breastfeeding from a natural, social and spiritual perspective rather than from a medical and technological perspective. Her seminal work, *Spiritual Midwifery,* published in 1975, propelled her into fame and respect and has been translated into at least six languages. This book inspired women to overcome pathological levels of fear of childbirth and became the guide for home birth midwives and mothers around the country and abroad. In 2003 she wrote *Ina May's Guide to Childbirth, a book* that speaks to a whole new generation, and she published *Ina May's Guide to Breastfeeding in 2009.* Ina May is the author of several medical and midwifery articles, and she and her partners produce numerous instructional videos. She promotes the Gaskin Maneuver, which is the first obstetrical maneuver to be named after a midwife. Ina May is co-founder and past president of the Midwives Alliance of North America, and she initiated the Safe Motherhood Quilt Project. Ina May has been involved in projects stateside and abroad to protect reproductive rights and to provide access to care for underserved women. In November 2009, the Faculty of Health and Human Sciences of Thames Valley University in London conferred her with the title "Honorary Doctor." Ina May and her husband have lived at The Farm for thirty-seven years. They had five children and have five grandchildren.

Diane Holzer, LM, CPM, PA-C has been attending births for almost thirty years, and her experience ranges from busy birth centers to home births. Diane loves to guide student midwives almost as much as she enjoys being with mothers during birth. She has spent a decade in El Paso, Texas, where she trained student midwives and ran birth centers. An activist at heart, Diane has volunteered thousands of hours to multiple causes including the Sanctuary Movement, immigrant rights and a shelter doing well-woman and prenatal care. Her most avid cause through the years has been the Midwives Alliance of North America (MANA). She served on the board of directors for twenty years, including two terms as president, and was an innovative leader and a major instrument for change. In 1991 Diane was a founding member of the Midwifery Education and Accreditation Council and served on its board for thirteen years. Diane served on the International Confederation of Midwives Board (ICM) as the regional representative for the Americas for six years, continues to be the liaison to the ICM for the Midwives Alliance, and was appointed ICM representative to the United Nations for a three-year term. Diane is an internationally known speaker, in particular, at one of her favorite venues, the 1995 Fourth World Conference on Women in Beijing. Diane teaches classes in women's health, natural family planning and well-woman care. Diane lives in northern California where she attends home births and works as a physician assistant at a rural health care family practice clinic.

Marsha Elaine Jackson, CNM, MSN, FACNM was told by a high school teacher in New Jersey that she would never make it through college. But Marsha did not let that statement cloud her vision. In 1974 she graduated Magna Cum Laude from Howard University with a baccalaureate degree in nursing, and in 1981 she became a Certified Nurse-Midwife and graduated with honors from Georgetown University receiving her master's degree. Marsha has worked in a newborn nursery, a neonatal unit, and as a nurse-clinician for maternal infant care functioning as a practitioner, teacher, consultant, and researcher. From 1981 to 1987 she operated a solo-home birth practice in Washington D.C., and worked with Cities-in-Schools, an adolescent pregnancy program. Marsha has the distinction of being the first nurse-midwife to have delivery privileges at Georgetown University Hospital. In 1987, she co-founded BirthCare & Women's Health, a full-scope midwifery practice providing home birth services and an accredited birth center serving the metropolitan Washington D.C. area. She is past chair of the American College of Nurse-Midwives' Home Birth Committee, past chair of the ACNM Nominating Committee, co-editor of the *ACNM Handbook: Home Birth Practice*, Board member of the ACNM Foundation, has published several articles related to home birth and received numerous awards. Marsha co-authored a chapter for *Varney's Midwifery*, and she was profiled in the Smithsonian Museum exhibition, *Reclaiming Midwives: Pillars of Community Support* that was on view from November 2005 through August 2006. Marsha is the mother of five, grandmother of six, and lives with her family in southern Maryland.

Jennie Joseph, LM, CPM was born and raised in England and received her midwifery education in London in 1981. For nearly thirty years Jennie has worked in hospitals, birthing centers and home birth settings along with teaching numerous student midwives in classrooms and clinical settings internationally. In 1994 Jennie was the first foreign-trained midwife to be licensed in Florida under the newly reopened Midwifery Practice Act. As Executive Director of The Birth Place, a freestanding birthing facility in Winter Garden, Florida, she cares for women from all walks of life. She developed The JJ Way™ maternal and child health care delivery model. It has shown such promising outcomes for indigent women that it has been funded for an ongoing research study. Her book entitled *Beautiful! Images of Health, Joy and Vitality in Pregnancy and Birth* depicts the results of her JJ Way™ program. Jennie launched the Nubian Health Network in 2004 in order to address the health care disparities being experienced by women of African descent and recently developed the "Save Our Babies" initiative. Jennie was nominated for the Orange County Black History Month Humanitarian Award in 2006 and received the prestigious Central Florida Women's Resource Summit Award in 2007. Jennie has provided expert commentary on pregnancy to numerous online and print media, local and national news channels, and talk radio stations. She was instrumental in initiating and running the School of Complementary Medicine's Midwifery Program from 1995-2000, and is the former Chair of Florida's Council of Licensed Midwifery. Jennie is the Executive Director of her own non-profit corporation, Commonsense Childbirth Inc. She has one child and is a grandmother of one.

Makeda Kamara, CNM, MPH was born at the mouth of the Chagres River in Gamboa, Panama, the last child of second generation immigrant parents from the Caribbean. She was raised in a very small tight-knit community. It was there that she was imbued with the essence of social responsibility and the importance of community, family, and women's ways of knowing. She migrated to the United States at the height of the Civil Rights and Black Power movements and got involved in the struggle for equal rights. Upon completion of her undergraduate studies, she left the United States to work in Tanzania, and it was there that she witnessed her first birth and was called to the honorable work of midwifery and women's health. She also worked in Uganda to combat *kwashiorkor* malnutrition. Upon return to the United States, Makeda earned a master's degree in public health while apprenticing with independent midwives and worked in the women's movement of the 1970s to establish feminist health centers. She later entered nursing school and received her Certified Nurse-Midwife degree. It was a difficult decision to go to nursing school. But Makeda felt that it was the only way she could reach her Afrikaan American sisters and be an effective voice in their struggle with the racist system they faced daily. Now more than twenty-five years later, she is still catching babies and working very diligently to effect changes and to improve the lives of women of Afrikaan descent. Makeda is the proud mother of two children, born at home and breastfed, and now young adults.

Abby J. Kinne, CPM began her family in 1963 and immediately became a La Leche League leader and local chapter president. Abby formed a support group for other parents who were equally frustrated with the status quo of childbirth in the 1960s. Many of these families invited her to share their home births, and soon thereafter her community identified her as a midwife. She is co-founder of the Center for Humane Options in Childbirth Experiences (CHOICE), a non-profit organization committed to providing educational services to couples seeking safe alternatives in childbirth and training programs for aspiring midwives. Abby is currently the Executive Director of CHOICE. In 1984 Abby co-founded the Ohio Midwives Alliance (OMA). She is currently OMA's President, a member of the Governing Board, and editor of the quarterly newsletter. In 1986 Abby became a licensed Advanced Emergency Medical Technician and provided Obstetrical Emergency training to EMTs for many years. Abby served the Midwives Alliance of North America as Statistics and Research Committee Chair from 1986-1988, Membership Chairperson from 1993-1995, Treasurer from 1995-2001, and First Vice President from 2001-2008. Abby contributed to the development of the North American Registry of Midwives (NARM) National Registry Exam, served on the NARM Certification Task Force as Skills Validation Chair, and was instrumental in developing NARM's national certification for midwives. In 1994, she became the first Certified Professional Midwife (CPM) in North America. She and her husband have been preparing for retirement by building their "dream home," a haven for themselves, their adult children and eleven grandchildren.

Kip Kozlowski, RN, CNM decided to become a nurse at the age of four, after treating her father for a headache. By age twenty-eight she had indeed become a nurse. By day she was employed in a busy hospital neonatal intensive care unit working in "the system." At night she did the radical work of educating women about choices, assisted at home births, became politically active in the birthing community and had her own babies at home. After years of living this dual existence, she gave up, and at age forty became a midwife. Kip has worked in several venues. After becoming a nurse-midwife, she established a short-lived hospital practice in 1985, worked in a home birth practice, and worked with a wild mountain male midwife in Colorado. She designed and taught classes, including "Mother-Daughter First Menstruation." She was owner of a women's bookstore and opened "Midwives Market," the famous midwifery bumper sticker business. In the late 1990s she joined a hospital-based midwifery practice for three years. In 2001 Kip felt she had to make one last attempt at her twenty-year dream of opening a freestanding birth center, and she solicited a handful of seasoned midwives to create this business with her. In 2003 Kip opened the Greenhouse Birth Center in mid-Michigan. The birth center offers full-scope midwifery care, massage therapy, childbirth classes, doula services, mother's support groups, mentoring for aspiring midwives, and community events. It is a place where families can have unbothered births in a quiet safe place. Kip is a wife, mother of four and grandmother of nine with twin grandbabies due any day.

Casey Makela is a Traditional Midwife, author, lecturer and artist. She is the founder of the Michigan School of Traditional Midwifery and the American College of Traditional Midwives. The Michigan School of Traditional Midwifery (www.traditionalmidwife.org), founded in the late 1980s, became the first licensed school in Michigan to offer midwifery as a vocational art and not a medical science. Casey's home birth practice, Gently Borne Midwifery, has served women and families in four states since 1985, primarily in Michigan. She has attended hundreds of births and currently serves "plain" Amish and Mennonite communities. Casey is passionate about educating midwives to increase the ranks in the profession and equally passionate about preserving birthing freedom for families. Casey is an author of books for both adults and children, has written birth-based articles for midwifery periodicals since the mid-1980s, and has done considerable lecturing and teaching. She is also an active advocate for unassisted birth about which she has written. Casey and her husband have raised their family in northern Michigan on Quaker Hill Farm (www.quakerfarm.com) where they have home schooled their children. Casey has had the honor of apprenticing several of her own daughters in the art of midwifery. Casey and her family were award-winning performing artists for a decade and recorded a children's music album in 1993. Casey was featured on a benefit album for the prevention of child abuse for which she won a national award in 1990s. Casey is currently working on her degree in Divinity and is a conservative plain Christian Quaker.

Linda McHale, CPM, EMT is a Certified Professional Midwife and an Emergency Medical Technician who has been a practicing midwife for over nearly thirty years. Linda received her early training with a study group and then through an apprenticeship. When she returned home from her apprenticeship, Linda went from being a Licensed Midwife in Texas to an illegal midwife in New Jersey. Later she assisted the efforts to get the CPMs legalized in New Jersey. Linda completed the Portfolio Evaluation Process (PEP) through the North American Registry of Midwives and became a CPM in 1995. Linda has been a guest speaker at numerous conferences, such as Midwifery Today, the Open Center in New York, the Midwives Alliance of North America (MANA), and the La Leche League, as well as a presenter at various schools, colleges and other birth-focused groups. Being interested in energy medicine, Linda became a Reiki practitioner and teacher. Linda has served on the Board of Directors of the Midwives Alliance of North America (MANA), as the Northeast Region Representative and Fundraising Chair. Linda currently serves on the Board of Directors of the Foundation for the Advancement of Midwifery (FAM) and as a member of the MANA/ACNM Liaison Committee. Linda has had the opportunity to work with many midwifery partners and apprentices over the years, including doulas, nurses, direct-entry midwives, Certified Professional Midwives (CPMs) and Certified Nurse Midwives (CNMs), and she is grateful for all of them. In April 2006 Linda married Dennis Glanfield. She has three children, two of them born at home, and one grandchild, also born at home.

Shafia M. Monroe was sixteen years old when her Muslim elders encouraged her to become an obstetrician. At age seventeen her uncle told her about the work of midwives, and she discovered the history of the Southern Black midwife and knew she wanted to become one. Shafia trained as an apprentice midwife and as a pre-med student at the University of Massachusetts where she studied the sciences necessary to provide a solid theoretical foundation for maternity care. In 1980 Shafia co-founded the Traditional Childbearing Group in Boston, the first non-profit Black home birth center in the country. She worked with thirteen midwives and apprentices to provide community-based direct services to African American families as well as midwifery apprenticeship training for young Black women. In 1991 Shafia moved to Portland, Oregon, and founded the International Center for Traditional Childbearing (ICTC), an organization devoted to infant mortality prevention, breastfeeding promotion and training for midwives. Shafia is the CEO of ICTC and has designed several training programs, including international cultural exchanges. In 2006 Shafia was featured on a community mural entitled "Women in Portland Who Made History" along with ten other women, and in 2007 she was featured as a "Living Treasure" in *Mothering* magazine. In 2007 Shafia published the *Black Midwives and Prenatal Providers Directory*, and she has been highlighted in numerous books. Shafia has received several awards and certificates for her leadership in reducing infant mortality. Shafia is married to Imam Mikal H. Shabazz, and together they are gifted with a blended family of sixteen children and fourteen grandchildren with one more on the way.

Sister Angela Murdaugh, CNM, MSN, FACNM is a Franciscan Sister of Mary and a native Arkansan. Sr. Angela is a daring voice for the profession, a talented administrator, a master clinician, a pioneer in birth center care, a sought-after speaker and a midwife with a vision of hope for the future. In 1972 she established the first freestanding birth center in Texas as part of a migrant health clinic. A decade later she established Holy Family Services and Birth Center near the Texas-Mexico border, a private, non-profit model that brings quality nurse-midwifery care to a population of underserved and impoverished women. Throughout her career Sr. Angela served as clinical faculty for nurse-midwifery students nationwide. In 1981 Sr. Angela was elected President of the American College of Nurse-Midwives. She also served in offices or on committees of the National Association of Childbearing Centers (NACC), her local chapter of ACNM and statewide Consortium of Texas Certified Nurse-Midwives. She has given testimony before various legislative committees and was instrumental in obtaining a Texas Attorney General's opinion that clearly defined the legal basis for nurse-midwifery practice. In 1985 Sr. Angela served on the State Department of Health committee that wrote the Texas Birth Center Regulations. She assisted in the writing of NACC's Standards for Birth Centers. She is a Distinguished Fellow of the American College of Nurse-Midwives, and in September of 2002, she was named to the Texas Women's Hall of Fame. Although semi-retired since 2007, Sr. Angela continues to be a presence at professional gatherings and is currently a regional Chapter Chair of ACNM.

Carol Nelson, LM, CPM-TN is a midwife, social and environmental activist, researcher and preceptor. She is in a partnership with five other midwives at The Farm Midwifery Center in Tennessee. Carol graduated as a nurse in 1968, became a Florida Licensed Midwife in1982 and received her Certified Professional Midwife (CPM) credential in 1995. Since the mid-1990s, Carol has been actively involved with the inception, development and implementation of the Certified Professional Midwife (CPM) credential through the North American Registry of Midwives (NARM), the certification agency for the CPM. She has served on the NARM Board as Treasurer since 1997 and as Director of the NARM Applications Department since 2003. Carol is co-author of the American Public Health Association (APHA) position papers, *Increasing Access to Out-of-Hospital*

Maternity Care Services Through State-Regulated and Nationally-Certified Direct-Entry Midwives, adopted in 2001, and *Safe Motherhood in the United States: Reducing Maternal Mortality and Morbidity*, adopted in 2003. Since 1997, Carol has held several positions in the APHA Maternal Child Health Section and on the APHA Governing Council. Carol has been Chair of the Midwifery Education and Advocacy Committee of the Midwives Alliance of North America since 1994. Carol has served on the Board of Directors of Plenty International, a non-profit alternative Relief and Development Organization affiliated with the United Nations, and is a founding mother of Swan Conservation Land Trust in the Western Highland Rim of Tennessee. Carol lives in Summertown, Tennessee, with Don Nelson, her husband of thirty-three years. She is the mother of four children and grandmother of seven.

Yeshi Neumann, MA, CNM, MPH is a midwife, international speaker and trainer, advocate for social justice, and facilitator of diversity work in health care and educational institutions. Gazing into the eyes of her newborn in 1970, she knew without a doubt that she would become a midwife. Yeshi moved to a hippie commune near the Salmon River of northern California where she and another woman became the midwives. She learned that birth was inseparable from the rhythm of the wind, the turn of the earth, and the surges of the river. After four years of attending births in the mountains, Yeshi moved to the San Francisco Bay Area and apprenticed herself to an experienced home birth midwife. In 1980 Yeshi became a Certified Nurse-Midwife (CNM) so she could attend births in the hospital where 99% of women in the United States give birth. She wanted to be able to provide childbirth care to different kinds of women including women without the social, educational or economic resources and those who do not desire to birth at home. She worked for many years as a staff midwife in inner city hospitals. Her disappointment and frustration with the kind of care she was able to give in the managed care obstetric paradigm impelled her to create Homestyle Midwifery. Homestyle Midwifery is Yeshi's way of providing unhurried, hands-on, soul-satisfying care to childbearing families in a hospital setting. It is her way of having women be welcome at their own births and babies be welcomed into this world. Yeshi lives in northern California. She has two daughters, two grand-daughters and many godchildren.

Debbie Pulley, CPM has a home birth practice in Atlanta, Georgia. Attending births since 1981, she has been blessed to have witnessed about 1,000 births and has reached the point in her career that she is the midwife for babies of the babies she assisted into the world. Midwifery is Debbie's passion. She is active in Georgia midwifery politics and is currently president of Georgia Midwifery Association. In 1998 the Secretary of State recognized her for "Significant Contributions to Health Care." She is the liaison between the local midwives and the State Department of Health, Vital Records, and Children's First program. Debbie is a leader in midwifery advocacy and public education at professional conferences each year, including the National Conference of State Legislatures, the largest annual gathering for state policymakers, and the American Public Health Association. Debbie serves on the North American Registry of Midwives (NARM) Board as Secretary and Director of Public Education & Advocacy. She has been involved with NARM since 1995 and was one of the first midwives nationwide to receive CPM certification by the organization. Debbie is the Legislative Committee Chair for the Midwives Alliance of North American and a member of the MANA/ACNM Liaison Committee. Debbie is also the owner/moderator of the Atlanta-ITP Freecycle group, an international organization that promotes reuse and keeping good stuff out of landfills. She has been married for thirty-five years and has two grown children and three beautiful grandchildren. For fun and relaxation Debbie plays and hosts tournaments in Gin to Win, an online Gin Rummy league.

Arisika Razak, RN, CNM, MPH is currently an Associate Professor in the Women's Spirituality Program at the California Institute of Integral Studies (CIIS) in San Francisco, and is the CIIS Director of the Integrative Health Studies Program. Arisika has worked for over thirty years in the fields of Women's Spirituality, Women's Studies, and Women's Health, providing academic, public health, clinical, artistic and healing services. She has served as health care advocate, abortion counselor, lay midwife, hospital based nurse-midwife, health care administrator and health educator. Arisika provided full-scope midwifery care to mainstream, marginalized and vulnerable women in the San Francisco Bay Area. After working with community organizations that demanded better obstetric services to combat high levels of infant mortality among African American women, she was chosen to direct Alameda County's Highland Hospital Nurse-Midwifery Service. She was a founding member of the Oakland Perinatal Health Project that successfully used midwives to lower perinatal morbidity and infant mortality among populations demographically at risk for perinatal loss. Arisika has led healing workshops for women for over two decades. Her dance and performance work celebrates women's bodies along with the blood mysteries of childbirth, menstruation, sexuality and menopause. Her teachings are based on spiritual traditions from around the world, scientific knowledge of women's health, and diverse liberation movements. Arisika has achieved local, national and international recognition as an educator, artist, and practitioner. She has three film credits, has contributed to several books, and presents at conferences on subjects of multiculturalism and diversity, women's health and healing, and embodied spirituality and movement. Arisika is the mother of one, grandmother of one and godmother of two.

Geradine Simkins, DEM, CNM, MSN is an activist, midwife, author and visionary who, in 1976, discovered midwifery when she was pregnant with her first child. Over the course of three decades, Geradine has walked in the shoes of a lay, direct-entry and nurse-midwife. She has worked as a home birth midwife, provided midwifery care in a bilingual clinic for Hispanic migrant farmworkers, was co-founder and staff midwife at a freestanding birth center, and has worked as a women's health consultant for American Indian organizations co-managing maternal and child health care programs. She was a founding mother of the Michigan Midwives Association in 1978, its first president, and co-designed MMA's apprenticeship and certification programs in the 1980s. Since 1998 Geradine has served on the Board of Directors of the Midwives Alliance of North America (MANA) as the Midwest Regional Representative, Second Vice President, and currently as President. In 2010 she was hired as MANA's first Interim Executive Director. She served on the Board of Directors of the Foundation for the Advancement of Midwifery. Geradine authored a chapter in the book, *From Calling to Courtroom,* and is a contributing author to *Our Bodies, Ourselves: Pregnancy and Birth.* She co-authored *Speaking with One Voice,* position papers on maternal and child health among American Indians and Native Hawaiians, and co-designed of the National Institutes of Health *Healthy Native Babies* curriculum on SIDS risk reduction for American Indian/Alaska Native communities. Occasionally, Geradine is a staff midwife at the Greenhouse Birth Center in mid-Michigan but concentrates on sustaining the midwifery profession and mentoring younger midwives. Geradine has three wonderful grown children and is the director of Birthways Midwifery in rural northern Michigan.

Saraswathi Vedam, RM, CNM, MSN, SciD(hc) is an Indian woman who grew up in both India and the United States and has been a practicing midwife, midwife educator, and academic midwife. She has been observing and caring for women for over thirty-five years. By the time she was a teenager, Saraswathi had witnessed the care of women in a variety of settings, including the Bombay slums, rural settings, tertiary care hospitals, and maternity centers. For over twenty-five years, Saraswathi has cared for families in home and out-of-home sites, including a large-volume hospital HMO practice in New York and her own private home and hospital midwifery practices in San Francisco, Indianapolis and Connecticut. Saraswathi has been active is setting birth policy. She was an expert consultant to the Hungarian Health Ministry and Alternatal Foundation. She served as Chair of the American College of Nurse Midwives' (ACNM) Homebirth Section and contributed to writing and editing several of the ACNMs' foundational documents on home birth practice. She also is the Senior Advisor for the Midwives Alliance of North America's Division of Research. She has authored national clinical practice guidelines and articles on evidence-based midwifery practice and has taught midwifery and medical students in schools across the United States and Canada. Saraswathi has served as consultant on advisory panels for diversity and cultural competency in education, and has presented internationally on midwifery care for diverse populations. Saraswathi is the mother of four biracial and bicultural daughters. She is currently the Director of the Midwifery Program at the University of British Columbia in Vancouver, British Columbia, Canada.

LIST OF WORKS CITED

Introduction

1. McCool, William, and Sandi J. McCool. "Feminism and Nurse-Midwifery: Historical Overview and Current Issues." *J Nurse-Midwifery* 34. (1989): 323-34.

2. Block, Jennifer. *Pushed: The Painful Truth About Childbirth and Modern Maternity Care*. Cambridge: Da Capo Press, 2007, 213.

3. Wertz, Richard W. and Dorothy C. Wertz. *Lying-in: A History of Childbirth in America*. New York: Schocken, 1977.

4. Jordan, Brigitte. *Birth in Four Cultures: A Cross-Cultural Investigation of Childbirth in Yucatan, Holland, Sweden and the United States*. Prospect Heights: Waveland Press, 1993.

5. Jordan, Brigitte, *Birth in Four Cultures*, 4.

6. Leavitt, Judith Walzer. *Brought to Bed: Childbearing in America, 1750-1950*. New York: Oxford University Press, 1986.

7. Wertz, Richard W., and Dorothy C. Wertz. *Lying-in: A History of Childbirth in America*. New York: Schocken Books, 1977, 6. Print.

8. Ettinger, Laura Elizabeth. *Nurse-Midwifery: The Birth of a New American Profession*. Columbus: Ohio State University Press, 2006, 8.

9. Wertz and Wertz, *Lying-in*.

10. Ettinger, *Nurse-Midwifery*, 8.

11. Leavitt, *Brought to Bed*, 54-58.

12. Leavitt, *Brought to Bed*.

13. Wertz and Wertz, *Lying-in*.

14. Leavitt, *Brought to Bed*.

15. Ettinger, *Nurse-Midwifery*, 8.

16. Leavitt, *Brought to Bed*.

17. Wertz and Wertz, *Lying-in*.

18. Wertz and Wertz, *Lying-in*.

19. Sears, William, and Martha Sears. *The Birth Book*. New York: Little, Brown and Company, 1994, 18.

20. Leavitt, *Brought to Bed*.

21. Wertz and Wertz, *Lying-in*.

22. Ettinger, *Nurse-Midwifery*, 10.

23. Wertz and Wertz, *Lying-in*.

24. Sears and Sears, *The Birth Book*, 17-22.

25. Perkins, Barbara Bridgman. *The Medical Delivery Business: Health Reform, Childbirth, and the Economic Order*. New Brunswick: Rutgers University Press, 2004.

26. Perkins, *The Medical Delivery Business*.

27. DeClercq, Eugene R., Carol Sakala, Maureen P. Corry, and Sandra Applebaum. *Listening to Mothers II: Report of the Second National Survey of Women's Childbearing Experiences*. New York: Childbirth Connection, 2006.

28. Sakala, Carol and Maureen P. Corry. *Evidence-Based Maternity Care: What It Is and What It Can Achieve*. New York: Milbank Memorial Fund, 2008, 10.

29. Centers for Disease Control and Prevention, National Center for Health Statistics. National Vital Statistics Report 57.12 (2008). Accessed December 2009. <http://www.cdc.gov/nchs/data/nvsr/nvsr57/nvsr57_12.pdf>.

30. CDC, National Center for Health Statistics, 2008.

31. DeClercq et al., *Listening to Mothers II*.

32. DeClercq et al., *Listening to Mothers II*, 29, 33.

33. DeClercq et al., *Listening to Mothers II*, 32.

34. DeClercq et al., *Listening to Mothers II*, 31, 84.

35. DeClercq et al., *Listening to Mothers II*, 35, 84.

36. Hamilton, B.E., J.A. Martin, and S.J. Ventura. "Births: Preliminary Data for 2006." National Vital Statistic Report 56(7). Hyattsville: National Center for Health Statistics, 2007. Available at: <http://www.cdc.gov/nchc/data/nvsr/nvsr56/nvsr56_007.pdf>.

37. Sakala and Corry, *Evidence-Based Maternity Care*, 10.

38. World Health Organization. "The World Health Report: Make Every Mother and Child Count," 2005. Available at: <http://www.who.int.whr/2005/en>.

39. Centers for Disease Control and Prevention, National Center for Health Statistics, Accessed Dec 2009. <http://www.cdc.gov/nchs/data/databriefs/db09.htm>.

40. World Health Organization, "The World Health Report", 2005.

41. Centers for Disease Control and Prevention. "Maternal Mortality—United States, 1982-1996", Morbidity and Mortality Weekly Report 47.34, 1998.

42. Centers for Disease Control and Prevention. "Safe Motherhood, Promoting Health for Women Before, During and After Pregnancy", 2008. Accessed December 2009. <http://www.cdc.gov/NCCDPHP/publications/aag/pdf/drh.pdf>.

43. Janssen, Patricia. A. "Outcomes of Five Years of Planned Home Birth Attended by Regulated Midwives Versus Planned Hospital Birth in British Columbia." Proceedings of the Seventh Annual General Meeting of the Canadian Association of Midwives, November 1-3, 2007. Vancouver: Canada.

44. Perkins, *The Medical Delivery Business*.

45. Agency for Healthcare Research and Quality, 2008. HCUPnet, Healthcare Cost and Utilization Project. Rockville: AHRQ. Available at: <http://hcupnet.ahrq.gov/>.

46. Sakala and Corry, *Evidence-Based Maternity Care*.

47. Hamilton, B.E., J.A. Martin, and S.J. Ventura. Births: Preliminary data for 2007." National Vital Statistics Reports 57(12). Hyattsville: National Center for Health Statistics, Released March 18, 2009. Available from: http://www.cdc.gov/nchs/data/nvsr/nvsr57/nvsr57_12.pdf.

48. Agency for Healthcare Research and Quality, 2008.

49. Sakala and Corry, *Evidence-Based Maternity Care*.

50. Sakala and Corry, *Evidence-Based Maternity Care*.

51. Cowan, C.A. and M. B. Hartman. 2005. "Financing Healthcare: Businesses, Households and Governments", 1987-2003. Health Care Financing Review 1(2): 126, web exclusive. Available at: <http://www.cms.hhs.gov/NationalHealth/Expend/Data/downloads/bhg-articles-04.pdf>.

52. Declercq et al., *Listening to Mothers II*.

53. Declercq et al., *Listening to Mothers II.*

54. Block, Pushed, 265.

55. Davis-Floyd, Robbie E., Lesley Barclay, Betty-Anne Daviss, and Jan Tritten. *Birth Models That Work*, Berkley: University of California Press, 2009.

56. Sakala and Corry, *Evidence-Based Maternity Care.*

57. Simonds, Wendy, Barbara Katz Rothman and Bari Meltzer Norman. *Laboring On: Birth in Transition in the United States*, New York: Routledge, 2007.

58. Budin, Wendy C., and Judith A Lothian, eds. "Advancing Normal Birth." Supplement of *Journal of Perinatal Education* 16.1 (2007): I-96S.

59. Rothman, Barbara Katz. *In Labor: Women and Power in the Birthplace,* Revised Ed. New York: W.W. Norton, 1991 [1982].

60. Davis-Floyd, Robbie E. *Birth as an American Right of Passage,* Berkeley: University of California Press, 1992.

61. Davis-Floyd, *Birth as an American Right of Passage.*

62. Ettinger, *Nurse-Midwifery,* 16-18.

63. Davis-Floyd, Robbie & Christine Barbara Baldwin, eds. *Mainstreaming Midwives: The Politics of Change.* New York: Routledge, 2006.

64. Chester, Penfield. *Sisters on a Journey.* New Brunswick: Rutgers University Press, 1997.

65. Leavitt, *Brought to Bed.*

66. Smith, Margaret Charles and Linda Janet Holmes. *Listen to Me Good: The Life Story of an Alabama Midwife.* Columbus: Ohio University Press, 1996.

67. Rude, Anna E. "The Midwifery Problem in the United States." *Journal of the American Medical Association* 81(12), September 22, 1923, 987-92.

68. American College of Nurse Midwives. "Become a Midwife". Accessed December 2009. Available at: <http://www.acnm.org/>.

69. North American Registry of Midwives. "Certification Process". Accessed December 2009. Available at: <http://www.narm.org/>.

70. Wachdorf, Cecilia M. "Midwifery, Bridging the Gap: A Study of Paradigms and Values." Ph.D. dissertation. ProQuest Digital Dissertations database. Publication No. AAT 3116447. Tampa: University of South Florida. 2003.

Afterword

1. Janssen, Patricia A., Angela D. Henderson, and Saraswathi Vedam. "The Experience of Planned Home Birth: Views of the First 500 Women." *Birth, Issues in Perinatal Care* 36.4 (2009): 297-304.

2. Christiaens, Wendy, and Piet Bracke. "Place of Birth and Satisfaction with Childbirth in Belgium and the Netherlands." *Midwifery* 25.2 (2009): e11-e19. Epub ahead of print 2007.

3. Lindgren, H.E., Ingela Radestad, K. Christensson, K. Wally-Bystrom, and Ingegerd Hildingsson. "Perceptions of Risk and Risk Management among 735 Women Who Opted for a Home Birth." *Midwifery* (2008). Epub ahead of print.

4. Janssen, Patricia A., E. Carty, and B. Reime . "Satisfaction with Planned Place of Birth among Midwifery Clients in British Columbia." *J Midwifery Women's Health* 51.2 (2006): 91-97.

5. Hildingsson, Ingegerd, Ulla Waldenstrom, and Ingela Radestad. "Swedish Women's Interest in Home Birth and In-Hospital Birth Center Care." *Birth* 30.1 (2003): 11-22.

6. Banyana, J.M., and R. Crow. "A Qualitative Study of Information about Available Options for Childbirth Venue and Pregnant Women's Preference for a Place of Delivery." *Midwifery* 19 (2003): 328-36.

7. Cunningham, J.D. "Experiences of Australian Mothers Who Gave Birth Either at Home, at a Birth Centre, or in Hospital Labour Wards." *Social Science & Medicine* 36.4 (1993): 475-483.

8. Soderstrom, B., P.J. Stewart, C. Kaitell, and M. Chamberlain. "Interest in Alternative Birthplaces among Women in Ottawa-Carleton." *CMAJ Canadian Medical Association Journal* 142.9 (1990): 963-969.

9. Rothman, Barbara Katz. *Two Models of Maternity Care: Defining and Negotiating Reality*. New York: New York University, 1979.

10. Rothman, Barbara Katz. *In Labor: Women and Power in the Birthplace*. Rev. ed. New York: W. W. Norton, 1991 [1982].

11. Davis-Floyd, Robbie. *Birth as an American Rite of Passage*. Berkeley: University of California Press, 1992.

12. Rooks, Judith. *Midwifery and Childbirth in America*. Philadelphia: Temple University Press, 1997.

13. Davis-Floyd, Robbie. "The Technocratic, Humanistic, and Holistic Paradigms of Childbirth." *International Journal of Gynecology and Obstetrics* 75.S1 (2001): S5-S23.

14. Perkins, Barbara Bridgman. *The Medical Delivery Business: Health Reform, Childbirth, and the Economic Order*. Piscataway, NJ: Rutgers University Press, 2004.

15. Simonds, Wendy, Barbara Katz Rothman, and Bari Meltzer Norman. *Laboring On: Birth In Transition in The United States*. New York: Routledge, 2007.

16. Boston Women's Health Book Collective, *Our Bodies, Ourselves: Pregnancy and Birth*. New York: Simon and Schuster, 2008.

17. Jordan, Brigitte. *Birth in Four Cultures: A Cross-Cultural Investigation of Childbirth in Yucatan, Holland, Sweden and the United States*. Prospect Heights: Waveland Press, 1993.

18. Romalis, Shelley, ed. *Childbirth: Alternatives to Medical Control*. Austin: University of Texas Press, 1982.

19. Cook, Katsi. "Center for Community Change." *First Environment Newsletter* 1.1 (Spring 1992): 2.

20. Sakala, Carol, and Maureen P. Cory. *Evidence-Based Maternity Care: What It Is and What It Can Achieve*. New York: Milbank Memorial Fund, 2008, 10-20.

21. World Health Organization. *The World Health Report*. Geneva: WHO, 2005.

22. AbouZahr, C. World Health Organization. *Maternal Morality in 2000: Estimates Developed by WHO, UNICEF and UNFPA*. Geneva: WHO, 2004.

23. Davis-Floyd, Robbie E. *Normal Childbirth: Evidence and Debate*. Soo Downe, ed., Oxford: Churchill Livingstone, 2004.

24. DeClercq, Eugene R., Carol Sakala, Maureen P. Corry, and Sandra Applebaum. *Listening to Mothers II: Report of the Second National Survey of Women's Childbearing Experiences*. New York: Childbirth Connection, 2006.

25. Enkin, Murray et al. *A Guide to Effective Care in Pregnancy and Childbirth*. Oxford: Oxford University Press, 2000: 362.

26. *Birthing the Future*. Dir. Suzanne Arms, 2003. Film. <http://www.birthingthefuture.com>

27. Klaus, Marshall, John Kennell, and Phyllis Klaus. *Bonding: Building the Foundation for Secure Attachment and Independence*. Reading: Addison-Wesley, 1995.

28. "When the Bough Breaks." *Unnatural Causes: Is Inequality Making Us Sick?* Series produced by California Newsreel with Vital Pictures, Exec. Producer Larry Adelman. Presented by the National Minority Consortia. Public Engagement Campaign in Association with the Joint Center for Political and Economic Studies Health Policy Institute, 2008. PBS documentary series, 2009. Transcript: <http://www.pbs.org/unnaturalcauses/assets/resources/when_bough_breaks_transcript.pdf>.

29. Jackson, Fleda Mack. "Race, Stress, and Social Support: Addressing the Crisis in Black Infant Mortality." *Joint Center for Political and Economic Studies.* Washington, DC: Health Policy Institute, 2007.

30. Smedley, Brian D., Adrienne Y. Stith, and Alan R. Nelson, Eds., Institute of Medicine. *Unequal Treatment: Confronting Racial and Ethnic Disparities in Healthcare.* Washington DC: National Academies Press, 2003.

31. Lockwood C. J., and E. Kuczynski. "Markers of Risk for Preterm Delivery." *Journal of Perinatal Medicine* 27.4 (1999): 245-9, 1999.

32. Creedy, Debra K., Ian M. Shochet, and Jan Horsfall. "Childbirth and the Development of Acute Trauma Symptoms: Incidence and Contributing Factors." *Birth* 27.2 (2001): 104-11.

33. Beck, Cheryl Tatano. "Birth Trauma: In the Eye of the Beholder." *Nursing Research* 53.1 (2004): 28-35.

34. Bailham, S. Joseph. "Post-Traumatic Stress Following Childbirth: A Review of the Emerging Literature and Directions for Research and Practice." *Psychology, Health & Medicine* 8.2 (2003): 159-168.

35. Czarnocka, J., and J. Slade. "Prevalence and Predictors of Post-Traumatic Stress Symptoms Following Childbirth." *British Journal of Clinical Psychology* 39.1 (2000): 35-51(17).

36. American Psychiatric Association. "Post Traumatic Stress Disorder, Criteria 309.81." *Diagnostic and Statistical Manual of Mental Disorders IV (DSM-IV),* Fourth Edition, Chicago: R.R. Donnelley & Sons Company, 2000.

37. DeClercq, Eugene R., *Listening to Mothers II.*

38. Korten, David. "We Are Hard-Wired to Care and Connect." *Yes! Magazine* 47 (2008): 48-51.

39. King, Martin Luther, Jr. *Letter from the Birmingham Jail,* April 16, 1963. Birmingham, Alabama, 1963. Harper Collins 1994 [1963].

40. Sakala, Carol, and Maureen P. Cory. *Evidence-Based Maternity Care.*

41. Coalition for Improving Maternity Services. "The Mother-Friendly Childbirth Initiative," 1996. Website accessed Dec 2009. <http://www.motherfriendly.org>.

42. Blanchette, H. "Comparison of Obstetric Outcome of a Primary-Care Access Clinic by Certified Nurse-Midwives and a Private Practice of Obstetricians in the Same Community." *American Journal of Obstetrics and Gynecology* 172.6 (1995): 1864-1868.

43. Davidson, M.R. "Outcomes of High-risk Women Cared for by Certified Nurse-Midwives." *Journal of Midwifery and Women's Health* 45.5 (2002): 378-383.

44. Mahoney, S.F., and L.H. Malcoe. "Cesarean Delivery in Native American Women: Are the Low Rates Explained by Practices Common in Indian Health Service?" *Birth* 32.3 (2005): 170-178.

45. Johnson, K.C., and Betty-Anne Daviss. "Outcomes of Planned Homebirths with Certified Professional Midwives. Large Prospective Study in North America." *BMJ* 333.7505 (2005): 1416.

46. Janssen, Patricia A., V.L. Holt, and S.J. Myers. "Licensed Midwife-Attended, Out-of-Hospital Births in Washington State: Are They Safe?" *Birth* 21.3 (1994): 141-148. 1994.

47. World Health Organization. "Care in Normal Birth: A Practical Guide", 1996. Available at: <http://www.who.int/making_pregnancy_safer/documents/who_frh_msm_9624/en/>.

48. American Public Health Association, "Supporting Access to Midwifery Services in the United States," (Position Paper). *American Journal of Public Health*, 91.3 (2001).

49. Dower, C.M., J.E. Miller, E.H. O'Neil, and the Taskforce on Midwifery. *Charting a Course for the 21st Century: The Future of Midwifery*. San Francisco: Pew Health Professions Commission and the UCSF Center for the Health Professions, 1999.

50. Walker, Alice. *Sent by Earth: A Message from the Grandmother Spirit after the Attacks on the World Trade Center and Pentagon*. Open Media Pamphlet Series, Greg Ruggiero, ed. Canada: Seven Stories Press First Edition, 2001.

51. Somé, Sobonfu E. *Welcoming Spirit Home: Ancient African Teachings to Celebrate Children and Community*. Novato: New World Library, 1999.

EDITOR'S NOTE
———————————————————

The midwives chosen for this anthology are all women, and throughout the book midwives are referred to as women. Because pregnancy and childbearing are exclusively female functions, until more recently, the events of women's procreative lives have been shaped and managed by women. We are aware that there are men who practice as midwives and who contribute to the profession. We honor their work in the field and support young men who are considering midwifery as a career.

RESOURCE ORGANIZATIONS

American College of Nurse-Midwives (ACNM)
8403 Colesville Rd. Suite 1550
Silver Spring, MD 20910
www.acnm.org
info@acnm.org

American College of Nurse-Midwives Foundation (ACNMF)
8403 Colesville Rd. Suite 1550
Silver Spring, MD 20910-6374
www.midwife.org/support.cfm
240-485-1850

American Midwifery Certification Board (AMCB)
849 International Dr. Suite 205
Linthicum, MD 21090
www.amcbmidwife.org
410-694-9424

Association of Midwifery Educators (AME)
24 S High St.
Bridgton, ME 04009
www.associationofmidwiferyeducators.org
207-647-5968

Citizens for Midwifery (CfM)
PO Box 82227
Athens, GA 30608-2227
info@cfmidwifery.org
www.cfmidwifery.org
888-CfM-4880

Foundation for the Advancement of Midwifery, Inc. (FAM)
2020 Pennsylvania Ave. NW , Box 720
Washington, DC 20006
info@formidwifery.org
www.formidwifery.org
877-594-9996

International Center for Traditional Childbearing (ICTC)
2823 N. Portland Blvd.
Portland, OR 97217
ictc@blackmidwives.org
www.blackmidwives.org
503-460-9324

Midwifery Business Network (MBN)
www.midwiferybusinessnetwork.com

Midwifery Education Accreditation Council (MEAC)
PO Box 984
La Conner, WA 98257
info@meacschools.org
www.meacschools.org
360-466-2080 (phone)
480-907-2936 (fax)

Midwives Alliance of North America (MANA)
611 Pennsylvania Ave. SE
Washington, DC 20003-4303
www.mana.org
www.mothersnatually.org
info@mana.org
888-923-MANA (6262)

National Association of Certified Professional Midwives (NACPM)
243 Banning Road
Putney, VT 05346
www.nacpm.org
800-704-9844

North American Registry of Midwives (NARM)
5257 Rosestone Dr.
Lilburn, GA 30047
www.narm.org
info@narm.org
888-842-4784

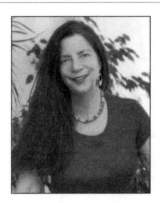

Geradine Simkins, CNM, MSN has been an activist since childhood. She is a midwife, author and visionary leader in midwifery, maternal and child health care, and social justice arenas. She is currently President of the Midwives Alliance of North America and the organization's Interim Executive Director. She has three extraordinary young adult children, owns and operates Birthways Consulting, is inspired by her journeys to foreign lands and cultures, and enriched daily by the natural beauty of living in rural northern Michigan.